W. X. Schneider · A.M. Owen · J. Duncan (Eds.)

Executive Control and the Frontal Lobe: Current Issues

Springer
Berlin
Heidelberg
New York
Barcelona
Hong Kong
London
Milan
Paris
Singapore
Tokyo

Werner X. Schneider · Adrian M. Owen
John Duncan (Eds.)

Executive Control and the Frontal Lobe: Current Issues

With 47 Figures and 21 Tables

Springer

Werner X. Schneider

Allgemeine und Experimentelle Psychologie
Institut für Psychologie, Ludwig-Maximilians-Universität
Leopoldstrasse 13, 80802 München, Germany
email: wxs@psy.uni-muenchen.de

Adrian M. Owen
John Duncan

MRC Cognition and Brain Sciences Unit
15, Chaucer Road, Cambridge CB2 2EF, United Kingdom
email: adrian.owen@mrc-cbu.cam.ac.uk
email: john.duncan@mrc-cbu.cam.ac.uk

The front cover image was kindly provided by Dr. Krish Singh, Magnetic Resonance and Image Analysis Research Centre, Liverpool University, and generated using Brain Tools, MRI3d Software.

ISBN 3-540-67676-7 Springer-Verlag Berlin Heidelberg New York

Library of Congress Cataloging-in-Publication Data
Executive control and the frontal lobe: current issues / W.X. Schneider, A.M. Owen, J. Duncan, eds. p.cm. "Second issues of material from 'Experimental brain research: special issue', pub. June 2000." Includes bibliographical references.
ISBN 3-540-67676-7
1. Prefrontal cortex. 2. Frontal lobes. 3. Cognition. I. Schneider, Werner X. II. Owen, Adrian M. III. Duncan, John. QP383.17.E96 2000 612.8'25-dc21 00-057361

Springer-Verlag Berlin Heidelberg New York
a member of BertelsmannSpringer Science+Business Media GmbH

Cover-Design: Design & Production, Heidelberg, Germany
Typesetting, printing and bookbinding: Stürtz AG, Würzburg, Germany

Printed on acid-free paper. SPIN: 10772007 27/3130 ih - 5 4 3 2 1 0

Contents

Adrian M. Owen · Werner X. Schneider
John Duncan

Executive control and the frontal lobe: current issues

Published online: 6 May 2000

While the importance of the prefrontal cortex for 'higher-order' cognitive functions is largely undisputed, no consensus has been reached regarding precise specification of these functions. For example, although some degree of regional specialization within the frontal lobe seems inevitable, by and large, most attempts to map specific cognitive functions onto neuroanatomical and/or cytoarchitectonic subdivisions have been disappointing. This is true, not only for data derived from human neuropsychological studies, but also from lesion and electrophysiological studies in the monkey and, more recently, from functional neuroimaging experiments in man. That is not to say, of course, that associations have never been drawn between specific cognitive functions and particular regions of the prefrontal cortex, but only that the level of consistency across different studies is often rather lower than for investigations focussing on more posterior cortical areas. This lack of consensus about functional segregation is compounded further by terminology; many of the concepts currently used to describe aspects of normal frontal-lobe functioning, such as 'executive control', 'monitoring and manipulation within working memory', 'temporal structuring of behaviour' and 'control of behaviour by context' remain rather non-specific and require more precise definition. In short, although a high degree of functional specialization probably exists within the frontal cortex, it seems increasingly likely that the structural organization of this system does not relate, in any straightforward way, to contemporary models of cognition.

It was with these issues in mind that we organised a workshop entitled 'Executive Control and the Frontal Lobe: Current Issues' at the Hanse Institute for Advanced Study in Delmenhorst, Germany, between 1 and 3 December, 1998. The following scientists accepted our invitation and acted either as speakers or discussants during the 3-day meeting: Jonathan D. Cohen, Rudolf Cohen, Mark D'Esposito, Adele Diamond, Stefan Everling, Paul C. Fletcher, Joaquin Fuster, James V Haxby, Glyn Humphreys, John D. Gabrieli, Rainer Goebel, Bernhard Hommel, Richard Levy, Hans Markowitsch, Earl K. Miller, Elisabeth A. Murray, Richard E. Passingham, Tomas Paus, Stefan Pollmann, Michael Petrides, Angela C. Roberts, Trevor W. Robbins, Brigitte Rockstroh, Ruediger J. Seitz and Tim Shallice. The papers presented in this issue (Vol. 133, No. 1) are based directly on talks given at the workshop in Delmenhorst and we are most grateful to Carlo Marzi for allowing us to publish them in this Special Issue of *Experimental Brain Research*. In all cases, the manuscripts were reviewed by at least two anonymous referees who were, to a large extent, recruited from among the workshop participants.

A major consideration in inviting speakers to the meeting was to ensure that a variety of methodological approaches and theoretical positions were well represented. Although not all of the attendees elected to contribute to this volume, we feel that what is presented here faithfully reflects that variability. Accordingly, several of the authors have focussed on behavioural and/or imaging data acquired from patients with discrete frontal-lobe lesions (Humphreys and Riddoch; Markowitsch and Kessler). Others describe the results of lesion studies in the monkey that have attempted to shed light on both the anatomical and functional organisation of the prefrontal cortex (Petrides; Levy and Goldman-Rakic; Passingham, Toni and Rushworth). Several papers consider functional neuroimaging studies of frontal-lobe functions in healthy control volunteers, either through meta-analysis (Koski and Paus), or by focussing on specific aspects of working memory (Pollmann and von Cramon; D'Esposito, Postle and Rypma; Owen), motor planning and motor programming (Seitz) or associative leaning (Passingham, Toni and Rushworth). Finally, two papers take a more

A.M. Owen (✉) · J. Duncan
Medical Research Council Cognition and Brain Sciences Unit, 15 Chaucer Road, Cambridge CB2 2EF, UK
e-mail: adrian.owen@mrc-cbu.cam.ac.uk
Tel.: +44 1223 355294 ext. 700, Fax: +44 1223 359062

W.X. Schneider
Department of Experimental Psychology, Ludwig-Maximilians University, Munich, Germany

global methodological approach to the study of frontal-lobe functions, highlighting its role in arbitrary visuomotor mapping (Murray, Bussey and Wise), and cross-temporal action control (Fuster), while in one chapter the interactions between the neuromodulatory executive systems of the reticular core and the frontal lobe are described (Robbins).

The workshop was financed in its entirety by the Hanse Institute for Advanced Study in Delmenhorst, who also hosted the event perfectly by creating a stimulating and enjoyable atmosphere for talks and discussions. We are very grateful to all of the staff at the Institute, but particularly to Marita Baumgarten and Beatrice Riewe and to Gerhard Roth, the Director. As those who were there will testify, the Delmenhorst meeting was remarkable, not only for the sheer breadth of work discussed, but also for the widely differing approaches and opinions of some of those presenting it. We hope that this Special Issue of *Experimental Brain Research* captures much of that same flavour and will provide the reader with up-to-date information from some of the leading figures in frontal-lobe research.

Mark D'Esposito · Bradley R. Postle · Bart Rypma

Prefrontal cortical contributions to working memory: evidence from event-related fMRI studies

Published online: 20 May 2000

Abstract Working memory refers to the short-term retention of information that is no longer accessible in the environment, and the manipulation of this information, for subsequent use in guiding behavior. In this review, we will present data from a series of event-related functional magnetic-resonance-imaging (fMRI) studies of delayed-response tasks that were designed to investigate the role of different regions of the prefrontal cortex (PFC) during different working-memory component processes. From these data, we conclude that: (1) lateral PFC is anatomically organized according to the types of cognitive operations that one performs when attempting to temporarily maintain and manipulate information; and (2) consistent with the picture that has emerged from the monkey electrophysiological literature, human lateral PFC is involved in several encoding- and response-related processes as well as mnemonic and nonmnemonic processes that are engaged during the temporary maintenance of information. Thus, lateral PFC activity cannot be ascribed to the function of a single, unitary cognitive operation.

Key words Working memory · Prefrontal cortex · Functional MRI

Introduction

Working memory refers to the short-term retention of information that is no longer accessible in the environment, and the manipulation of this information, for subsequent use in guiding behavior. An interacting set of processes can be recruited to maintain information in working memory and to perform operations on it. Working memory makes important contributions to many cognitive functions, such as reasoning, language comprehension, planning, and spatial processing. Important evidence for the neural basis of working memory was initially provided from animal studies (for a review, see Owen et al. 1999). For example, electrophysiological studies of awake behaving monkeys have used delayed-response tasks to study working memory. In these tasks, the monkey must keep "in mind", or actively maintain, a representation of the target stimulus [or of the anticipated probe stimulus (Rainer et al. 1999; Watanabe 1996)] over a short delay. During such tasks, neurons within the lateral prefrontal cortex (PFC) have been found to be persistently activated during the delay period when the monkey is maintaining information in memory prior to a making a motor response that is contingent on this information (Funahashi et al. 1989; Fuster and Alexander 1971). The necessity of this region for active maintenance of information over short delays has been demonstrated in monkey studies showing that lesions of the lateral PFC impair performance on these tasks (Bauer and Fuster 1976; Funahashi et al. 1993).

Using event-related functional magnetic-resonance-imaging (fMRI) designs, groups have begun to demonstrate that lateral PFC in humans is also engaged during the active maintenance of information over short delays in delayed-response tasks (Courtney et al. 1997; Zarahn et al. 1999). These studies, however, have not assessed the role of PFC during other processes that are engaged during delayed-response tasks, such as encoding processes at the time of stimulus presentation and retrieval processes at the time of probe presentation. Electrophysiological studies in monkeys performing delayed-response tasks, however, have revealed that PFC neurons can also be active during many non-delay portions of the task, and it is well established that PFC neurons can respond during any combination of target, delay, and response periods (Chafee and Goldman-Rakic 1998; Funahashi et al.

M. D'Esposito (✉) · B. Rypma
Helen Wills Neuroscience Institute
and Department of Psychology,
3210 Tolman Hall, University of California,
Berkeley, CA 94720–1650, USA
e-mail: despo@socrates.berkeley.edu
Tel.: +1-510-6433340, Fax: +1-510-6425293

B.R. Postle
Department of Psychology,
University of Wisconsin-Madison,
1202 W. Johnson St, Madison, WI 53706–1611, USA

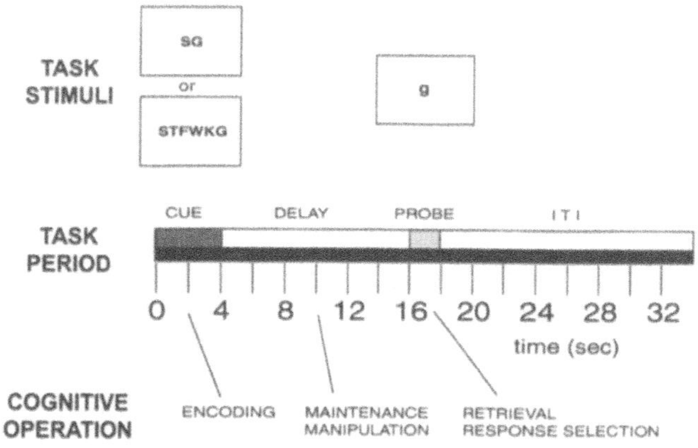

Fig. 1 Schematic illustration of a prototypical delayed-response task with proposed cognitive processes that may be engaged at each task period. *ITI* Intertrial interval

1989; Fuster et al. 1982). Thus, in addition to active maintenance, the PFC appears to be involved in processes that may include stimulus encoding, sustained attention to stimuli, manipulation of information being actively maintained, decision about a probe, preparation for a motor response, and execution of the motor response itself.

In this review, we will present data from a series of event-related fMRI studies of delayed-response tasks that were designed to investigate the role of different regions of the PFC during different component processes engaged when information is stored and temporarily manipulated during delayed-response performance (Fig. 1). This was achieved by examining the temporal dynamics of PFC activity over the course of a single trial, and isolating the variance in the fMRI signal attributable to the theoretically dissociable components of the trial [i.e., target, delay, probe (Zarahn et al. 1997)]. This capability represents an important methodological advance, because it permits direct measurement of the PFC contribution to the different processes that can contribute to working memory performance. As our review will demonstrate, event-related fMRI designs have emerged as a powerful method for the studies of human cognition that are analogous to awake, behaving monkey physiological studies.

Previously, fMRI and positron emission tomography (PET) investigations of working memory have employed blocked experimental designs that require the integration of a neuroimaging signal across entire blocks of each type of trial in an experiment. This approach has at least three important limitations. First, its temporal resolution is inherently poor, typically on the order of tens of seconds, and is thus ill-suited for direct measurement of working-memory-related processes, which operate on the order of seconds or milliseconds. Second, it often requires the pairing of the assumption of "pure insertion" (Sternberg 1969) with application of the logic of "cognitive subtraction" (Posner et al. 1988), a combination that may yield unreliable results (Friston et al. 1996; Zarahn et al. 1997). For example, a blocked experimental design may contrast performance on a delayed-response task (comprised of stimulus presentation, delay, and probe components) with performance on a visual matching task (comprised of only stimulus presentation and probe components), with the subtraction of neuroimaging signal from these two conditions intended to reveal the brain regions contributing to cognitive processes *not* shared by the two – in this case, delay-related processes. The assumption guiding this design is that the *insertion* of the delay period will not interact with the stimulus presentation and probe components of the trial. Such a design was featured in the early, influential neuroimaging investigations of Jonides, Smith, and colleagues (Jonides et al. 1993; Smith et al. 1995). It has been demonstrated empirically, however, that PFC voxels that are *not* active during the delay-period of a delayed-response task can evince greater probe-related activity when the response is preceded by a delay period than when it is immediately preceded by stimulus presentation (Zarahn et al. 1997). That is, the insertion of a delay period into a visual matching task can have interactive effects on nonmnemonic parts of the task, and a conventional block-design analysis would incorrectly identify such a voxel as having delay-period activity.[1] A third limitation of blocked neuroimaging studies is that inferences derived from them are usually based on aggregate task performance and fMRI activation data. This approach has been useful for mapping the contributions of various brain regions to working memory, but does not permit the investigation of relations between behavioral (e.g., reaction time, accuracy) and physiological indices (e.g. fMRI activation) associated with working-memory task performance. In this review, we will also present data that address relations between individual differences in performance and individual differences in cortical activity.

Maintenance versus manipulation processes

In some behavioral contexts, information must be maintained in the state in which it was encoded (as when one remembers a telephone number when walking from the phone book to the telephone). Other circumstances require the manipulation of this remembered information (as when one simultaneously performs mental calculations and remembers the intermediate products). Presumably, these manipulations or additional operations entail the recruitment of additional cognitive processes not required for simple maintenance of information. One systems neuroscience model encompassing this view proposes that the ventrolateral PFC (primarily the inferior

[1] Note that event-related designs can also rely on cognitive subtraction, as, for example, when comparing delay-period activity associated with the retention of three items versus delay-period activity associated with retention of six items, a design we will discuss in a subsequent section. A more detailed consideration of different types of neuroimaging experimental designs can be found in: Aguirre GK, D'Esposito M (1999) Experimental design for brain fMRI; in: Moonen CTW, Bandettini PA (eds) Functional MRI. Springer, Berlin Heidelberg New York, pp 369–380.

frontal gyrus, Brodmann's areas 47, 44, 45) is the site where information is initially received from posterior association areas and where organization of information held in working memory is performed, whereas dorsolateral PFC (primarily the middle frontal gyrus, areas 9 and 46) is additionally recruited only when monitoring and manipulation of information within working memory is required (Petrides 1989, 1994). Empirical support for such a dorsal/ventral organization in human PFC came from a PET study contrasting PFC activation associated with several different spatial working-memory tasks that varied manipulation and monitoring demands (Owen et al. 1996). The results were consistent with the Petrides model and have been replicated in subsequent fMRI (Owen et al. 1998) and PET (Owen et al. 1999) experiments. Interpretation of these results is complicated, however, by the complex set of subtractions and comparisons required to partial out the relative contributions of tests of delayed-response, span, self-ordered choosing, and n-back utilized in these studies – and of the control task associated with each – to measures of PFC activation. In addition to the concerns about interpreting results produced by a cognitive subtraction analysis, the blocked designs of these studies also prevented direct inference as to whether the additional monitoring-related neuroimaging signal in dorsolateral PFC was attributable to neural activity arising during encoding, delay, or probe portions of such tasks. Thus, although these studies represent important initial tests of this processing model of the anatomical organization of working memory function in PFC, they left many important questions unresolved.

We have performed two event-related fMRI studies designed to investigate the proposed neural dissociation between processes required for the active maintenance of information in working memory and the processes engaged when this information is manipulated. In the first study (D'Esposito et al. 1999a), the behavioral paradigm was a delayed-response task in which a set of five letters was presented simultaneously, in a randomly determined order, followed immediately by an instruction cue ("FORWARD" or "ALPHABETIZE"), followed by an 8-s delay, during which only a fixation cross appeared on the screen, followed by a probe that prompted the subject to make a button-press response. Thus, subjects were presented with two types of trials (in random order) in which they were required either to: (1) *maintain* a randomly ordered sequence of five letters across a delay period, or (2) *manipulate* a comparable sequence of letters by arranging them into alphabetical order during the delay period. In both conditions, the probe consisted of a letter and a number. In the *maintenance* condition, subjects were instructed to determine whether the letter was in the ordinal position represented by the number. This condition, therefore, simply required retention of the letters in the same format as presented at the beginning of the trial. In the *manipulation* condition, subjects were instructed to determine whether that letter would be in the ordinal position represented by the number if the items in the memory set were rearranged into alphabetical order. This condition, therefore, required subjects to transpose the order of the five items presented at the beginning of the trial during the delay period.

In each subject, activity during the delay period was found in both dorsolateral and ventrolateral PFC in both types of trials. Additionally, in each subject, dorsolateral PFC activity was significantly greater in trials during which information held in working memory was manipulated (Fig. 2). Thus, our results were broadly consistent with a hierarchical processing model of the organization of working memory function in PFC, in that they revealed a consistently greater contribution of dorsal PFC to manipulation processes than of ventral PFC.

These results differed importantly from those of previous studies (Awh et al. 1996; Owen et al. 1996, 1998, 1999; Smith et al. 1998), however, in that they provided evidence for dorsolateral PFC contribution to working-memory maintenance trials. Although our maintenance task differed methodologically from some of those of Owen and colleagues, for example, in that it may not have required "monitoring" operations to the same extent, such differences would only be expected to *lessen* the extent to which our tasks would recruit dorsolateral PFC. The results discussed here are consistent with those of at least five other studies that have shown, with several different types of stimuli, that active maintenance in working memory recruits dorsolateral PFC (Cohen et al. 1997; Courtney et al. 1997; Postle and D'Esposito 1999; Postle et al. 1999; Zarahn et al. 1999). The finding that dorsolateral PFC is engaged during active maintenance as well as during manipulation processes is the first piece of evidence that we marshal in support of our view that lateral PFC subserves several discrete working-memory-related cognitive processes.

A second event-related fMRI experiment, utilizing a variation of the same task, replicated the results of the first in that it also provided evidence for dorso- *and* ventrolateral PFC activity during the delay-period of working-memory maintenance trials, but consistently greater activity during alphabetization trials only in dorsolateral PFC (Postle et al. 1999). This second study also extended our earlier results in two important ways. First, it might have been argued the greater activity of dorsolateral PFC associated with the alphabetize condition in the earlier study (D'Esposito et al. 1999a) was due to the greater difficulty of this condition rather than to the additional mental processes required by this task. In this second experiment, however, performance on "Forward 5" (maintenance) and "Alphabetize 5" (manipulation) tasks was equivalent, thereby removing the difficulty confound from these data. (For these analyses we operationalized difficulty as performance accuracy.) We could thus unequivocally attribute to alphabetization-related processes to the increased activity that we observed in dorsolateral PFC.

The second advance represented by this task was the inclusion of a condition requiring maintenance of two letters, a modification that permitted investigation of working-memory load effects. We found delay-specific load effects in dorsolateral PFC in only two of the five subjects participating in the experiment, and, importantly, no evidence of delay-period load effects in any voxels that evinced greater manipulation than maintenance activity (Postle et al. 1999). We did find, in contrast, consistent delay-period load effects in all subjects in left posterior perisylvian cortex. Group analyses revealed a double-dissociation, with greater load-than-alphabetization activity in left posterior perisylvian regions, and greater alphabetization-than-load activity in PFC, indicating that the neurophysiological factors underlying manipulation and storage differed qualitatively, not just quantitatively (Postle et al. 1999). These results, therefore, provide the first evidence that the manipulation-related processes ascribed to dorsolateral PFC are fundamentally nonmnemonic in nature. That is, whereas they play an important role in the exercise of executive control of working memory, they do not govern the maintenance or storage per se of the information held in working memory. We believe that many manipulation-related processes may also be recruited to support non-working-memory behaviors. This result has implications not only for hierarchical processing models of the organization of working-memory function in PFC, but also for the interpretation of "load effects" observed in PFC in experiments that parametrically manipulate the number of items maintained in an n-back task (Braver et al. 1997; Cohen et al. 1997; Jonides et al. 1997), suggesting that these effects may be attributable to nonmnemonic processes contributing to performance of these tasks and not the to information-storage or -maintenance processes. This last proposal received support from the results of the next study we will describe, an examination of load-effects in item-recognition working memory.

The effect of load on encoding, maintenance, and retrieval processes

Recently, two studies have shown that dorsolateral PFC recruitment increases in parallel to increased memory load during performance of tasks with no overt requirements to manipulate information held in working memory (Manoach et al. 1997; Rypma et al. 1999). For exam-

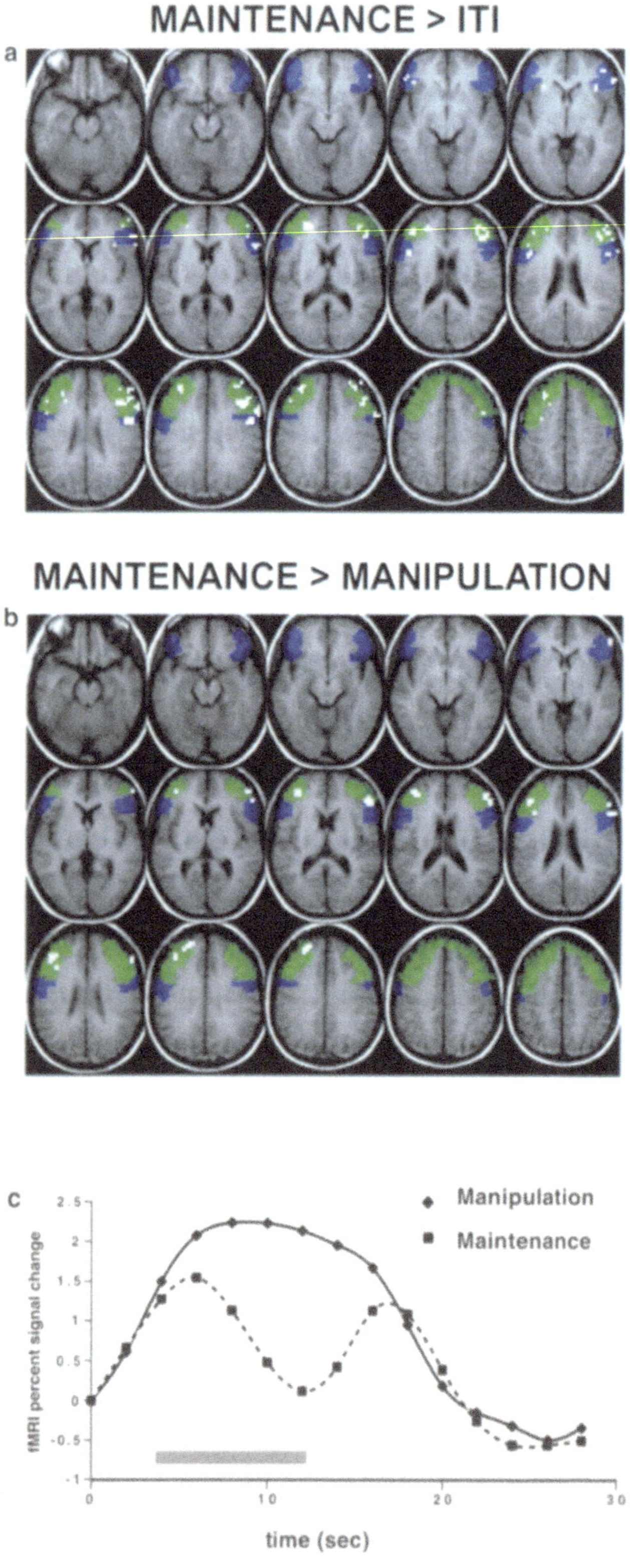

Fig. 2 **a** Representative subject *t*-map illustrating the voxels demonstrating significant delay-period activity (versus baseline) during maintenance trials, during which the subject maintained a representation of five letters in the order in which they were presented. **b** A *t*-map from the same subject illustrating the voxels demonstrating significantly greater delay-period activity during manipulation ("alphabetize 5 letters") than maintenance trials. The *green-shaded* ROI represents ventrolateral PFC (inferior frontal gyrus) and the *blue-shaded* ROI represents dorsolateral PFC (middle frontal gyrus). Maintenance-related activity (**a**) is seen in both ventrolateral and dorsolateral PFC, whereas manipulation activity is greater than the maintenance activity only in dorsolateral PFC (**b**). **c** The trial-averaged time series from the voxels highlighted in **b**. Note the two peaks in the maintenance condition correspond to the stimulus presentation and the probe periods of the trial. In the manipulation condition, in contrast, these voxels maintained a high level of activity throughout the delay period. The *solid bar* along the horizontal axis represents the duration of the delay period

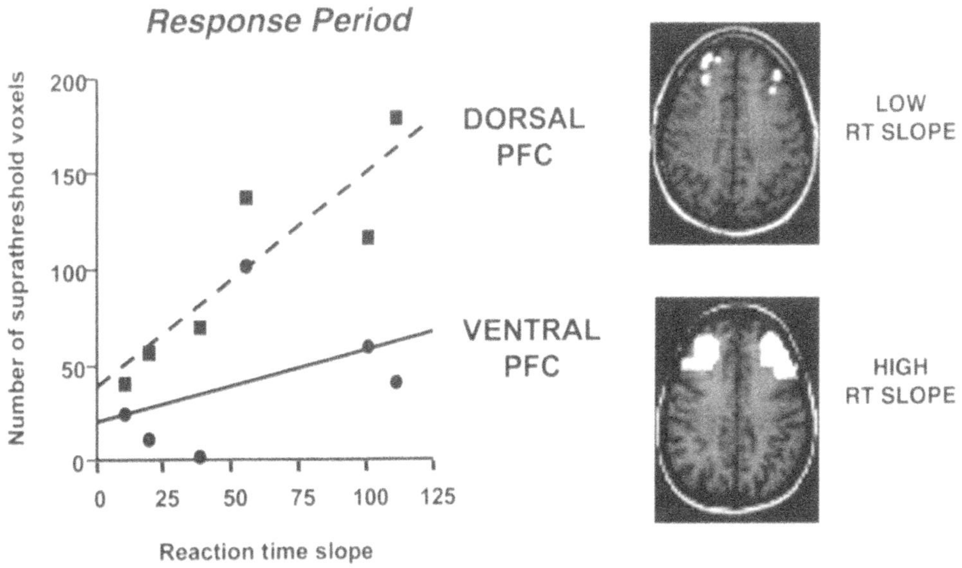

Fig. 3 A scatter plot of the numbers of suprathreshold voxels during the "Response Period" of a delayed response task in dorsal prefrontal cortex (PFC; *dotted line, squares*; slope =1.34, r^2=0.76, P<0.05) and ventral PFC (*solid line, circles*; slope =0.36, r^2=0.18) plotted against reaction-time slopes. Also shown are axial slices of activation patterns in the two representative subjects with the lowest and highest reaction-time (*RT*) slopes

ple, Rypma and colleagues (1999) observed activation in dorsolateral PFC in a Sternberg-type item-recognition task in which subjects were required to maintain one, three, or six letters in working memory for 5 s. When subjects were required to maintain three letters in working memory, relative to one letter, activation in frontal regions was limited to left ventrolateral PFC (BA 44). However, when subjects were required to maintain six letters, relative to one letter, the additional activation of dorsolateral PFC was observed. Rypma and colleagues proposed that dorsolateral PFC may be recruited during maintenance tasks in which subjects must actively maintain information loads that approach or exceed short-term memory capacity. According to this view, the same dorsolateral PFC circuits important for manipulation of information in working memory may be recruited for the mediation of strategic processes necessary for the maintenance of a high load of information. Alternative interpretations of the Rypma et al. (1999) and Manoach et al. (1997) results were possible, however, because both featured blocked designs that didn't permit identification of the specific component processes that were sensitive to the load manipulation.

In an event-related fMRI study intended to elucidate the relative contributions of target, delay, and probe task periods to PFC activation in item-recognition working-memory performance, we asked subjects to maintain either two or six letters across an unfilled delay period and found that the effects of increased memory load were observed only in dorsolateral PFC, lateralized to the right hemisphere, and were observed only in the *encoding* period of the task (Rypma and D'Esposito 1999). Consistent with the results of Postle et al. (1999), described earlier, *delay*-period load effects were only seen in left posterior cortex. These results suggested that the load-sensitive processes in dorsolateral PFC that were identified in earlier block design studies (Manoach et al. 1997; Rypma et al. 1999) contribute to encoding processes, but not to the maintenance of information in working memory. It may be that initial encoding of information requires cognitive operations (e.g., monitoring the contents of working memory, updating and coordination of multiple memory buffers) that are similar to those required in the "manipulation" tasks described previously. Additional experiments are required to test this possibility.

Because we observed considerable inter-subject variability in fMRI signal magnitude and activation extent, we performed additional analyses to explore possible relations between individual differences in PFC physiological measures and task performance. For this analysis, we operationalized performance of each individual subject in terms of their memory retrieval *rate*, the interpolated slope obtained when plotting reaction time (RT) against memory load (two- vs. six-letter trials). The RT slope is believed to index memory-retrieval (or "scanning") rate when subjects must make a yes/no judgment about the membership of a probe stimulus to the memory set (Sternberg 1966). Further, memory-retrieval rate may vary with the efficiency of memory-scanning processes. We operationalized PFC activity as the number of voxels identified with a load-independent contrast selective for voxels evincing delay-period activity during two-letter and six-letter trials. Linear-regression analyses were then applied to data from each trial component and from two PFC regions of interest (e.g., dorsolateral and ventrolateral) to test for relationships between performance and activity.

The results of these individual differences analyses indicated that, in the dorsolateral PFC, retrieval rate and fMRI activation were positively correlated (r^2=0.76; P<0.05), but only at the time of response (Fig. 3). This correlation corresponded to an increase of 1.34 activated voxels per millisecond of increase in retrieval rate and accounted for 76% of the variance (Rypma and D'Esposito 1999). These results suggest two conclusions. First, because increased retrieval rate corresponds to less efficient working-memory scanning, poorer performers on this task may have recruited broader networks within dorsolateral PFC to compensate for inefficient working-memory scanning processes. Second, the finding of a significant brain-behavior link only in dorsolateral PFC (and not ventrolateral PFC), and only during response (and not during other task periods), suggests that this region of PFC represents an important substrate of memory scanning, a retrieval process that is initiated with the onset of the probe stimulus.

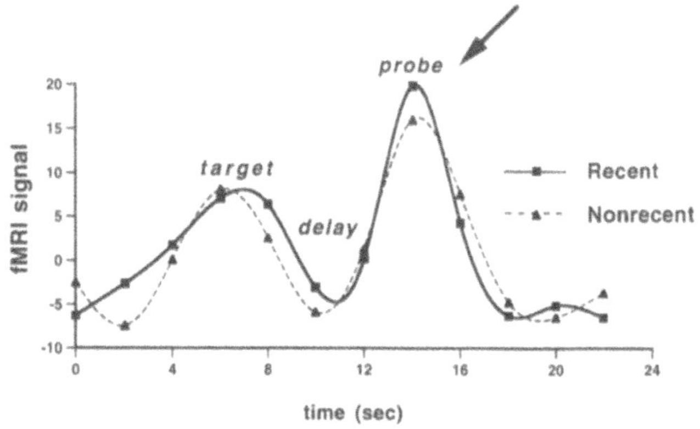

Fig. 4 The trial-averaged time series data for a representative subject extracted from voxels within the left inferior frontal gyrus (Brodmann's area 45) demonstrating a main effect for the probe period across both "Recent Negative" and "Nonrecent Negative" trials. Activity in the two conditions differed statistically only during the probe portion of the task (*arrow*)

The effect of proactive interference on encoding, maintenance, and retrieval processes

Although the previously described study characterized the neural substrate of one component process (or set of processes) recruited in association with the onset of the probe stimulus in a delayed-response task, there are certainly many other processes engaged during this portion of the task, candidates among them including: shifting attention among items held in working memory (Garavan 1998; McElree 1998); inhibition of prepotent responses (Diamond 1990); mediation of proactive interference (Jonides et al. 1998); coordination of multiple task performance (D'Esposito et al. 1995); response preparation (D'Esposito et al. 2000); and motor execution. An important empirical question is the extent to which each of these theoretically dissociable, probe-related processes relies on the same neural substrate. To begin to approach this problem, we chose to focus on another memory-related phenomenon, proactive interference (PI), whose existence is measured by RTs. Like the previous study, this experiment illustrates the advantages of the *temporal resolution* of an event-related experimental design over that of a block design.

Using event-related fMRI, we scanned subjects as they performed a four-letter item-recognition task, during which they judged whether or not the probe was from the target set of four consonant letters. The task was designed such that we controlled the amount of PI associated with the probe stimulus on each trial. Two types of trials were of greatest interest: those with "Recent Negative" probes that matched a letter from the target set of the two previous, but not the present trial (and thus featured a high level of PI), and those with "Nonrecent Negative" probes that did not match a target letter from any of these trials. We hypothesized that a correct response to a "Recent Negative" probe would engage interference-resolution processes, possibly inhibition of the tendency to respond "yes" based on the sheer familiarity of the probe (which had been rehearsed extensively on the two previous trials). A correct response to a "Nonrecent Negative" probe, by contrast, would minimize demands on interference resolution, reflecting the absence of PI from the previous trials. We predicted that interference-resolution processes associated with "Recent Negative" trails would manifest themselves in brain activation and behavioral data. A previous study indicated that "Recent Negative" trials are associated with an RT cost believed to reflect the operation of a process or set of processes that detect and resolve PI (Jonides et al. 1998), and behavioral results from our study also revealed a small, but reliable RT effect.

The Jonides et al. (1998) study was a PET study that found that Brodmann's area 45 in left ventrolateral PFC demonstrated greater activation in association with "Recent Negative" trials. Because this study used a blocked design that averaged signals across all components of trials in each condition of the delayed-response task, however, it was unsuitable for investigation of temporal dynamics of the inhibitory processes ascribed to the observed PFC activation. For example, rather than reflecting a temporally discrete response-related process that was sensitive to PI, this neuroimaging effect could have occurred during stimulus presentation, delay, or retrieval components of trials in which PI was present, or in any combination of these three. Importantly, the PI-related activity reported by Jonides and colleagues (1998) could have also reflected a state-dependent mental "set" that persisted steadily during blocks of trials that featured high stimulus overlap, as might be expected if subjects adopted a different behavioral strategy for blocks that featured a high proportion of stimulus overlap across trials (Johnson et al. 1997). Our event-related design, in contrast, although employing a similar behavioral paradigm as Jonides et al. (1998), featured randomization of trial types that obviated the possible contamination of our data with context-dependent effects that can manifest themselves when trials representing a particular experimental treatment are blocked together.

The physiological data from our task confirmed that there were no differences in PFC between the two trial types in target presentation or delay-period activation, but that there was significantly greater probe-related activation for "Recent Negative" than "Nonrecent Negative" trials within left ventrolateral PFC, but not in other regions of PFC (Fig. 4). These findings spatially and

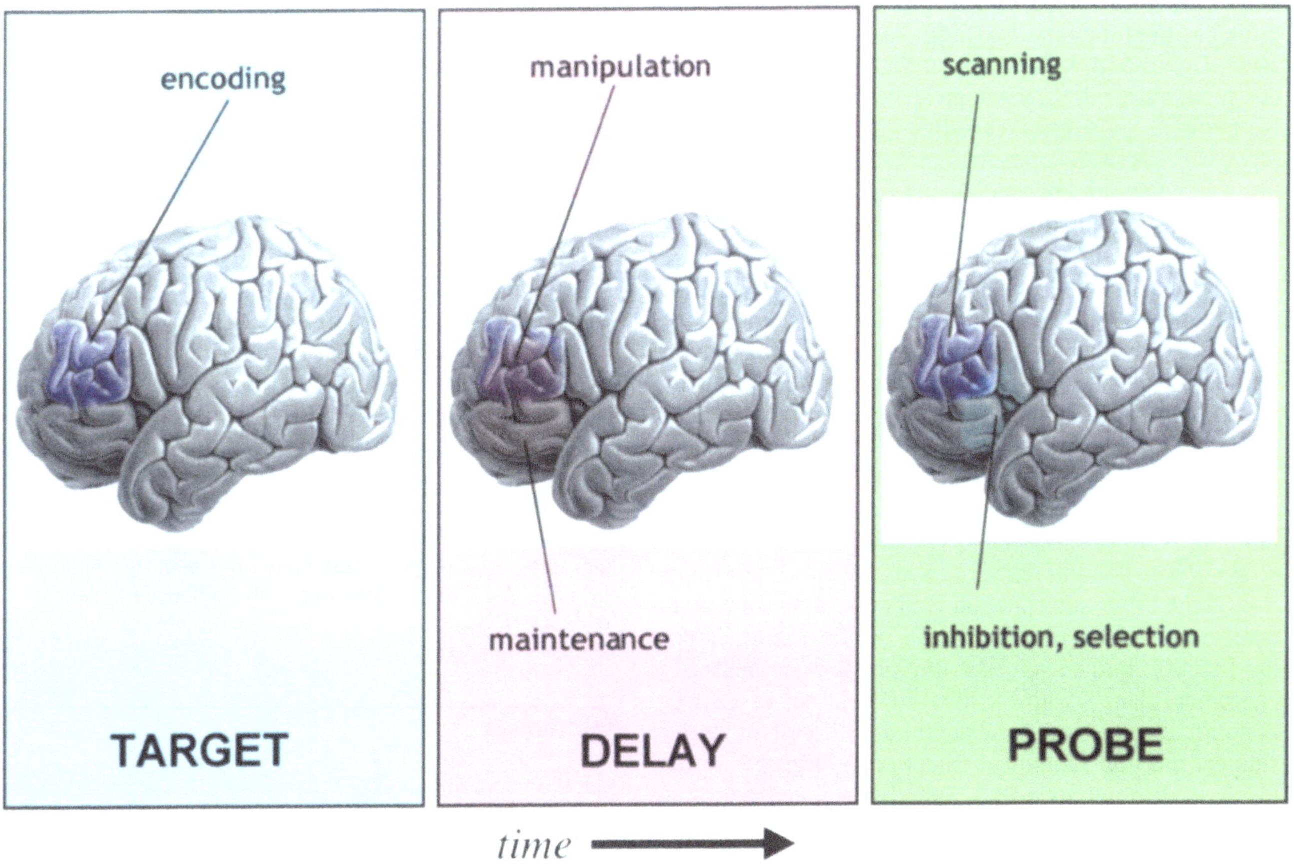

Fig. 5 Schematic illustration that summarizes the findings from the event-related functional magnetic-resonance-imaging (fMRI) studies presented in this paper

temporally characterized a physiological PI effect that was reliable across subjects, and that was associated with a mean RT cost of 32 ms produced by our PI manipulation. Further investigation of these effects needs to be carried out to determine whether the process(es) indexed by these effects are best characterized as response inhibition (Jonides et al. 1998), selection among candidate memoranda (Thompson-Schill et al. 1997), probe discrimination (McElree and Dosher 1987; Monsell 1978), or an as yet unarticulated alternative. But, regardless of what subsequent studies tell us about the computational nature of the processes underlying this PI effect, we have already established that it is supported by a different region of PFC than that which supports memory-scanning-related processes that are also associated with the probe/response component of working-memory-task performance.

Conclusions

Lateral PFC in humans is clearly recruited during many different cognitive processes that are engaged by the performance of delayed-response tasks. Moreover, lateral PFC seems to be functionally organized according to the types of cognitive operations that one performs when attempting to maintain and manipulate information over short periods of time. Figure 5 schematically summarizes the findings of the studies that were presented in this paper. When the amount of to-be-remembered information presented at the beginning of a delayed-response trial approaches or exceeds short-term memory capacity (e.g., Waugh and Norman 1965), dorsolateral PFC is preferentially engaged. Dorsolateral PFC-supported processes may facilitate the efficient encoding of information. During the subsequent delay interval, when no information is accessible to the subject, both ventro- and dorsolateral PFC are recruited. If manipulation of this information is additionally required during the delay period, dorsolateral PFC is recruited to an additional extent. Upon the presentation of the probe stimulus, when a subject is required to make a response based on what was presented at the beginning of the trial, dorsolateral PFC is again engaged, presumably as the subject scans the information that was retained across the trial and chooses an appropriate motor response. Furthermore, the extent of activation of dorsolateral PFC is correlated with the efficiency of this scanning process. That is, faster memory scanning results in less PFC activation. If, at the time of the probe, there is PI from previously remembered information, a more ventral region of left PFC is engaged to adjudicate the conflict caused by this interference. Together, the results of these studies highlight the temporal dynamics of PFC function during working memory task performance. One strong conclusion that can be drawn from these data is that lateral PFC activity cannot be ascribed to the function of a single, unitary cognitive operation. Consistent with the picture that has emerged from the monkey electrophysiological literature, human PFC is involved in several encoding- and response-related processes, as well as to mnemonic and nonmnemonic processes that are engaged during the temporary maintenance and manipulation of information.

It is important to emphasize the types of inferences that can be drawn from our review of functional MRI studies of PFC. It is the nature of all physiological studies of the nervous system (including single- and multiunit electrophysiology, EEG, MEG, measures of glucose metabolism, and, important for the present purposes, hemodynamic measures such as fMRI) that they support inferences about the *association* of a particular brain system with a cognitive process. Thus, functional neuroimaging is an *observational, correlative* method (Sarter et al. 1996). The inference of *necessity* of a brain region to a given cognitive function cannot be made without a demonstration that the inactivation of this region disrupts the function in question. But interpretation of neuropsychological data is subject to a different set of caveats. Among them, lesion localization is difficult in human studies, the interruption of fibers of passage by a brain insult is difficult to assess, and the lesioned area may contribute in a nonspecific way to the normal functioning of a distal region that is itself the true neural substrate of the function in question. When lesion and functional neuroimaging studies are combined, however, a stronger level of inference can result. One type of combination might be that: (1) lesions to a cortical area impair a given cognitive process, and that (2) the cognitive process evokes changes in neural activity in the same cortical area in intact subjects. The inference that the neuroanatomical area is computationally necessary for the cognitive process is now rendered less vulnerable to the limitations of either method in isolation.

Few studies of patients with focal lesions of PFC performing delayed-response tasks have been reported. In a recent review of such studies, we found that some groups of patients with PFC lesions can be impaired on delayed-response tasks, and that these deficits tend to be more prominent when patients perform delayed-response tasks that include distraction during the delay (D'Esposito and Postle 1999). We also found that patients with lateral PFC lesions are generally not impaired on tests of working-memory span [i.e., digit span and block (spatial) span (D'Esposito and Postle 1999)]. This evidence from human lesion studies, combined with the results from some of the fMRI studies that we have summarized in this review, allow us to draw several conclusions and form new hypotheses about the function of lateral PFC. First, lateral PFC does not seem to make a *necessary* contribution to simple working-memory storage. Second, lateral PFC, and specifically dorsolateral, is likely necessary for the manipulation of information. Third, dorsolateral PFC may only make necessary contributions to the maintenance of information when this information must be shielded from concurrent distracting stimuli (Chao and Knight 1998). Fourth, dorsolateral PFC makes an important contribution to working-memory encoding processes (Rypma and D'Esposito 1999). Finally, lateral PFC may make an important contribution to *probe*-related processes on tests of delayed response, among these memory scanning (Rypma and D'Esposito 1999) and interference resolution processes (D'Esposito et al. 1999b). Thus, the improved inferential power and the improved temporal resolution of event-related fMRI, combined with an analysis of the human neuropsychological literature, have permitted us to articulate a model of the organization of working memory functions of PFC (Fig. 5) that is more precise, at a mechanistic and at a temporal level, than currently existing models (e.g., Petrides 1989, 1994; Smith and Jonides 1999)

Acknowledgments This work was supported by NIH grants NS01762, AG13483, AG15793 and the American Federation for Aging Research.

References

Awh E, Jonides J, Smith EE, Schumacher EH, Koeppe RA, Katz S (1996) Dissociation of storage and rehearsal in verbal working memory: evidence from PET. Psychol Sci 7:25–31

Bauer RH, Fuster JM (1976) Delayed-matching and delayed-response deficit from cooling dorsolateral prefrontal cortex in monkeys. J Comp Physiol Psychol 90:293–302

Braver TS, Cohen JD, Nystrom LE, Jonides J, Smith EE, Noll DC (1997) A parametric study of prefrontal cortex involvement in human working memory. Neuroimage 5:49–62

Chafee MV, Goldman-Rakic PS (1998) Matching patterns of activity in primate prefrontal area 8a and parietal area 7ip neurons during a spatial working memory task. J Neurophysiol 79:2919–2940

Chao L, Knight R (1998) Contribution of human prefrontal cortex to delay performance. J Cogn Neurosci 10:167–177

Cohen JD, Perlstein WM, Braver TS, Nystrom LE, Noll DC, Jonides J, Smith EE (1997) Temporal dynamics of brain activation during a working memory task. Nature 386:604–607

Courtney SM, Ungerleider LG, Keil K, Haxby JV (1997) Transient and sustained activity in a distributed neural system for human working memory. Nature 386:608–611

D'Esposito M, Postle BR (1999) The dependence of span and delayed-response performance on prefrontal cortex. Neuropsychologia 37:89–101

D'Esposito M, Detre JA, Alsop DC, Shin RK, Atlas S, Grossman M (1995) The neural basis of the central executive system of working memory. Nature 378:279–281

D'Esposito M, Postle BR, Ballard D, Lease J (1999a) Maintenance versus manipulation of information held in working memory: an event-related fMRI study. Brain Cogn 41:66–86

D'Esposito M, Postle BR, Jonides J, Smith EE (1999b) The neural substrate and temporal dynamics of interference effects in working memory as revealed by event-related functional MRI. Proc Natl Acad Sci USA 96:7514–7519

D'Esposito M, Ballard D, Zarahn E, Aguirre GK (2000) The role of prefrontal cortex in sensory memory and motor preparation: an event-related fMRI study. Neuroimage (in press)

Diamond A (1990) The development and neural bases of memory functions as indexed by the A-not-B and delayed response tasks in human infants and infant monkeys. In: Diamond A (ed) The development and neural bases of higher cognitive functions. New York Academy of Sciences, New York, pp 267–317

Friston KJ, Price CJ, Fletcher P, Moore C, Frackowiak RSJ, Dolan RJ (1996) The trouble with cognitive subtraction. Neuroimage 4:97–104

Funahashi S, Bruce CJ, Goldman-Rakic PS (1989) Mnemonic coding of visual space in the monkey's dorsolateral prefrontal cortex. J Neurophysiol 61:331–349

Funahashi S, Bruce CJ, Goldman-Rakic PS (1993) Dorsolateral prefrontal lesions and oculomotor delayed-response performance: evidence for mnemonic "scotomas". J Neurosci 13: 1479–1497

Fuster JM, Alexander GE (1971) Neuron activity related to short-term memory. Science 173:652–654

Fuster JM, Bauer RH, Jervey JP (1982) Cellular discharge in the dorsolateral prefrontal cortex of the monkey in cognitive tasks. Exp Neurol 77:679–694

Garavan H (1998) Serial attention within working memory. Memory Cogn 26:263–276

Jonides J, Smith EE, Koeppe RA, Awh E, Minoshima S, Mintun MA (1993) Spatial working memory in humans as revealed by PET. Nature 363:623–625

Jonides J, Schumacher EH, Smith EE, Lauber E, Awh E, Minoshima S, Koeppe RA (1997) Verbal working memory load affects regional brain activation as measured by PET. J Cogn Neurosci 9:462–475

Jonides J, Smith EE, Marshuetz C, Koeppe RA, Reuter-Lorenz PA (1998) Inhibition of verbal working memory revealed by brain activation. Proc Natl Acad Sci USA 95:8410–8413

Manoach DS, Schlaug G, Siewert B, Darby DG, Bly BM, Benfield A, Edelman RR, Warach S (1997) Prefrontal cortex fMRI signal changes are correlated with working memory load. Neuroreport 8:545–549

McElree B (1998) Attended and non-attended states in working memory: accessing categorized structures. J Memory Lang 38: 225–252

McElree B, Dosher BA (1987) Serial position and set size in short-term memory: the time course of recognition. J Exp Psychol 118:346–373

Monsell S (1978) Recency, immediate recognition memory, and reaction time. Cogn Psychol 10:465–501

Owen AM, Evans AC, Petrides M (1996) Evidence for a two-stage model of spatial working memory processing within the lateral frontal cortex: a positron emission tomography study. Cereb Cortex 6:31–38

Owen AM, Stern CE, Look RB, Tracey I, Rosen BR, Petrides M (1998) Functional organization of spatial and nonspatial working memory processing within the human lateral frontal cortex. Proc Natl Acad Sci USA 95:7721–7726

Owen AM, Herrod NJ, Menon DK, Clark JC, Downey SP, Carpenter TA, Minhas PS, Turkheimer FE, Williams EJ, Robbins TW, Sahakian BJ, Petrides M, Pickard JD (1999) Redefining the functional organization of working memory processes within human lateral prefrontal cortex. Eur J Neurosci 11:567–574

Petrides M (1989) Frontal lobes and memory. In: Boller F, Grafman J (eds) Handbook of neuropsychology. Elsevier, Amsterdam New York, pp 601–614

Petrides M (1994) Frontal lobes and working memory: evidence from investigations of the effects of cortical excisions in non-human primates. In: Boller F, Grafman J (eds) Handbook of neuropsychology. Elsevier Science, Amsterdam, pp 59–84

Posner MI, Petersen SE, Fox PT, Raichle ME (1988) Localization of cognitive operations in the human brain. Science 240:1627–1631

Postle BR, D'Esposito M (1999) "What" – then – "where" in visual working memory: an event-related fMRI study. J Cogn Neurosci 11:585–597

Postle BR, Berger JS, D'Esposito M (1999) Functional neuroanatomical double dissociation of mnemonic and executive control processes contributing to working memory performance. Proc Natl Acad Sci USA 96:12959–12964

Rainer G, Rao SC, Miller EK (1999) Prospective coding for objects in primate prefrontal cortex. J Neurosci 19:5493–5505

Rypma B, D'Esposito M (1999) The roles of prefrontal brain regions in components of working memory: effects of memory load and individual differences. Proc Natl Acad Sci USA 96:6558–6563

Rypma B, Prabhakaran V, Desmond JE, Glover GH, Gabrieli JD (1999) Load-dependent roles of frontal brain regions in the maintenance of working memory. Neuroimage 9:216–226

Sarter M, Bernston G, Cacioppo J (1996) Brain imaging and cognitive neuroscience: toward strong inference in attributing function to structure. Am Psychol 51:13–21

Smith EE, Jonides J (1999) Storage and executive processes of the frontal lobes. Science 283:1657–1661

Smith EE, Jonides J, Koeppe RA, Awh E, Schumacher EH, Minoshima S (1995) Spatial versus object working memory: PET investigations. J Cogn Neurosci 7:337–356

Smith EE, Jonides J, Marshuetz C, Koeppe RA (1998) Components of verbal working memory: evidence from neuroimaging. Proc Natl Acad Sci USA 95:876–882

Sternberg S (1966) High-speed scanning in human memory. Science 153:652–654

Sternberg S (1969) The discovery of processing stages: extensions of Donders' method. Acta Psychol 30:276–315

Thompson-Schill SL, D'Esposito M, Aguirre GK, Farah MJ (1997) Role of left inferior prefrontal cortex in retrieval of semantic knowledge: a reevaluation. Proc Natl Acad Sci USA 94:14792–14797

Watanabe M (1996) Reward expectancy in primate prefrontal neurons. Nature 382:629–632

Waugh NC, Norman DA (1965) Primary memory. Psychol Rev 72:89–104

Zarahn E, Aguirre GK, D'Esposito M (1997) A trial-based experimental design for functional MRI. Neuroimage 6:122–138

Zarahn E, Aguirre GK, D'Esposito M (1999) Temporal isolation of the neural correlates of spatial mnemonic processing with fMRI. Cogn Brain Res 7:255–268

Stefan Pollmann · D. Yves von Cramon

Object working memory and visuospatial processing: functional neuroanatomy analyzed by event-related fMRI

Published online: 12 May 2000

Abstract We report an event-related functional magnetic-resonance-imaging (fMRI) experiment that investigates the relationship of transient visual object memory, visuospatial orienting, and object recognition. Delayed object matching and visuospatial orienting involved a highly overlapping network of brain areas. Common areas were the frontal eye fields (FEF), the pre-supplementary motor area (pre-SMA)/SMA complex, the precentral gyri, and the horizontal and descending branches of the intraparietal sulcus (IPS). Selective delay activation was observed anterior to the FEF and in the ascending part of the IPS. Right dorsolateral prefrontal cortex was involved in goal-directed visual search, but showed no delay activity.

Key words Attention · Memory · Object recognition · fMRI · Event-related

Introduction

Working memory has been defined as "the collection of mental processes that permit information to be held temporarily in an accessible state, in the service of some mental task" (Cowan 1998). According to this definition, most everyday activities would, to some degree, involve working memory. This central importance may explain the great number of studies which have been devoted to this topic in recent years.

Working memory can be subdivided into a memory component, holding information active for the current task, and a manipulation component, working on the activated information. It has been further subdivided according to the information it works on, into verbal versus nonverbal, spatial versus nonspatial, or verbal versus object memory. In this paper, we compare the functional neuroanatomy associated with holding object information accessible with a specific manipulation component, attention-demanding visual search. Using event-related functional magnetic-resonance imaging (fMRI), we investigated the timecourse of activation when an object (the cue) was held accessible over a short delay, followed by visual search for a target object that had to be matched to the cue. In this way, activations associated with holding object information accessible were discriminated from activations related to visuospatial orienting and object recognition, respectively.

S. Pollmann (✉) · D.Y. von Cramon
Max-Planck-Institute of Cognitive Neuroscience, Stephanstrasse 1a, 04103 Leipzig, Germany
e-mail: pollmann@cns.mpg.de
Tel.: +49-341-9940226, Fax: +49-341-9940221

Delayed matching

Many studies with nonhuman primates have used delayed-matching or delayed-response experiments to investigate working memory (Fuster and Alexander 1971; Funahashi et al. 1989). In delayed matching, the animal is presented with a cue stimulus, which is to be remembered. After a delay, alternative stimuli are presented, and the animal has to select the stimulus which matches the cue stimulus presented before the delay. Neurons in numerous brain areas have been found to respond selectively during the delay intervals, setting up a temporal contingency between stimulus presentation and match and/or response execution (Fuster 1985). Such delay activity has been reported in numerous brain areas in monkeys, e.g., in inferotemporal (Fuster and Jervey 1981, 1982) and parietal cortex (Koch and Fuster 1989; Chafee and Goldman-Rakic 1998). In prefrontal cortex, delay activity has been observed on both sides of the principal sulcus. It has been suggested that, in the monkey brain, neurons in ventrolateral prefrontal cortex preferentially display delay activity during visual object-memory tasks, whereas dorsolateral prefrontal cortex supports visuospatial working memory (Wilson et al. 1993). However, other studies have found prefrontal neurons that were responsive to the featural ("what") or spatial ("where") characteristics of a stimulus to be intermixed in the same area (Quintana et al. 1988). Furthermore, when the task requires object and location information to be processed, many prefrontal neurons have been shown to convey object information on the one hand and have highly localized memory fields on the other hand (Rainer et al. 1998).

Whereas in the monkey, ventrolateral and dorsolateral prefrontal cortex is separated by the principal sulcus, this structure does not exist in the human brain, complicating the search for homologous areas. It is commonly assumed that the superior and middle frontal gyrus [Brodmann areas (BA) 9, 46] represent human dorsolateral prefrontal cortex, whereas the homologue of ventrolateral prefrontal cortex would be found more ventrally, including the anterior portion of the inferior frontal gyrus (BA 47, 45). In recent reviews of positron emission tomography (PET) and fMRI working-memory studies, the locations of activation maxima in human prefrontal cortex, when plotted onto a standardized brain, did not show a spatial/non-spatial distinction (Owen 1997; Rushworth et al. 1997; D'Esposito et al. 1998). Neither were activations related to spatial tasks found more frequently in middle frontal gyrus nor were the locations of nonspatial activations more ventral (D'Esposito et al. 1998). Whereas the latter metaanalysis looked at activations located anterior to the vertical plane through the anterior commissure (VAC), covering "true" prefrontal cortex, a second metaanalysis (Smith and Jonides 1999) included more posterior activations (up to 25 mm posterior to the AC-plane), thus including the frontal lobes completely. Smith and Jonides found a dorsal-ventral difference with more dorsal activation foci for spatial working-memory tasks. In particular, they observed a cluster of "spatial" activations in *premotor* cortex, i.e., more posterior than for "nonspatial" activations. This again agrees with monkey data of Rainer et al. (1998), who found a majority of location-selective neurons in posterior locations near the arcuate sulcus, in the vicinity of the frontal eye fields.

Courtney et al. (1996, 1998) reported delay activity in a spatial delayed matching task along the superior frontal sulcus. This delay activation was located immediately anterior to the junction of the superior frontal sulcus and the precentral sulcus, which has been identified in a number of studies as the putative location of the human frontal eye field (FEF; Paus 1996; Luna et al. 1998). Courtney et al. (1998) also found activation at the junction of the superior precentral and superior frontal sulcus in a saccade-generation control task, confirming the location of the frontal eye fields (FEF). The delay activation was located immediately anterior to the saccade-related activation. Courtney et al. (1998) emphasized that the human FEF is found more posterior than the monkey FEF, and that spatial working-memory-related neurons, which are found immediately anterior to the FEF in the monkey, may also be shifted in the posterior direction in the human brain, maintaining its topographical relationship with the FEF. However, in a recent comparative cytoarchitectonic study, Petrides and Pandya (1999) came to the conclusion that in the monkey, as in the human brain, specifically spatial information processing would occur not in areas 9/46, but in the more posterior dorsolateral frontal areas 8 and rostral 6, which receive strong inputs from inferior parietal cortex and connect to the oculomotor system. The findings of Courtney et al. would, thus, fit the functional organization found in the monkey brain.

An area outside of the frontal lobes that consistently shows activation in imaging studies of working memory is posterior parietal cortex (PPC). In delayed matching studies, PPC was found to be active when spatial information had to be retained (Courtney et al. 1996; Smith et al. 1995), but also in delayed matching of objects (Baker et al. 1996; Smith et al. 1995). Since we focus on nonverbal tasks, verbal delayed matching-to-sample (DMS) studies are not discussed here (for an overview, cf. D'Esposito et al. 1998; Smith and Jonides 1999).

One difficulty with early PET-studies of delayed matching (Haxby et al. 1994) is that neurons in a given area respond not only during the delay, but also during stimulus presentation. Using event-related fMRI, it has been shown that the contribution of stimulus- and delay-associated activity gradually varies between visual areas in occipital cortex, e.g., posterior lingual and fusiform gyri (showing strong general perceptual activation) and mid-anterior fusiform gyrus (specific face-related activation), to prefrontal cortex, which showed a dominance of delay activity (Courtney et al. 1997).

Visuospatial orienting and visual search – commonalities with delayed matching

Many of the areas involved in DMS have also been found to be activated by tasks affording visuospatial orienting. Visuospatial orienting can proceed overtly, via eye-movements, or covertly, by attending to a peripheral location without changing fixation. In a series of imaging experiments, Corbetta and colleagues investigated the functional neuroanatomy of covert and overt orienting. They found a core network of brain structures involved in both kinds of orienting, consisting of posterior parietal areas, along the intraparietal sulcus and both lateral and medial areas of superior frontal cortex (Corbetta 1998). Less consistently, right inferior parietal and superior temporal cortex were activated, as well as anterior cingulate cortex (BA 24, 32). In a direct comparison (Corbetta et al. 1998), overt and covert orienting activated a largely overlapping set of structures, suggesting common mechanisms for the guidance of eye movements and covert attention shifts, as expected from behavioral data showing a tight coupling of the deployment of attention to the location of intended saccades (Deubel and Schneider 1995).

Among the frontal structures activated by both overt and covert shifts of attention were the putative locations of the human supplementary (SEF) and frontal eye fields (FEF, cf. Paus 1996; Luna et al. 1998; Petit et al. 1998). Since the area anterior to the FEF, along the superior frontal sulcus, has been found to be active during the delays of a spatial working-memory task (Courtney et al. 1998), one topic of our study was whether visual delayed matching and visual search lead to adjacent activations along the posterior part of the superior frontal sulcus. Other areas that are activated both by visual-orienting tasks and delayed-matching tasks are the precentral gyrus and posterior parietal cortex. Here, the question was whether we would be able to differentiate subregions within these areas that may be specific to transient object memory or visuospatial orienting.

Mostly, visuospatial orienting serves the purpose of identifying a stimulus at a particular location. This is the typical situation in visual-search tasks. In previous fMRI studies, we were able to show that attention-demanding visual search leads to activation of the same structures as discussed above for visual orienting (Pollmann et al. 1998). For parietal cortex, the similarity of activations related to "pure" visuospatial orienting and visual search had been demonstrated before by Corbetta et al. (1995). This similarity of activation patterns in visual orienting and search tasks is not surprising, as long as the search task is constructed in such a way that search for the target object has to proceed via saccades to different parts of the search display.

However, visual search for a given object goes beyond orienting to a specific location (which is usually denoted by a simple symbol like a dot or cross), in that there is additional processing of object information. In the present experiment, we varied the difficulty of object matching, in order to discriminate object recognition processes from visuospatial orienting and object memory.

Recent investigations of the temporal resolution of the blood oxygen-level-detection (BOLD) response have demonstrated that, within the same session, signal onset differences in the subsecond range can be discriminated reliably (Dymond et al. 1999; Menon et al. 1999). This enables us to differentiate the activations elicited by different cognitive processes within a trial. The advantages of having both delayed matching and visual search in close temporal succession lies in the elimination of several artifacts, which may affect comparisons between task blocks within an imaging session or, worse, different imaging experiments. The comparison of task blocks within an fMRI session may be confounded by factors such as signal drift or movement artifacts. Comparisons between fMRI sessions, even when the same subjects are repeatedly measured, are affected by the intraindividual variation of the BOLD response (Aguirre et al. 1998a). Comparisons between imaging experiments with different subject samples are, in addition, affected by the interindividual differences in the neuroanatomy, among other factors. We therefore chose to design an experiment that would allow the discrimination of delay- and search-related activity occurring subsequently within trials. Given the fact that, according to the literature, we expect an overlap between delay and search-related activation patterns, event-related fMRI seems to be the best way to detect subtle differences in activation.

Materials and methods

Subjects

Nine subjects (22–29 years old, five female), all students of the University of Leipzig, participated in this study. All were right-handed, as assessed with the Edinburgh Handedness Inventory (Oldfield 1971). The subjects gave written informed consents following institutional guidelines.

Cognitive task

The task that we used to discriminate between activations associated with object memory, visuospatial orienting, and object recognition was a delayed matching task with artificial, "paperclip"-like geometrical objects.[1]

In every trial, a unique "paperclip"-stimulus was presented and had to be matched, after a variable delay, to a target "paperclip", which was placed in a search display consisting of 11 "paperclips" (Fig. 1). The location of the target stimulus was marked by a frame, which differed in appearance from the frames of the distractor stimuli. In one half of the trials, the target frame was open on the left, whereas the distractor frames were closed (Fig. 1a). In the other half of trials, the target frame was closed and the distractor frames were open (Fig. 1b). There is a search asymmetry for these kinds of stimuli, in that search for a closed among open objects takes longer than the reverse (Treisman and Gormican 1988). The difficulty of object matching was varied by changing the viewpoint of cue and target object. When both were presented from the same viewpoint (Fig. 1b), match was easy. However, the object could also be rotated in the horizontal plane, making the match more difficult (Fig. 1a). This way of presentation enabled us to manipulate the difficulty of the search for the target location independent of the difficulty of object-recognition processes on the target stimulus, presented at this location (for a discussion of such "compound tasks", cf. Duncan 1985; Theeuwes 1992). Both invariant and changed views were presented in random sequence over the experiment, so that the difficulty of the match would not influence the encoding of the cue stimulus. In addition, subjects were alerted to the fact that the target stimulus may be presented from a different viewpoint than the cue and were asked to encode the cue as a three-dimensional object. The subjects indicated their matching decision by a forced choice (present/absent) button press.

Trials began with the presentation of the cue stimulus for 2 s. Cue presentation was followed by a blank screen of 2- to 8-s duration. The duration of this delay period was varied in exponentially declining frequency, so that the probability for the delay to end after a given duration was equivalent to the probability that it would end at one of the longer durations. In this way, subjects could not anticipate the duration of the delay. Following the delay, the search display was presented until the subject responded or for a maximum of 5 s. The search display was followed by presentation of a central fixation cross (intertrial interval) until the next trial began. The time for the presentation of the search display plus the following intertrial interval was always 10 s. In one half of the trials, the target location in the search display was characterized by a singular open or closed frame, respectively. Within the open and closed frame trials, the target location contained the cue object presented from the same viewpoint in one third of trials, the cue object rotated by 20° in another third, and a different object, randomly generated using the same parameter space as for the cues, in the remaining third of trials. For each trial, novel objects were generated.

Magnetic resonance imaging

Stimuli were displayed by an LCD projector on a back-projection screen mounted in the bore of the magnet behind the participants'

[1] We thank Prof. Nikos Logothetis (Max-Planck-Institute for Biological Cybernetics, Tübingen) for making the stimulus generation software available

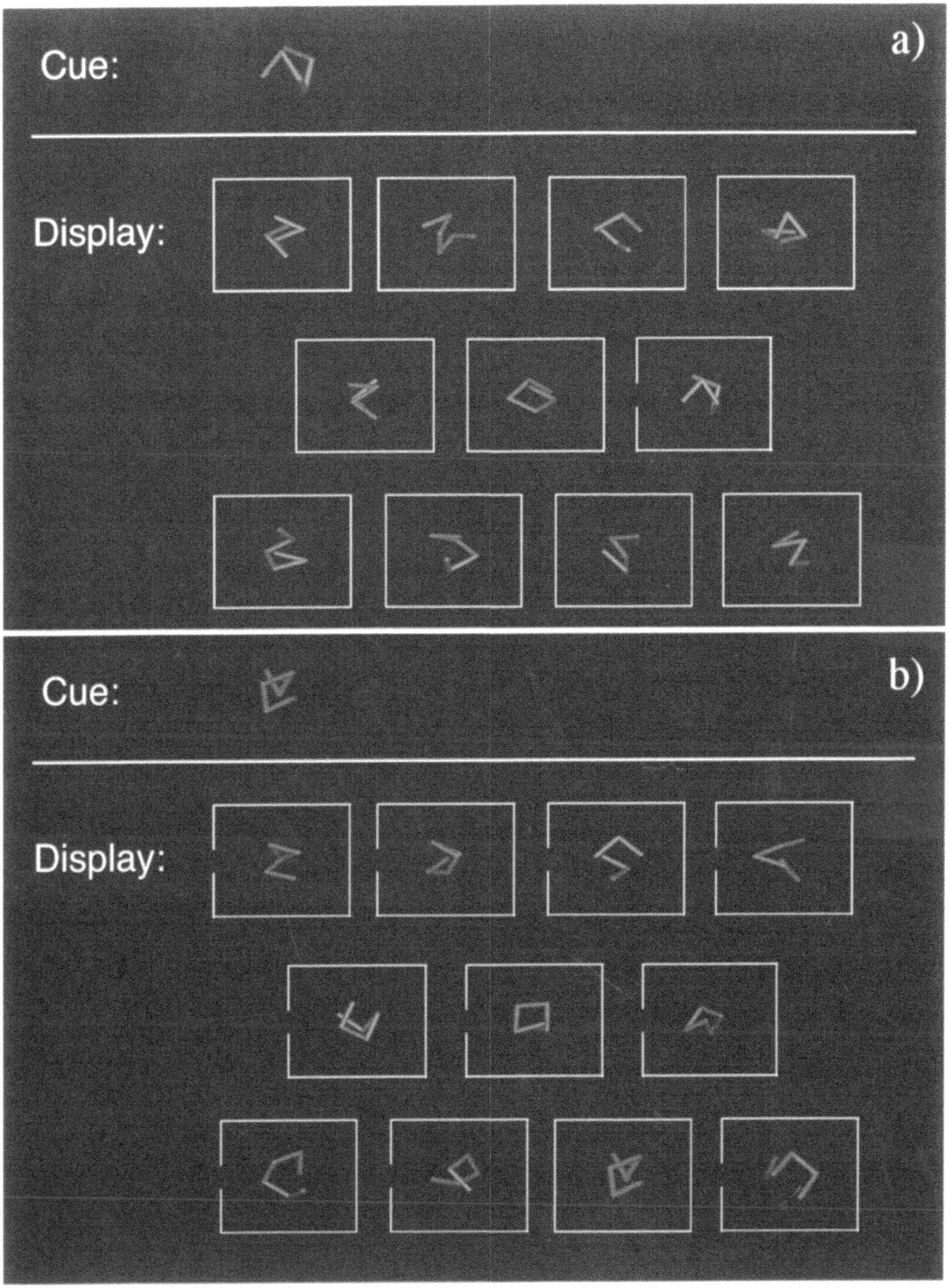
a)
Cue:
Display:
b)
Cue:
Display:

Table 1 Activation associated with visual search difficulty. All tables contain only activations >100 mm^3. *L* Left, *R* right

	Maximum	Location			
Superior frontal sulcus/superior precentral sulcus (FEF)	8.10	L	–27	–7	49
	14.58	R	37	0	39
preSMA	18.72	L	–7	11	45
Middle frontal gyrus	6.90	R	28	26	37
Precentral gyrus/sulcus	11.91	L	–45	–3	40
Postcentral gyrus	10.95	L	–33	–28	62
Intraparietal sulcus/ cuneus	15.18	L	–32	–55	50
	39.42	R	1	–79	13
Inferior parietal lobule	6.00	L	–47	–35	25
Insula	9.90	L	–36	9	15
	13.29	R	26	20	11

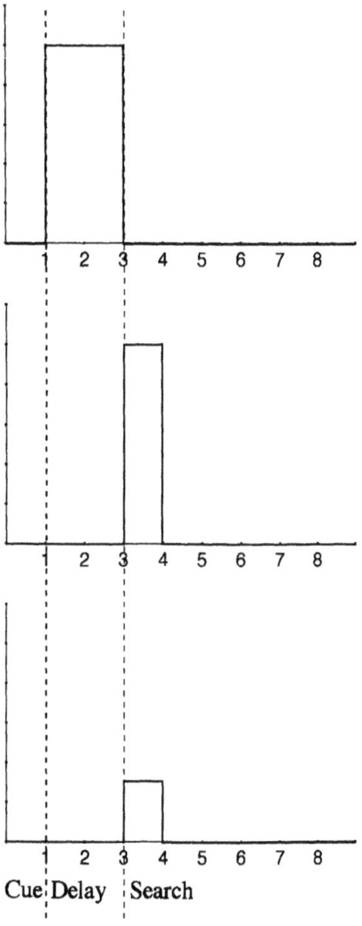

Fig. 2 Schematic description of the regressors for delay activation (*top*) and visual-search difficulty as well as object-recognition difficulty (*middle*: difficult condition, *bottom*: easy condition). The delay regressor followed the duration of the delay. Visual-search difficulty and object-recognition difficulty were varied orthogonally to each other

◀ **Fig. 1a, b** The combined delayed-matching/visual-search experiment. Subjects first had to memorize the cue object. After a delay of 2- to 8-s duration, they had to find the target location, indicated by a unique frame. Then, they had to decide whether the object at this location matched the cue. In case of a match, the object could be presented from the same (**b**) or a rotated (**a**) viewpoint. Unique open frames among closed frames (**a**) were detected faster than unique closed frames among open frames (**b**)

head. Participants viewed the screen wearing mirror glasses, which were equipped with corrective lenses if necessary.

The experiment consisted of six runs of 30 trials each, preceded and followed by 10 s of fixation. Functional images were acquired at 3T (Bruker 3T/100 Medspec, Bruker Medizintechnik GmbH, Ettlingen, Germany) using a gradient-recalled EPI sequence (TR=2000 ms, TE=40 ms, flip angle=90°). Forteen axial slices were acquired oriented along the AC-PC plane, with a field-of-view of 19.2 cm and an image matrix of 64×64. Slice thickness was 5 mm, interslice distance 2 mm, allowing whole-brain coverage.

Data analysis

Images were motion corrected with the algorithm of Friston et al. (1996) and gaussian filtered in the spatial domain with a FWHM= 3 mm. Data were analyzed in event-related fashion, using multiple regression. Activation was characterized as delay-activity when the time course of the BOLD-signal increased followed the variable delay durations over trials (corrected for the lag and dispersion of the hemodynamic response: lag=4.8 s, σ=1.8 s; cf. Clark et al. 1998). Orienting-related activation was characterized by high increases in difficult orienting trials (closed target frame), and low increases in easy orienting trials (open target frame), which were time-locked to the presentation of the search display (Fig. 2). Analogously, object-matching-related activation was characterized by high signal increases in difficult matching trials (changed viewpoint) and low signal increase in easy matching trials (invariant viewpoint).

Degrees of freedom were corrected for temporal autocorrelation of the BOLD-response (Worsley and Friston 1995). Average z-maps were computed, after registration with individual, three-dimensional anatomical images and normalization by linear scaling (Lohmann et al. 1999), by performing *t*-tests for known variance at corresponding voxels across participants (Bosch 2000). To correct for multiple comparisons, the significance criterion was set to α=0.000001.

Results and discussion

There was a high degree of overlap in the brain structures that showed delay activity as well as activity related to visuospatial orienting. Object-matching specific activation was mainly restricted to two areas, one in occipital cortex and the other in the pre- and postcentral gyri. Object recognition overlapped more with visuospatial orienting than with delay activity.

Frontal eye fields

A distinct bilateral activation during attentive search was found at the junction of the superior precentral and supe-

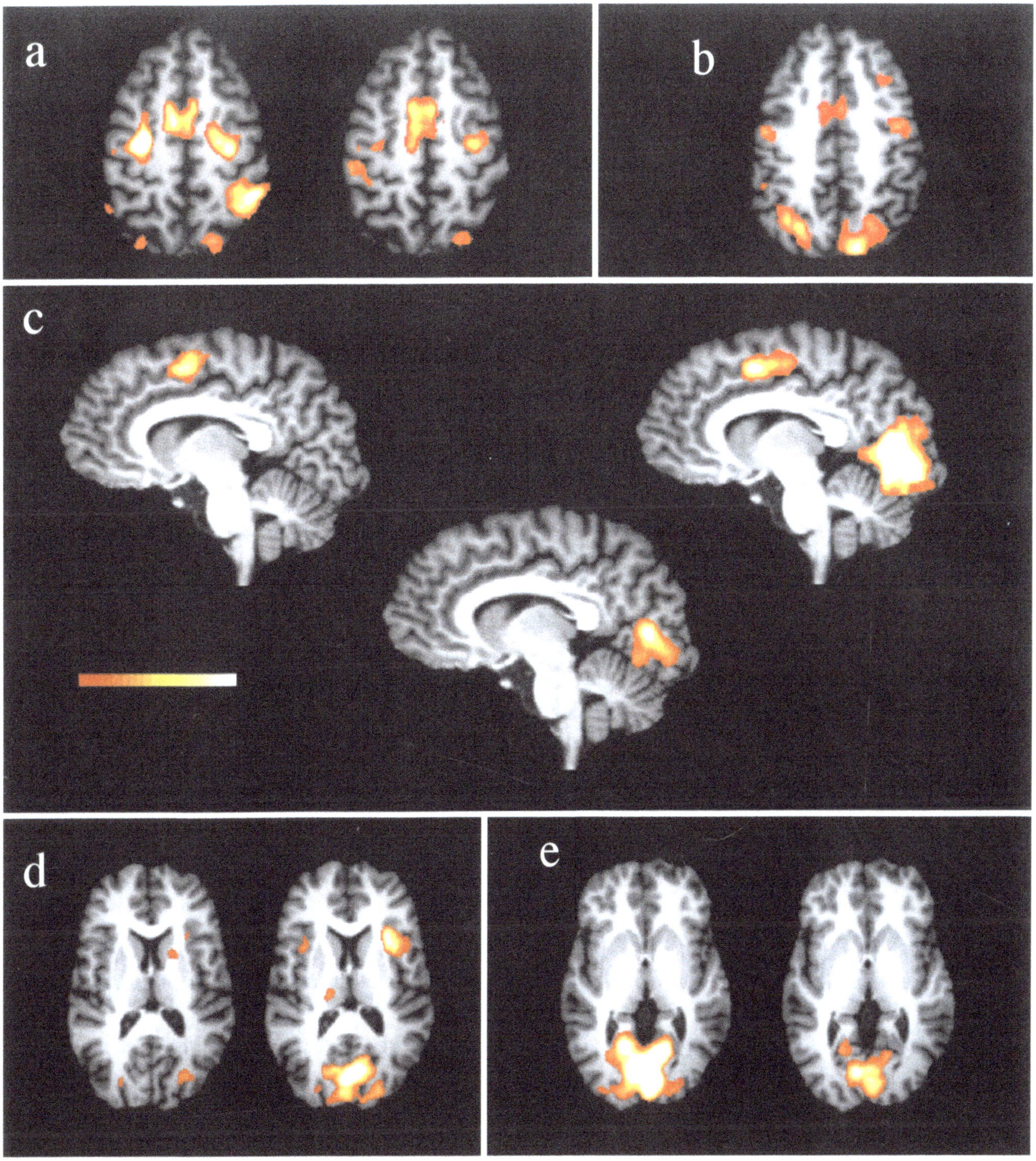

Fig. 3 **a** The junction of the precentral and superior frontal gyri was activated by visuospatial orienting (*right*), indicating the putative location of the frontal eye fields (FEF). Delay activity was observed at the same location (*left*), extending anteriorly along the superior frontal gyri. The left hemisphere is on the left in all figures. The *color scale* for all activations is given in **c**; it ranges from z=4.75–24. **b** The right middle frontal gyrus was selectively activated by visuospatial orienting. **c** Delay activity (*left*) in medial frontal cortex was observed anterior to the vertical plane through the anterior commissure (VAC), at the location of the pre-supplementary motor area (pre-SMA), whereas the activation elicited by visuospatial orienting (*right*) extended from the pre-SMA to the SMA proper, posterior to the VAC. Visual orienting led to strong activation over the entire medial aspect of the occipital lobes, whereas object recognition (*bottom*) was associated with activation in striate and peristriate cortex. **d** Delay activity was observed in right anterio-superior insula (*left*). Orienting-related activation (*right*) was seen bilaterally in the insula, dominantly in the right hemisphere. **e** Both visuospatial orienting (*left*) and object recognition (*right*) led to activation of the cuneus, reaching to the parieto-occipital fissure

Table 2 Activation associated with the delay period. *L* Left, *R* right

	Maximum	Location			
Superior frontal sulcus/superior precentral sulcus (FEF)	30.24	L	–27	–8	49
	15.36	R	17	1	57
preSMA	16.29	L	–11	4	59
Lateral precentral gyrus/ sulcus	13.29	L	–48	0	42
	18.48	R	43	2	31
Intraparietal sulcus	22.29	L	–47	–36	46
	19.29	R	17	–65	46
Middle temporal gyrus middle occipital gyrus	10.32	L	–40	–79	20
Middle temporal gyrus/ inferior temporal sulcus	8.34	L	–48	–57	–1
	10.53	R	48	–48	0
Insula	6.03	R	41	3	–3
Caudate nucleus/putamen	8.67	R	17	10	7

rior frontal gyri, the putative location of the human FEF (Fig. 3a, Table 1). This activation was expected because this area has been regularly found to be activated in tasks which afforded eye movements (Paus 1996; Petit et al. 1998; Luna et al. 1998). The junction of the superior precentral and superior frontal gyri was also active during the delay (Fig. 3a, Table 2). However, the delay activation was much larger than with orienting, extending anteriorly along the posterior superior frontal sulcus.

Thus, our data confirm that the area along the superior frontal sulcus, just anterior of the FEF, is involved in working memory. However, this area was previously found to be active during delayed matching of locations, but not during delayed matching of faces (Courtney et al. 1996, 1998). It was thus interpreted as being an area subserving spatial working memory. On first sight, this seems to contradict our data, since we used an object-memory task. However, there were several differences to previous delayed object-matching tasks. Our "paperclips" were artificial objects, not too closely resembling any known objects. In addition, each object was unique. This reduced the likelihood of a verbal or categorical labeling, which may have occurred in previous studies using faces or real objects. In contrast to previous studies using nonsense shapes, subjects knew that the object representations, which they had to compare with the cue object, could be presented from a different viewpoint, and they were instructed to encode the objects as three-dimensional structures. Since the three-dimensional structure of the "paperclips" is defined by the angles between the component rods, there was an important spatial component to this task. Thus, our data show quite clearly that the area along the posterior superior frontal sulcus is not only important for spatial working memory, but also for working memory for visual objects, at least when three-dimensional object characteristics have to be retained.

Dorsolateral prefrontal cortex

We did not find delay-associated activation in middle or inferior frontal gyrus, which has been reported in other object-DMS studies. Visuospatial orienting, however, elicited an activation in right middle frontal gyrus (Fig. 3b). Dorsolateral prefrontal cortex has been found to be reliably activated by tasks with high manipulation demands (D'Esposito et al. 1998). However, due to the separation of visuospatial search (for the target frame) and subsequent object-recognition processes, visual search processes in our experiment were not a manipulation of a working-memory content. Thus, the activation rather reflects a middle frontal gyrus contribution to attention-demanding search per se. The difference between difficult and easy search was that the target frame did not "pop-out" by a feature difference with the distractor items, but had to be searched in a top-down controlled manner. It is not unlikely that the right middle frontal gyrus was involved in this control process. A similar finding has been recently reported by Rosen et al. (1999). In their spatial cueing experiment, right middle frontal gyrus was active (in BA46) when endogenous cues (arrows at fixation) indicated the target location, but not when exogenous cues (brightening of boxes around the target location) were used. In behavioral studies, it has been shown that exogenous cues lead to fast, automatic shifts of attention to the target location, whereas endogenous cues facilitate processing at the target location more slowly, indicating effortful shifts of attention.

Supplementary motor area/pre-supplementary motor area

Delay- as well as orienting-associated activation was also found in frontomedian cortex (Fig. 3c). Medial wall delay activation was found in superior frontal cortex anterior to the vertical plane through the anterior commissure (VAC).

Activation associated with visuospatial orienting largely overlapped with delay activity. Only in the left hemisphere, did orienting-related activation extend posteriorly past the VAC. These data confirm recent findings of Petit et al. (1998), who investigated medial wall activations in delayed matching of faces and locations. Both in the spatial and the face-matching tasks, delay activity was observed mostly anterior to the VAC. Location of peak activity and extent of activation hardly differed

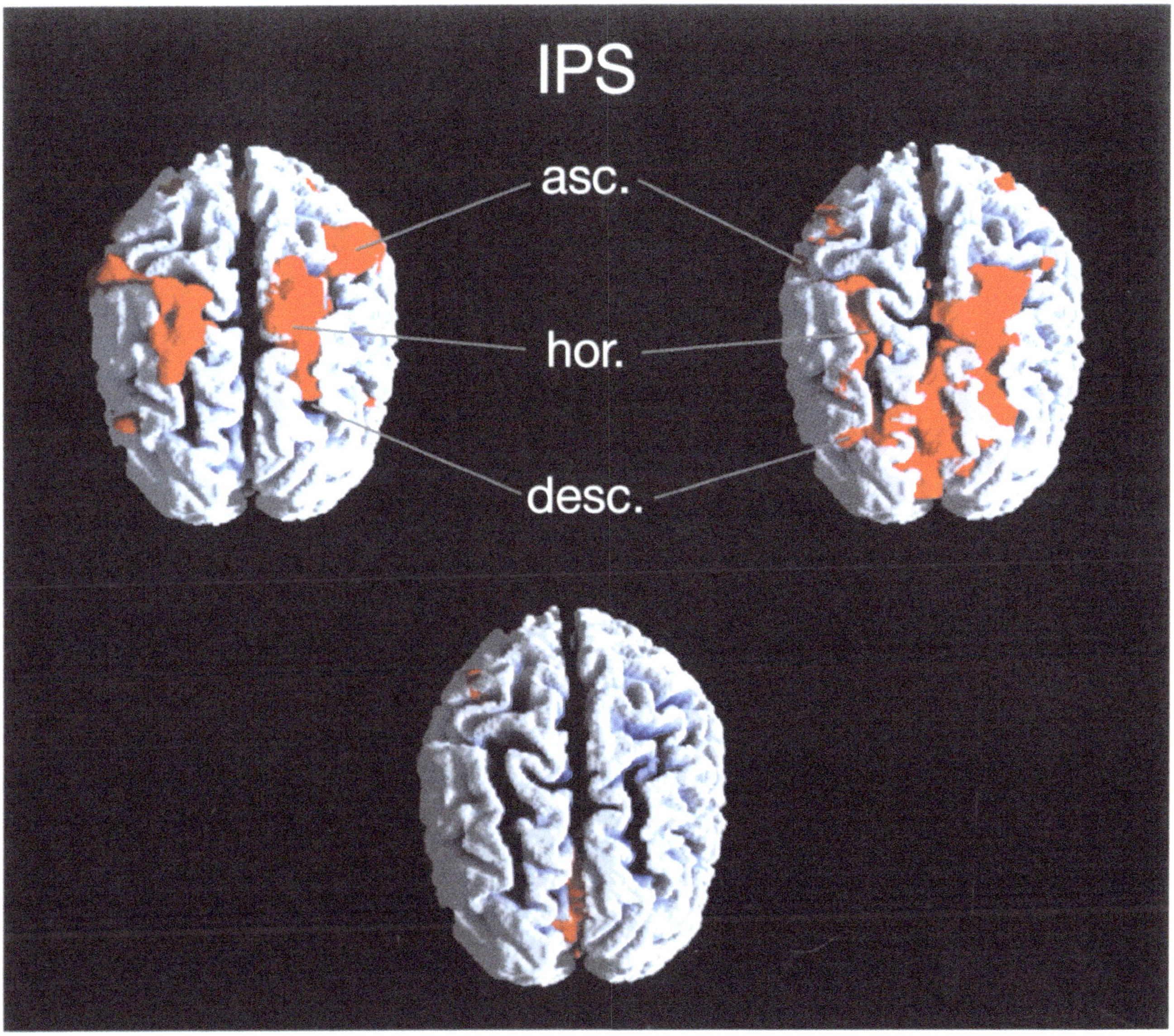

Fig. 4 Activation along the intraparietal sulcus (*IPS*). Delay activation (*left*) was observed along the ascending (*asc.*), horizontal (*hor.*), and descending (*desc.*) branches. Orienting-related activation (*right*) was mainly seen in the horizontal and descending branches

between face-matching and location matching. Petit et al. concluded that the sustained activation of the pre-supplementary motor area (pre-SMA) during working-memory delays, since it was independent of the content to be remembered (locations or faces), was most likely tied to the type of response, which was identical in both tasks. In their study, as in ours, subjects could not prepare a specific response. However, they knew that they had to respond after a short delay. Following Picard and Strick (1996), the VAC demarcates the border of SMA proper (posterior to VAC) and pre-SMA (anterior to VAC). They interpreted the pre-SMA delay activation as an indication of response-preparatory processes. In a motor control condition, when subjects had to execute a prespecified button press after a delay, the activation was found in SMA proper. This was interpreted as a preparation of the actual response execution. The similarity of the delay activation of Petit et al. and ours underlines the independence of this activation of the kind of stimuli which have to be retained during the delay (faces versus abstract objects).

Lateral premotor cortex

Delay activity and visuospatial orienting were associated with largely overlapping areas of bilateral activation in the precentral gyrus. The dorsal-ventral extent of both activations was confined to the height of the middle frontal gyrus. Broca's area, which has been found activated along with lateral premotor cortex in previous studies when verbal rehearsal was afforded by the task (Awh et al. 1996), was not activated in the present experiment. Although it is difficult to draw conclusions from a

Table 3 Activation associated with object-recognition difficulty. *L* Left, *R* right

	Maximum	Location			
Postcentral gyrus	10.29	L	–33	–28	62
Precentral sulcus	6.81	R	38	–1	39
Striate cortex	11.91	L	–10	–82	14
Cuneus	7.56	R	6	–66	23

null effect, the activation pattern is certainly fitting for our experiment, where verbal labeling (and thus verbal rehearsal) was discouraged by the use of novel artificial objects in every trial. Object recognition was associated with a right precentral activation at the same location as for the delay and orienting conditions.

Insula

Orienting strongly activated the superior portion of the anterior gyrus brevis of the insula, bilaterally, but dominantly in the right hemisphere. Delay activity was limited to the right insula (Fig. 3d). Courtney et al. (1997) also reported a bilateral activation of the anterior insula in their delayed matching experiment. In their study, mostly delay activity contributed to this activation, while unspecific visual stimulation or face-specific perceptual processes contributed less to insular activation. Our data replicated delay activation in this area. In addition, they show that the antero-superior insula, especially in the right hemisphere, contributes even more to attentive visual search than to the "bridging of the delay" for object matching.

Posterior parietal cortex

Delay activation was bilaterally detected along the banks of the intraparietal sulcus (IPS), from the ascending over the horizontal to the descending branch (Fig. 4). Orienting-associated activation was mostly confined to the horizontal, descending branches of the IPS, overlapping with the delay activation. Orienting-associated activation was more pronounced in the right IPS. The pattern of delay activation, covering the entire extent of the IPS, with especially pronounced activation in the ascending and descending branches, resembles the activation pattern for the location memory task in the study of Courtney et al. (1996). The function of the area along the ascending branch of the IPS in working memory remains to be investigated. However, although the reported coordinates are variable, previous studies of covert attention show a cluster of activations along the horizontal and descending branches of the IPS (Nobre et al. 1997; Rosen et al. 1999), whereas spatial delayed matching studies consistently reported activations in BA 40, near the anterior end of the IPS (Smith et al. 1995; Courtney et al. 1996). An exception is the study of Corbetta et al. (1998), who found orienting-related activations at the anterior and posterior end of the IPS. The difference between this study and "classical" spatial cueing experiments may be the more complex task used by Corbetta et al., with sequential shifts of attention between locations of varying eccentricity. Correct shifts of attention between different peripheral locations are likely to require more spatial working memory than the usual shift between fixation and a single location in each hemifield.

Occipital cortex

From the descending part of the IPS, orienting-associated activation continued into the intraoccipital sulcus and occipital cortex, where it extended to both cuneus and striate/extrastriate areas. High object recognition demands led to foci of activation in the cuneus bilaterally, which extended to the parieto-occipital fissure and into lingual and right fusiform gyrus (Fig. 3c, e; Table 3). Thus, with the exception of a right precentral and a left postcentral spot of activation, object recognition was restricted to ventral visual areas, in agreement with imaging studies on object recognition (Kanwisher et al. 1997; Aguirre et al. 1998b).

Conclusions

We observed a large overlap of brain areas that showed delay activity and activation related to visuospatial orienting. The activations were in line with previous reports of separate studies of delayed object matching and visuospatial orienting. Differences between delay activity and visuospatial orienting were found in the exact localization of activation within anatomical structures. Within the frontal lobe, the FEF showed the expected orienting-related activation. We were also able to replicate delay activity in the same area, which extended anteriorly along the posterior superior frontal sulcus, but also included the area activated by visuospatial orienting. This activation shows that the cortex along the posterior superior frontal sulcus contributes not only to spatial working memory, but also to object working memory. Whether this superior frontal activation is seen in object working-memory tasks may depend on the nature of the objects, especially on the demands on three-dimensional object memory.

We observed delay activity in the pre-SMA, in line with previous data from face- and location-matching tasks. Our data thus confirm previous reports that imply that the pre-SMA is activated independently of the stimulus characteristics of the task. The pre-SMA, instead, seems to be involved in a response preparatory set, when the subject knows that a response will soon be required without knowing the exact response to be carried out. In contrast, the SMA contralateral to the responding hand may be involved in the programming of the actual response, indicated by its response-associated activation timecourse.

Dorsolateral prefrontal cortex (DLPFC) was not significantly involved in holding object information accessible. However, right DLPFC was activated by top-down-controlled visuospatial orienting. Together with a report of right DLPFC activation in endogenous spatial cueing, this suggests a role of right DLPFC in the voluntary control of spatial orienting.

Acknowledgements We thank Joachim Wiese for programming support and two anonymous reviewers for their helpful comments on a previous version of this paper.

References

Aguirre GK, Zarahn E, D'esposito M (1998a) The variability of human, BOLD hemodynamic responses. Neuroimage 8:360–369

Aguirre GK, Zarahn E, D'Esposito M (1998b) An area within human ventral cortex sensitive to 'building' stimuli: evidence and implications. Neuron 21:373–383

Awh E, Jonides J, Smith E, Schumacher E, Koeppe R, Katz S (1996) Dissociation of storage and rehearsal in verbal working memory: evidence from positron emission tomography. Psychol Sci 71:25–31

Baker SC, Frith CD, Frackowiak RSJ, Dolan RJ (1996) Active representation of shape and spatial location in man. Cereb Cortex 6:612–619

Bosch V (2000) Statistical analysis of multi-subject fMRI data: the assessment of focal activations. J Magn Reson 11:61–64

Chafee MV, Goldman-Rakic PS (1998) Matching patterns of activity in primate prefrontal area 8a and parietal area 7ip neurons during a spatial working memory task. J Neurophysiol 79:2919–2940

Clark VP, Maisog JM, Haxby JV (1998) fMRI study of face perception and memory using random stimulus sequences. J Neurophysiol 79:3257–3265

Corbetta M (1998) Frontoparietal cortical networks for directing attention and the eye to visual locations: identical, independent, or overlapping neural systems? Proc Natl Acad Sci USA 95:831–838

Corbetta M, Shulman GL, Miezin FM, Petersen FE (1995) Superior parietal cortex activation during spatial attention shifts and visual feature conjunction. Science 270:802–805

Corbetta M, Akbudak E, Conturo TE, Snyder AZ, Ollinger JM, Drury HA, Linenweber MR, Petersen SE, Raichle ME, Van Essen DC, Shulman GL (1998) A common network of functional areas for attention and eye movements. Neuron 21: 761–73

Courtney SM, Ungerleider LG, Keil K, Haxby JV (1996) Object and spatial visual working memory activate separate neural systems in human cortex. Cereb Cortex 6:39–49

Courtney SM, Ungerleider LG, Keil K, Haxby JV (1997) Transient and sustained activity in a distributed neural system for human working memory. Nature 386:608–611

Courtney SM, Petit L, Maisog JM, Ungerleider LG, Haxby JV (1998) An area specialized for spatial working memory in human frontal cortex. Science 279:1347–1351

Cowan N (1998) Visual and auditory working memory capacity. Trends Cogn Sci 2:77–78

D'Esposito M, Aguirre GK, Zarahn E, Ballard D, Shin RK, Lease J (1998) Functional MRI studies of spatial and nonspatial working memory. Brain Res Cogn Brain Res 7:1–13

Deubel H, Schneider WX (1995) Saccade target selection and object recognition: evidence for a common attentional mechanism. Vision Res 36:1827–1837

Duncan J (1985) Visual search and visual attention. In: Posner M, Marin O (eds) Attention and performance XI. Erlbaum, Hillsdale, pp 85–106

Dymond R, Norris DG, Pollmann S, Zysset S (1999) Application of double voxel functional spectroscopy to event-related cognitive experiments. Magn Reson Med 41:217–223

Friston KJ, Williams S, Howard R, Frackowiak RSJ, Turner R (1996) Movement-related effects in fMRI time-series. Magn Reson Med 35:346–355

Funahashi S, Bruce CJ, Goldman-Rakic PS (1989) Mnemonic coding of visual space in the primate dorsolateral prefrontal cortex. J Neurophysiol 61:331–349

Fuster JM (1985) The prefrontal cortex and temporal integration. In: Peters A, Jones EG (eds) Cerebral cortex, Vol 4. Plenum, New York, pp 259–329

Fuster JM, Alexander GE (1971) Neuron activity related to short-term memory. Science 173:652–654

Fuster JM, Jervey JP (1981) Inferotemporal neurons distinguish and retain behaviorally relevant features of visual stimuli. Science 212:952–955

Fuster JM, Jervey JP (1982) Neuronal firing in the inferotemporal cortex of the monkey in a visual memory task. J Neurosci 2:361–375

Haxby JV, Horwitz B, Ungerleider LG, Maisog JM, Pietrini P, Grady CL (1994) The functional organization of human extrastriate cortex: a PET-rCBF study of selective attention to faces and locations. J Neurosci 14:6336–6353

Kanwisher N, McDermott J, Chun M (1997) The fusiform face area: a module in human extrastriate cortex specialized for face perception. J Neurosci 17:4302–4311

Koch KW, Fuster JM (1989) Unit activity in monkey parietal cortex related to haptic perception and temporary memory. Exp Brain Res 76:292–306

Lohmann G, Müller K, Bosch V, Hessler S, Mentzel H, Cramon D von (1999) Lipsia – a software package for the evaluation of functional MRI data. Technical report, Max-Planck-Institute of Cognitive Neuroscience, Leipzig

Luna B, Thulborn KR, Strojwas MH, McCurtain BJ, Berman RA, Genovese CR, Sweeney JA (1998) Dorsal cortical regions subserving visually guided saccades in humans: an fMRI study. Cereb Cortex 8:40–47

Menon R, Luknowsky D, Gati J (1998) Mental chronometry using latency-resolved functional MRI. Proc Natl Acad Sci USA 9518:10902–10907

Nobre AC, Sebestyen GN, Gitelman DR, Mesulam MM, Frackowiak RSJ, Frith CD (1997) Functional localization of the system for visuospatial attention using positron emmission tomography. Brain 120:515–533

Oldfield RC (1971) The assessment and analysis of handedness: the Edinburgh Inventory. Neuropsychologia 9:97–113

Owen A (1997) The functional organization of working memory processes within human lateral frontal cortex: the contribution of functional neuroimaging. Eur J Neurosci 9:1329–1339

Paus T (1996) Location and function of the human frontal eye field: a selective review. Neuropsychologia 34:475–483

Petit L, Courtney SM, Ungerleider LG, Haxby JV (1998) Sustained activity in the median wall during working memory delays. J Neurosci 18:9429–9437

Petrides M, Pandya DN (1999) Dorsolateral prefrontal cortex: comparative cytoarchitectonic analysis in the human and the macaque brain and corticocortical connection patterns. Eur J Neurosci 11:1011–1036

Picard N, Strick PL (1996) Motor areas of the medial wall: a review of their location and functional activation. Cereb Cortex 6:342–353

Pollmann S, Wiggins CJ, Norris DG, Cramon DY von, Schubert T (1998) Use of short intertrial intervals in single-trial experiments: a 3T fMRI-study. Neuroimage 8:327–339
Quintana J, Yajeya J, Fuster JM (1988) Prefrontal representation of stimulus attributes during delay tasks. I. Unit activity in cross-temporal integration of sensory and sensory-motor information. Brain Res 474:211–221
Rainer G, Asaad WF, Miller EK (1998) Memory fields of neurons in the primate prefrontal cortex. Proc Natl Acad Sci USA 95:15008–15013
Rosen AC, Rao SM, Caffara P, Scaglioni A, Bobholz JA, Woodley SJ, Hammeke TA, Cunningham JM, Prieto TE, Binder JR (1999) Neural basis of endogenous and exogenous spatial orienting: a functional MRI study. J Cogn Neurosci 11:135–152
Rushworth MFS, Nixon PD, Eacott MJ, Passingham RE (1997) Ventral prefrontal cortex is not essential for working memory. J Neurosci 17:4829–4838
Smith EE, Jonides J (1999) Storage and executive processes in the frontal lobes. Science 283:1657–1661
Smith EE, Jonides J, Koeppe RA, Awh E, Schumacher EH, Minoshima S (1995) Spatial versus object memory: PET investigations. J Cogn Neurosci 7:337–356
Theeuwes J (1992) Perceptual selectivity for color and form. Percept Psychophys 51:599–606
Treisman A, Gormican S (1988) Feature analysis in early vision: evidence from search asymmetries. Psychol Rev 95:15–48
Wilson FAW, O'Scalaidhe SP, Goldman-Rakic PS (1993) Dissociation of object and spatial processing domains in primate prefrontal cortex. Science 260:1955–1958
Worsley KJ, Friston KJ (1995) Analysis of fMRI time-series revisited – again. Neuroimage 2:173–181

Richard Levy · Patricia S. Goldman-Rakic

Segregation of working memory functions within the dorsolateral prefrontal cortex

Published online: 20 May 2000

Abstract It is now widely accepted that the prefrontal cortex (PFC) plays a critical role in the neural network subserving working memory (WM). At least three related questions are still under debate: (1) is the PFC critical for all constituent processes of WM (i.e., short-term storage, manipulation, and utilization of mental representations) or only in one or a few of them? (2) Is there segregation of function among different cytoarchitectonic subdivisions of the PFC? (3) If this be the case, is this segregation based on the nature of the information being processed or on the type of cognitive operation performed? The present review article describes findings in the monkey supporting a modular "domain-specific" model of PFC functional organization with respect to WM operations. In this model, the dorsolateral prefrontal cortex (DLPFC) is composed of several subregions, based primarily on the nature of the information being processed in WM. Storage and processing functions are integrally related in each area. Future studies designed to map as yet uncharted areas of prefrontal cortex with refined anatomical and physiological approaches may provide a critical test of the model and evaluate the extent to which it applies generally or, instead, mainly to visual domains or only to dorsolateral convexity areas.

Key words Working memory · Cognition · Prefrontal cortex · Rhesus monkey

Introduction

It is widely accepted that the prefrontal cortex plays a major role in the most complex aspects of human thought, such as reasoning and planning. A set of elemental processes, including the maintenance, manipulation, and utilization of mental representations, has been postulated to constitute an operational working-memory (WM) system, which greatly contributes to these higher cognitive functions (Baddeley 1986; Goldman-Rakic 1987). WM involves both a short-term storage capacity for maintaining mental representations in an active state and a capacity for processing or manipulating information held in the WM "buffer", often referred to as the "central executive" (Baddeley 1986) or supervisory attentional systems (Shallice 1982). Experimental studies both in monkeys and humans have clearly demonstrated the critical role played by the prefrontal cortex (PFC) in the neural network subserving WM (Goldman-Rakic 1987; Fuster 1997; Smith and Jonides 1999). In consequence, there is remarkable consensus in the field regarding the association between prefrontal mechanisms and WM capacity. Much less agreement, however, exists on the issue of how the "two-tier" modular model of WM described above is instantiated at the level of brain organization. In particular, a major question pertains to whether the PFC participates in all constituent processes of WM or only in one or a few of them. Moreover, as the PFC is a large territory (including multiple cytoarchitectonic areas), it is of interest to determine the specific contribution to WM of particular areas and subareas within this region. If there is segregation of function among different cytoarchitectonic subdivisions of the PFC, as seems biologically reasonable, is this segregation based on the nature of the information being processed or on the type of cognitive operation performed? The answer to this question holds the key to the general features of the functional architecture of cognition.

This short review article describes findings in the monkey that may contribute to a coherent model(s) of anatomical and functional organization of the PFC for WM. In the following sections, we will review some of the data that has lead to a modular "domain-specific" model of PFC functional organization with respect to WM operations (Goldman-Rakic 1987). This model pos-

R. Levy · P.S. Goldman-Rakic (✉)
Section of Neurobiology, Yale University School of Medicine, 333 Cedar Street, New Haven, CT 06510, USA
e-mail: patricia.goldman-rakic@yale.edu
Fax: +1-203-7855263

Present address:
R. Levy, Fédération de Neurologie and INSERM U.289, Hôpital de la Salpêtrière, 75013 Paris, France

tulates that the dorsolateral prefrontal cortex (DLPFC) is composed of several subregions, based on the sensory nature of the information being processed in WM, regardless of the level of processing. In this view, the cortex surrounding the principal sulcus (Walker's area 46 in the primate) is thought to be specialized for visual-spatial processing, whereas cortex on the inferior convexity below area 46 (Walker's areas 12 and 45) is involved in nonspatial visual (e.g., object/face) processing within WM. Further, sensory input may be only one dimension by which these areas differ; other associated features, such as intrinsic circuitry and efferent mechanisms, may more fully characterize areal specializations. Although several lines of evidence support domain specificity for the rhesus monkey, some caveats are in order: (1) the modular segregation of the visual memory system in the DLPFC may not generalize to other sensory domains; (2) other areas of the prefrontal cortex may play supramodal integrative multiple domain functions; (3) this model might not apply without significant modification to the organization of the human DLPFC; and (4) the model does not specify the type of WM operation processed within each domain-specific module. To place the domain-specific hypothesis in a wider theoretical context, we will briefly describe alternative models of anatomical and organization of the DLPFC vis a vis WM and discuss findings that are not congruent with the domain-specific model.

Evidence for the "domain-specific" model

Anatomical definitions

As this review focuses on anatomical and functional relationships, it is important to define the main regions of interest and their connectivity. Our reference for PFC subdivisions is Walker's (1940) cytoarchitectonic map, recognizing that it may be only an approximation to functional subdivisions being established by contemporary neurophysiological methods. Area 9 represents the most superior and dorsal part of the DLPFC. It has both a lateral and a medial aspect within the prefrontal cortex. For purposes of this review, we refer to this area as "dorsomedial" (DM). Area 46 is entirely included in the DLPFC. It lies beneath area 9, and it encompasses the principal sulcus, the major sulcus in the DLPFC. It is noteworthy that this area has been the most-studied part of the DLPFC (Goldman-Rakic 1987; Fuster 1997), and we refer to it as "dorsolateral" (DL). Areas in the inferior part of the DLPFC, beneath area 46 and above the lateral orbital prefrontal cortex, are Walker's area 12 and 45, referred to here as the "inferior convexity" (IC). Two other areas, Walker's area 8 and a part of 10 (the frontal pole) occupy the lateral aspect of the prefrontal cortex. Area 8 should be briefly mentioned. It is subdivided into area 8A, in the arcuate concavity, caudal to area 46, and area 8B, dorsomedial and caudal to area 9. The most caudal part of the principal sulcus merges with the anterior extension of area 8A. Thus, numerous lesions or electrophysiological studies focused on the principal sulcus region have also included the most anterior part of area 8A. The frontal eye field (FEF) is generally not included in this anterior cortex, as it is located more caudally within the rim and fundus of the arcuate sulcus (Goldberg and Bushnell 1981).

Extrinsic connections

The extrinsic connections of the PFC provide essential information regarding the issue of regionalization of function. Numerous anatomical studies have shown that DL and IC prefrontal cortices receive differential connections from posterior association cortices. The dorsolateral areas receive dense projections from the inferior parietal association cortex (Mesulam et al. 1977; Petrides and Pandya 1984; Andersen et al. 1985; Barbas and Mesulam 1985; Cavada and Goldman-Rakic 1989), a region involved in visuospatial processing (Pohl 1973; Batuev et al. 1985; Friedman and Goldman-Rakic 1994; Chafee and Goldman-Rakic 1998). By contrast, IC cortex is networked with the inferotemporal association cortex (Kuypers et al. 1965; Jones and Powell 1970; Chavis and Pandya 1976; Jacobsen and Trojanowski 1977; Kawamura and Neito 1984; Shiwa 1987; Barbas 1988; Seltzer and Pandya 1989; Ungerleider et al. 1989; Distler et al. 1993; Webster et al. 1994; Bullier et al. 1996), a region involved in the representation of visual objects (Bruce et al. 1981; Fuster and Jervey 1981; Perret et al. 1982; Desimone et al. 1984; Baylis et al. 1985; Fuster 1990; Miller et al. 1991, 1993; Rodman et al. 1993). The fact that DL and IC prefrontal cortices are the recipients of differential projections from areas that are themselves specialized visual processing areas (spatial vs. feature) is highly suggestive of a parallel organization of domain-specific modules within the PFC. It would be reasonable to expect, and we have proposed, that regions receiving these differential visual system inputs are functionally related to and are extensions of the dorsal and ventral visual-processing streams with which they are selectively connected (Goldman-Rakic 1987, 1996).

Selective lesions and behavior

The delayed-response (DR) tasks have been a primary instrument for assessing WM capacity in the nonhuman primate. Their main feature is that they require monkeys to maintain a mental representation during a delay period and then use this representation to guide the choice of response at the end of the delay (Hunter 1913). DR tasks can be formatted to examine WM for various informational domains (e.g., spatial DR, spatial or object delayed alternation, object/color delayed matching or nonmatching to sample, oculomotor DR). For this reason, they have long been used to study the possible areal specializations of the prefrontal cortex (for a review, see

Goldman-Rakic 1987). Lesions of the DLPFC, and more specifically those restricted to the principal sulcus or the middle third of its sulcus, are sufficient to produce a deficit as severe as larger PFC lesions in performance on spatial-DR and spatial-alternation tasks (Mishkin and Pribram 1955; Butters and Pandya 1969; Butters et al. 1971, 1972; Goldman-Rakic 1987; Fuster 1997). An important point is that the deficits which follow dorsolateral lesions are not necessarily modality-specific, i.e., the stimuli to be recalled need not be visual. Delayed-response tasks with spatial auditory cues or somatic stimulation as memoranda may also be impaired after lesions of the DLPFC cortex (Shindy et al. 1994). The spatial deficits are also independent of the mode of response. Thus, in an oculomotor analog of the classical spatial DR tasks, Funahashi and colleagues (Funahashi et al. 1993a) demonstrated that a unilateral lesion of DLPFC, sparing the FEF area, disrupted performance of memory-guided eye movements to spatial cues in the visual field contralateral to the hemisphere in which the lesion was placed. The deficit was delay-dependent and not present in a sensory-guided version of the task. Finally, monkeys with DLPFC are unimpaired in nonspatial DR tasks in which the physical features (patterns, shapes, or colors) of objects are the behaviorally relevant memoranda. Thus, monkeys with DL prefrontal lesions perform as well as intact monkeys in performance on delayed object alternation and object or color matching or nonmatching-to-sample tasks (Stamm and Rosen 1973; Passingham 1975; Mishkin and Manning 1978; Bachevalier and Mishkin 1986). Thus, there is little evidence to indicate a role of the DL prefrontal sector in object recognition or in basic short-term memory for object features. The fact that so many studies clearly indicate that one given subregion of the PFC – the principal sulcal area – is specialized in the processing of one given sensory domain – the visuospatial domain – provides strong evidence for the concept of a domain-specific module within the PFC, even if lesion studies have not yet shown the same degree of specialization for other PFC areas (for instance, see Mishkin et al. 1969). Taken together, these findings attest to the critical role played by the principal sulcal region in the most elementary WM operation, i.e., the "on-line" maintenance and utilization of mental representations of visuospatial coordinates within the spatial domain.

By contrast to DL, lesions of IC cortex cause impairments in tasks based on the identity or features of object rather than their spatial location. This impairment is seen in classical WM tasks, such as delayed object alternation (Mishkin and Manning 1978) and "recognition memory" like the object/color delayed matching or non-matching-to sample tasks (Iversen and Mishkin 1970; Passingham 1975; Mishkin and Manning 1978; Kowalska et al. 1991), tasks which include a short-term memory component. The impairment produced by IC lesions on the non-matching tasks is sometimes described as small and transient (Passingham 1975; Bachevalier and Mishkin 1986; Kowalska et al. 1991), unlike the severe impairment in these tasks after ventromedial prefrontal lesions (Bachevalier and Mishkin 1986; Meunier et al. 1997). Thus, in a recent study, Rushworth et al. (1997) have found that lesions restricted to the anterior part of IC cortex (Walker's area 12) were without lasting effect on the relearning of various cognitive tasks based on color and shape discrimination (visual pattern association, delayed, or simultaneous color matching to sample tasks). However, larger lesions incorporating the caudal IC (Walker's area 45A) and the lateral orbital prefrontal cortex produced impairments of various degree on these tasks. Although the nature of the underlying impairment after such lesions remains unclear, a deficit specific to features of objects could account for the behavioral impairments observed after inferior prefrontal lesions. Moreover, some studies have shown that neither spatial DR or delayed alternation tasks are impaired following IC lesions (Mishkin and Manning 1978; Passingham 1985). However, impairments on spatial DR tasks have occasionally been observed following large IC lesions (e.g., Mishkin et al. 1969). These deficits have been long been attributed to nonsensory difficulties in shifting-response strategies rather than to sensory processes per se (Mishkin 1964). Indeed, selective deficits on spatial tasks have never been demonstrated in monkeys with IC lesions. It is also possible that deficits on spatial tasks arise from inadvertent damage to portions of the inferior arcuate sulcus, affecting a portion of the spatial system. One should thus acknowledge that, though there is a strong case from lesion and single-unit-recording studies favoring a specific role of IC cortex in "object-cognition", no clear-cut double dissociation (as the one evidenced in DL cortex for "spatial cognition") has yet been demonstrated. Consequently, the precise role of IC cortex with respect to WM domains deserves further examination. Single-unit-recording studies designed to map this region more precisely should provide a clearer basis for future lesion studies.

The DM, or superior portion of the prefrontal promontory, is the least understood of its main divisions. Performance on the classical spatial DR, delayed alternation, and delayed non-matching to sample tasks is not impaired following DM lesions (Goldman et al. 1971; Levy and Goldman-Rakic 1999). Moreover, in more complex spatial or nonspatial WM tasks, the involvement of DM cortex remains in question (see discussion below).

In summary, in the visual domain, lesion studies in the non-human primate provide compelling evidence for a model of anatomical and functional segregation of the PFC, based at least in part on sensory processing, in which the DL prefrontal cortex (i.e., Walker's area 46 including the principal sulcus) is specialized for spatial cognition involving a WM process, whereas the IC/ventrolateral prefrontal (i.e., Walker's area 12/45) plays a role in object cognition involving WM. The DM and the prearcuate regions do not seem to participate in this domain-specific processing within WM.

Single-unit-recording studies

The "domain-specific" model is also supported by a wealth of single-unit-recording studies. Recordings of area 46/8a neurons during spatial DR, spatial alternation, or memory-guided oculomotor-saccades and anti-saccades tasks have demonstrated that a significant proportion of these neurons is engaged in short-term spatial-mnemonic functions (Fuster and Alexander 1971; Kubota and Nikki 1971; Kojima and Goldman-Rakic 1982; Funahashi et al. 1989, 1990, 1991; Carlson et al. 1990, 1997; Wilson et al. 1993). Indeed, many DL neurons have receptive fields ("memory field") depending on the spatial location of relevant stimuli (Funahashi et al. 1989). These memory fields can be defined as maximal and constant (from trial to trial) firing of a neuron to the representation of a visual target in one or a few locations of the visual field (Goldman-Rakic 1996). Although many DL neurons may respond to various sensory stimuli (visual, somatosensory, auditory) (Tanila et al. 1992, 1993; Carlson et al. 1997; Rao et al. 1997), the large number of DL neurons engaged in DR tasks seem to be exclusively responsive to maintenance of spatial information in short-term memory (Funahashi et al. 1993b; Carlson et al. 1997). By contrast, it appears that neurons tuned specifically to the identity or features of objects are very few in DL area compared with other PFC areas (Wilson et al. 1993; O'Scalaidhe et al. 1997; Rao et al. 1997), as might be expected from the fact of the preferential dorsal pathway input to DLPFC. Moreover, a recent study (Romo et al. 1999) has shown that neurons engaged in a vibrotactile WM task without a visuospatial component are located in the IC cortex; importantly, none of these neurons were found in the DL region. Neuronal responses to vocalizations are currently being mapped in this laboratory, and preliminary evidence is revealing circumscribed territories dedicated to auditory processing in the vicinity of the object processing areas of IC cortex (Romanski and Goldman-Rakic 1999). Wilson et al. (1993) have recorded single units in DL and IC regions while monkeys performed two different oculomotor DR tasks varying with respect to pattern or location as relevant cues. Differential neuronal activity during the delay depended on site of recording within the DLPFC, i.e., neurons in DL cortex were responsive to spatial, whereas neuronal activities in IC cortex were related to object features. Finally, in a recent mapping of PFC, covering Walker's areas 8, 9, 12, 45 and 46, O'Scalaidhe et al. (1999) tested over 2000 neurons and discovered that a subset of these neurons responded selectively to monkey faces – visual stimuli that may be considered prototypical of object vision. Careful reconstruction of electrode tracks in each of three monkeys located these neurons to the IC cortex and the lateral orbital prefrontal region; none were found in the principal sulcal region (O'Scalaidhe et al. 1999).

Taken together, the combined data obtained from anatomy, lesions, and electrophysiological studies in the rhesus monkey support a model of anatomical and functional segregation of the DLPFC in the non-human primate, based on the sensory domain of the information processed in WM.

Other models of anatomical and functional organization of the PFC

Although it is widely accepted that the PFC is involved in WM functions, and generally that its functional organization is modular as we have proposed, there is disagreement as to the particulars of this organization . For example, Petrides and Owen have postulated a segregation within the PFC based on the nature of processing within WM rather than a sensory domain-specific modularity (Petrides 1995; Owen et al. 1996a, 1998, 1999; Owen 1997). In this model, the PFC is divided into two subregions: the superior convexity, or – as they have referred to it – the "mid-dorsolateral" cortex (the cortex above the principal sulcus-Walker's area 9 and upper 46), and the IC, referred to as " ventrolateral " cortex (cortex below the principal sulcus-Walker's areas 12/45 and lower 46). According to Owen (1997), the ventrolateral prefrontal cortex is "concerned with the active organization of sequences of responses based on conscious, explicit retrieval of information and active comparison about stimuli held in short-term memory". By contrast, the mid-dorsolateral region is viewed as an executive processor that allows active manipulation and monitoring of information within WM. This view differs from the "domain-specific model" in that different subregions are devoted to storage and processing, respectively, and each processes several sensory domains, whereas in the "domain-specific" model one given subregion processes only one informational domain (be it visual, auditory, or somatic spatial input), but subserves both storage and processing operations. Although recent functional-imaging studies in humans have been interpreted as supportive of the Owen/Petrides model (Petrides et al. 1993a; Owen et al. 1996a, 1996b, 1998; Owen 1997), evidence for this model from experimental studies in monkeys is sparse. Indeed, only one study in the monkey (Petrides 1995) may support this hypothesis. In this study, monkeys were trained to perform self- or externally ordered tasks and, thereafter, were subject to lesions either of the superior convexity (Walker's area 9 and upper 46) or the prearcuate regions (Walker's area 8). Monkeys with bilateral superior-convexity lesions were profoundly impaired in re-learning a three-object self-ordered task, suggesting that lesions in this region disrupt performance on tasks requiring the monitoring of nonspatial visual information in WM. However, our recent attempt to replicate this finding (in monkeys with DM lesions trained on an similar nonspatial and three-item self-ordered task) produced a different result, which we discuss below in comparison with the Petrides et al. study.

Another model of DLPFC functional organization that needs to be considered is that of a unitary association cortex that integrates information in a supra-modal fashion. Fuster and co-authors have shown that cooling the principal sulcal region produced both spatial and nonspatial short-term memory deficits and also impairment on a delayed matching task with cross-modal (visual and somesthetic sensory modalities) contingencies (Fuster and Bauer 1974; Bauer and Fuster 1976; Quintana and Fuster 1993). However, as recognized by the authors (Fuster 1989, p 77), this method could not rule out a functional dissociation within the DLPFC because of the large area of the PFC cooled in these studies. Several authors have found neuronal activation in the DLPFC in response to nonspatial stimuli (Tanila et al. 1992, 1993; Bodner et al. 1996; Carlson et al. 1997; Rao et al. 1997). Moreover, some neurons throughout the DLPFC are activated by both spatial and nonspatial visual stimuli during WM tasks if these stimuli are presented within central vision (Quintana et al. 1988; Rao et al. 1997; Rainer et al. 1998; Miller 1999). Neuronal responses in DLPFC for both spatial and nonspatial items are not necessarily inconsistent with a domain-specific model for several reasons. The nonspatial stimuli may, by prior association, immediately signify the spatial response to be made at the end of the delay, so that the neuronal response may actually be related to the impending movement rather than to the features of the stimulus. Again, it must be stressed that the domain-specific hypothesis is not a modality-specific hypothesis: several sensory modalities feed into the perceptual/mnemonic mechanisms related to spatial WM. Further, the specificity of the DL region for spatial WM operations could be relative and some neurons within this area may be linked with other domain-specific regions. Finally, the presence of such responses apparently does not specify their functional importance for that area. Lesion studies emphasize this concept: DL lesions consistently produce a deficit restricted to visuo-spatial cognition (for a review, see Goldman-Rakic 1987). Rarely, if ever, have monkeys with DL lesions exhibited strong or permanent impairments on object-based tasks.

Association of storage and processing within the visuo-spatial domain

Regarding the functional specialization of the different subregions of the DLPFC with respect to their spatial and nonspatial specificity or to their involvement in simpler or more complex aspects of WM (e.g., maintenance versus processing and/or monitoring functions), we have undertaken a study to determine the degree of anatomic segregation for WM functions within the DLPFC in the rhesus monkey (Levy and Goldman-Rakic 1999). The monkeys were trained to perform several WM tasks according to two dimensions: sensory modality (visual spatial and nonspatial modalities) and level of processing (low vs. high executive demand within WM). Tasks with low executive demand within WM were considered to be represented by the conventional DR format, in which monkeys store and use only one item of information. WM tasks with higher executive processing demand were self-ordered (SO) tasks (Petrides and Milner 1982; Petrides et al. 1993a; Petrides 1995) (Fig. 1). The SO tasks require the same basic WM processes engaged by the DR tasks (i.e., maintenance and utilization of internal representations), but impose a larger memory load (three items versus one) than do the DR tasks and also require the monkey to compare his current choice with previous choices, i.e., to serially self-order internal representations. This additional monitoring process is conceptually an important upgrade in the level of processing over the classical DR tasks, requiring as it does a supplementary executive operation. In the present study, we employed a nonspatial SO task (OBJ-SO) based on Petrides (1995) and designed a new spatial version (POS-SO) expressly for this study (Fig. 1). Once the tasks were learned, one group of monkeys was given a bilateral resection of Walker's areas 9/8B, namely the dorsomedial (DM) aspect of the PFC, whereas a second group received a bilateral lesion of Walker's area 46/8A, namely the dorsolateral (DL) aspect of the PFC. We reasoned that, if a "modality-specific" model prevailed, DL lesions would produce a selective spatial WM deficit. Alternatively, if areal segregation were based on the nature of operation performed, regardless of the sensory information processed, then DM and/or DL lesions should produce a supra-modal impairment (in both the spatial and nonspatial domain), particularly in the SO tasks with high executive demand.

In fact, lesions of DL region produced a significant and stable impairment in the two spatial WM, but little or no impairment in the two nonspatial WM tasks. As the spatial SO task requires the same basic WM processes as the spatial DR task, it is not possible to determine, from this study, the contribution to this deficit of the components that differentiate the SO task from the DR task. Therefore, two interpretations of this result are possible: (1) the DL area is involved both in elementary WM operations (maintenance) and in more executive operations (self-ordering) and indeed, the maintenance of single items in short-term memory is a constituent operation of sequential processing; or (2) the DL region is mainly involved in storing spatial information (for both DR and SO tasks), while still another area of the PFC may be selectively involved in the executive aspects of WM. If this were the case, it would be necessary to demonstrate that there exists a cortical area, damage to which causes deficits on the spatial SO task, but not the DR task. No such executive area has yet been discovered in monkeys and the requisite double dissociation remains to be demonstrated. At present, a parsimonious interpretation of our data is that the storage and processing components of WM are inextricable within informational domains. It is, thus, reasonable and appealing that each prefrontal module, networked with sensory, motor, limbic, and association areas (Selemon and Goldman-Rakic 1988), can support domain-specific executive operations. And, indeed, a wide range of operations integral to WM, including preparation, inhibition, or sequencing of motor responses and context-contingencies, have been consis-

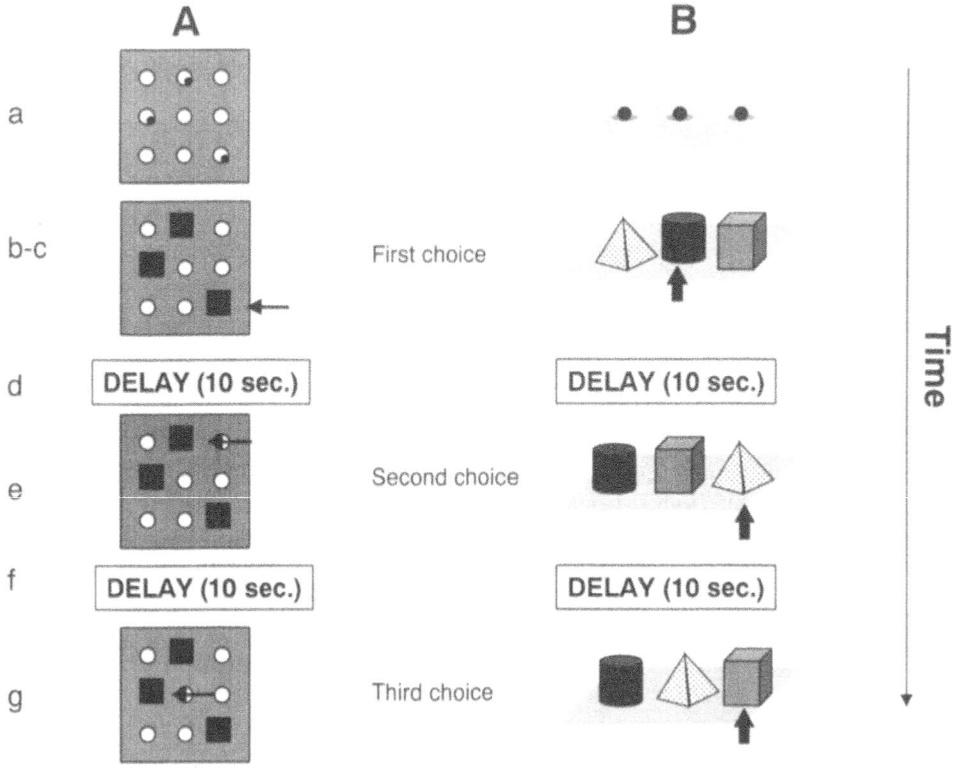

Fig. 1A,B The spatial (POS-SO) and object (OBJ-SO) self-ordered tasks. **A** The POS-SO task. The monkey views a testing tray with nine foodwells (*a*), three of which are covered by identical blue plaques (*b*), each plaque covering a reward; the monkey is allowed to displace any one of the three plaques to retrieve a reward (*c*); an opaque screen is lowered for a 10-s delay period, during which the plaque is replaced over the empty well (*d*). After this first delay, the monkey is allowed to make his second choice by displacing any of the three plaques (*e*); however, to receive a reward, he must choose one of the two remaining plaques that cover baited wells. After the second choice, the opaque screen is again lowered for a second 10-s delay period (*f*). To complete the trial, the monkey has to displace the one remaining plaque over the foodwell that still contains a reward (*g*). The trial is completed only when the monkey has found all rewards. Thus, a trial could consist of a minimum of three choices, but choice of an incorrect foodwell prolongs the current trial until all rewards are retrieved (all choices being separated from each other by a 10-s delay). Monkeys received ten trials a day. Positions of plaques were pseudo-randomly distributed in order to discourage the monkeys from adopting spatial strategies. **B** The OBJ-SO task. The testing procedure is similar to the POS-SO task except that: (1) the position of the object is changed following a pseudorandom order during the delay periods; (2) the test tray contains three foodwells, each covered by an object distinctive for shape, color, and size and containing a reward. New sets of three objects were used on each trial. Monkeys received ten trials a day

tently observed in DL cortex (Funahashi et al. 1993b, 1997; Williams and Goldman-Rakic 1995; Watanabe 1996). Thus, the intrinsic neuronal circuitry within the DL area provides for a spectrum of functions compatible with all levels of WM operations, including executive operations.

Monkeys with DM lesions were not impaired either on spatial or nonspatial WM tasks, whether the task engaged a higher executive component or not. Our failure to demonstrate impairment in the spatial SO task following DM lesions (areas 9 and 8B) indicates that this region is no more essential for self-ordering spatial information than it is for the simple maintenance of spatial information. These results are in accord with a study by Passingham (1985), in which monkeys were taught to retrieve rewards hidden behind 25 small doors without returning to the same location twice, thus engaging self-monitoring and serial organization of mental representations. Yet, lesions of the principal sulcus produced a marked impairment in this task, whereas dorsomedial frontal convexity lesions (similar to our DM lesions and to the mid-frontal lesion of Petrides) failed to do so.

The fact that neither DL nor DM lesions produced impairments on the nonspatial SO task suggests that neither subregion is critical for accomplishing this task. This result differs from those obtained by Petrides (1995), in which monkeys with "mid-frontal" lesions were profoundly impaired on a non-spatial SO task similar to that used in the present study. It appears that no formal explanation can be provided so far to explain the differences between the two studies. It should be noted that our tripartite separation of the lateral prefrontal cortex (DM-area 9/8B, DL-46/8A, and IC-12/45) differs from Petrides's approach, in which the lateral prefrontal cortex is subdivided into a dorsolateral (above the principal sulcus) and a ventrolateral (below the principal sulcus) parts. Nevertheless, the resection in the Petrides (1995) study corresponds closely to our DM lesion, as it removed mainly areas 9 and 8B and largely spared the principal sulcus in two of three animals. An alternative explanation of the difference between our study and Petrides' may arise from the different types of stimuli used in the two studies. In Petrides' study, the same three stimuli were used from trial to trial, whereas, in our study, a different set of objects was used from trial to trial. However, this difference would have been more than offset by the fact that, in Petrides' study, monkeys were given only one trial a day in order to reduce intertrial interference.

In summary, our study demonstrated a functional dissociation between the dorsomedial and dorsolateral prefrontal cortex with respect to WM processes: only lesions of dorsolateral areas 46/8A impaired WM processes, whereas lesions of the dorsomedial areas 9/8B were without lasting consequences. Second, the deficit following the dorsolateral lesion was confined to the spatial domain and did not encompass object WM. The present finding of a dissociation of deficits on nonspatial and spatial tasks after DL lesions, and the marked impairment observed in both simple and complex spatial WM tasks, confirm and extend the evidence for a specialization in DL cortex for spatial WM, regardless of the level of processing within this domain. Finally, the findings revealed that dorsolateral cortical areas are no less critical for tasks with low WM demand than for more complex sequential processing with higher WM load. These results support an anatomical-functional segregation of the PFC for WM based on the type of information being processed rather than on the nature of the operations performed. Although the present study does not specify a particular area for nonspatial WM processing, several studies indicate that the inferior convexity (mainly Walker's area 12/45) may be specialized for nonspatial processing (see discussion above).

Do experimental studies in humans support the "domain-specific" model?

By adapting tasks conceptually derived from the DR tasks used in monkeys, functional-imaging studies of human cognition have repeatedly shown significant increases of activity in the DLPFC in WM tasks (for a review, see Owen et al. 1997; Ungerleider et al. 1998; Smith and Jonides 1999), confirming that this region plays a crucial role in WM processes in humans. The issues of anatomical-functional segregation and the specific role played by the DLPFC in WM have been, of course, raised using functional imaging as a tool. Although several studies by Petrides, Owen, and their collaborators suggest a division of the lateral frontal cortex based on the level of operation performed, according to the two-stage model described above (Petrides et al. 1993a; Owen et al. 1996a, 1998). Thus, Petrides and colleagues (1993a, 1993b) reported that self-ordering tasks activate BA 9/46 (mid-dorsolateral region), whether they require monitoring of verbal or visuospatial materials. In addition, Owen (1997) performed a meta-analysis of activation studies that employed both spatial and nonspatial WM tasks and failed to dissociate peaks of activation for these tasks within the DLPFC. Owen and colleagues have also reported the engagement of different PFC regions with different levels of executive demand (Owen et al. 1998, 1999). However, for each of the negative findings in the literature, there are numerous functional-imaging studies that strongly support a domain-based segregation of function within the PFC (Smith et al. 1995, 1996; Courtney et al. 1996, 1997, 1998; McCarthy et al. 1996; Belger et al. 1998; Kelley et al. 1998; Kohler et al. 1998; Smith and Jonides 1999; R. Adcock, T. Constable, J. Gore, and P.S. Goldman-Rakic, unpublished observations). For instance, Courtney and colleagues have found that object WM activates an inferior frontal region, whereas activation for spatial WM activated a caudal portion of the superior frontal gyrus (Courtney et al. 1996, 1998). Others have reported double dissociations between loci of activation within the prefrontal cortex based on hemispheric lateralization, the right PFC being predominantly activated by spatial WM tasks and the left PFC by object WM tasks (Smith et al. 1995; McCarthy et al. 1996). Although disparities exist between studies with respect to the exact loci for different tasks, the main point is that tasks equated for WM demand, but formatted for different domains activated different areas in these studies. The visuospatial and feature domains may be particularly difficult to dissociate as tasks described as "spatial" often can be performed as "object" if stimuli are presented foveally, as is commonly the case. Further, the spatial/temporal resolution of fMRI may yet not be sufficient to detect segregation in closely adjacent areas. Clearly, more studies are indicated to overcome the technical and design issues in this difficult area. However, clear evidence for domain specificity comes from studies on WM for verbal material. A number of studies have demonstrated that Broca's area (left BA 45/47) is crucial for verbal WM and especially for subvocal rehearsal (Cohen et al. 1994, 1997; Demb et al. 1995; Awh et al. 1996; Smith et al. 1996, 1998; Wexler et al. 1999). Broca's area and other areas related to semantic processing are distant and distinct from activation peaks found in most studies of spatial WM (see Owen 1997). That verbal-, spatial-, and object-based WM each depend on a distinct area(s) within the PFC provides evidence for the predicted homology in functional architecture of the DLPFC in humans and monkeys and for "domain-specificity".

References

Andersen RA, Essick GK, Siegel MR (1985) The encoding of spatial location by posterior parietal neurons. Science 230:456–458

Awh E, Jonides J, Smith EE, Schumacher EH, Koeppe RA (1996) PET evidence for a dissociation between the storage and rehearsal components of verbal working memory. Psychol Sci 7:25–31

Bachevalier J, Mishkin M (1986) Visual recognition impairment follows ventromedial but not dorsolateral prefrontal lesions in monkeys. Behav Brain Res 20:249–261

Baddeley A (1986) Working memory. Clarendon Press, Oxford

Barbas H (1988) Anatomic organization of basoventral and mediodorsal visual recipient prefrontal regions in the rhesus monkey. J Comp Neurol 276:313–342

Barbas H, Mesulam MM (1985) Cortical afferent input to the principalis region of the rhesus monkey. Neuroscience 15:619–637

Batuev AS, Shaefer VI, Orlov AA (1985) A comparative characteristics of unit activity in the prefrontal and parietal areas during delay performance in monkeys. Behav Brain Res 16:57–70

Bauer RH, Fuster JM (1976) Delayed-matching and delayed-response deficit from cooling dorsolateral prefrontal cortex in monkeys. J Comp Physiol Psychol 90:293–302

Baylis GC, Rolls ET, Leonard CM (1985) Selectivity between faces in the responses of a population of neurons in the cortex in the superior temporal sulcus of the monkey. Brain Res 342:91–102

Belger A, Puce A, Krystal JH, Gore JC, Goldman-Rakic PS, McCarthy G (1998) Dissociation of mnemonic and perceptual processes during spatial and nonspatial working memory using fMRI. Hum Brain Map 6:14–32

Bodner M, Kroger J, Fuster JM (1996) Auditory memory cells in dorsolateral prefrontal cortex. Neuroreport 7:1905–1908

Bruce CJ, Desimone R, Gross CG (1981) Visual properties of neurons in a polysensory area in the superior temporal sulcus of the macaque. J Neurophysiol 46:369–384

Bullier J, Schall JD, Morel A (1996) Functional streams in occipito-frontal connections in the monkey. Behav Brain Res 76:89–97

Butters N, Pandya DN (1969) Retention of delayed-alternation: effect of selective lesion of sulcus principalis. Science 165: 1271–1273

Butters N, Pandya D, Sanders K, Dye P (1971) Behavioral deficits in monkeys after selective lesions within the middle third of sulcus principalis. J Comp Physiol Psychol 72:132–144

Butters N, Pandya D, Stein D, Rosen J (1972) A search for the spatial engram within the frontal lobes of monkeys. Acta Neurobiol Exp 32:305–329

Carlson S, Tanila H, Pertovaara A, Lahteenmaki A (1990) Vertical and horizontal coding of space in the monkey dorsolateral prefrontal cortex. Brain Res 527:145–149

Carlson S, Rama P, Tanila H, Linnankoski I, Mansikka H (1997) Dissociation of mnemonic coding and other functional neuronal processing in the monkey prefrontal cortex. J Neurophysiol 77:761–774

Cavada C, Goldman-Rakic PS (1989) Posterior parietal cortex in rhesus monkey. II. Evidence for segregated corticocortical networks linking sensory and limbic areas with the frontal lobe. J Comp Neurol 287:422–445

Chafee MV, Goldman-Rakic PS (1998) Matching patterns of activity in primate prefrontal area 8a and parietal area 7ip neurons during a spatial working memory task. J Neurophysiol 79:2919–2940

Chavis DA, Pandya DN (1976) Further observations on corticofrontal connections in the rhesus monkey. Brain Res 117:369–386

Cohen JD, Forman SD, Braver TS, Casey BJ, Servan-Schreiber D, Noll DC (1994) Activation of the prefrontal cortex in a nonspatial working memory task with functional MRI. Hum Brain Map 1:293–304

Cohen JD, Perlstein WM, Braver TS, Nystrom LE, Noll DC, Jonides J, Smith EE (1997) Temporal dynamics of brain activation during a working memory task. Nature 386:604–608

Courtney SM, Ungerleider LG, Keil K, Haxby JV (1996) Object and spatial working memory activate separate neural system in human cortex. Cereb Cortex 6:39–49

Courtney SM, Ungerleider LG, Keil K, Haxby JV (1997) Transient and sustained activity in a distributed neural system for human working memory. Nature 386:608–611

Courtney SM, Petit L, Maisog JM, Ungerleider LG, Haxby JV (1998) An area specialized for spatial working memory in human frontal cortex. Science 279:1347–1351

Demb JB, Desmond JE, Wagner AD, Vaidya CJ, Glover GH, Gabrieli JDE (1995) Semantic encoding and retrieval in the left inferior prefrontal cortex: a functional MRI study of task difficult and process specificity. J Neurosci 15:5870–5878

Desimone R, Albright TD, Gross CG, Bruce C (1984) Stimulus selective properties of inferior temporal area TEO in macaque monkeys. J Neurosci 4:2051–2062

Distler C, Boussaoud D, Desimone R, Ungerleider LG (1993) Cortical connections of inferior temporal area TEO in macaque monkeys. J Comp Neurol 334:125–150

Friedman HR, Goldman-Rakic PS (1994) Coactivation of prefrontal cortex and inferior parietal cortex in working memory tasks revealed by 2DG functional mapping in the rhesus monkey. J Neurosci 14:2775–2788

Funahashi S, Bruce CJ, Goldman-Rakic PS (1989) Mnemonic coding of visual space in the monkey's dorsolateral prefrontal cortex. J Neurophysiol 61:331–349

Funahashi S, Bruce CJ, Goldman-Rakic PS (1990) Visuospatial coding in primate prefrontal neurons revealed by oculomotor paradigm. J Neurophysiol 63:811–831

Funahashi S, Bruce CJ, Goldman-Rakic PS (1991) Neuronal activity related to saccadic eye mouvements in the monkey's dorsolateral prefrontal cortex. J Neurophysiol 65:1464–1483

Funahashi S, Bruce CJ, Goldman-Rakic PS (1993a) Dorsolateral prefrontal lesions and oculomotor delayed-response performance: evidence for mnemonic "scotomas". J Neurosci 13: 1479–1497

Funahashi S, Chafee MV, Goldman-Rakic PS (1993b) Prefrontal neuronal activity in rhesus monkeys performing a delayed anti-saccade task. Nature 365:753–756

Funahashi S, Inoue M, Kubota K (1997) Delay-period activity in the primate prefrontal cortex encoding multiple spatial positions and their order of presentation. Behav Brain Res 84: 203–223

Fuster J (1989) The prefrontal cortex. Raven press, New York

Fuster J (1997) The prefrontal cortex. Raven press, New York

Fuster JM (1990) Inferotemporal units in selective visual attention and short-term memory. J Neurophysiol 64:681–697

Fuster JM, Alexander GE (1971) Neuron activity related to short-term memory. Science 173:652–654

Fuster JM, Bauer RH (1974) Visual short-term memory deficit from hypothermia of frontal cortex. Brain Res 81:393–400

Fuster JM, Jervey JP (1981) Inferotemporal neurons distinguish and retain behaviorally relevant features of visual stimuli. Science 212:952–955

Goldberg ME, Bushnell MC (1981) Behavioral enhancement of visual responses in monkey cerebral cortex. II. Modulation in frontal eye fields specifically related to saccades. J Neurophysiol 46:773–787

Goldman-Rakic PS (1987) Circuitry of primate prefrontal cortex and regulation of behavior by representational memory. In: Plum F, Mountcastle F (eds) Handbook of Physiology, Vol 5. The American Physiological Society, Washington DC, pp 373–517

Goldman-Rakic PS (1996) Regional and cellular fractionation of working memory. Proc Natl Acad Sci USA 93:13473–13480

Goldman PS, Rosvold HE, Vest B, Galkin TW (1971) Analysis of the delayed-alternation deficit produced by dorsolateral prefrontal lesions in the rhesus monkey. J Comp Physiol Psychol 77:212–220

Hunter WS (1913) The delayed reaction in animals and children. Behav Monogr 2:1–86

Iversen SD, Mihskin M (1970) Perseveration interference in monkeys following selective lesions of the inferior prefrontal convexity. Exp Brain Res 11:376–386

Jacobson S, Trojanowski JQ (1977) Prefrontal granular cortex of the rhesus monkey. I. Intrahemispheric cortical afferents. Brain Res 132:209–233

Jones EG, Powell TPS (1970) An anatomical study of converging sensory pathways within the cerebral cortex of the monkey. Brain 93:793–820

Kawamura K, Neito J (1984) Corticocortical projections to the prefrontal cortex in the rhesus monkey investigated with horseradish peroxidase technique. Neurosci Res 1:89–103

Kelley WM, Miezin FM, McDermott KB, Buckner RL, Raichle ME, Cohen NJ, Ollinger JM, Akbudak E, Conturo TE, Snyder

AZ, Petersen SE (1998) Hemispheric specialization in human dorsal frontal cortex and medial temporal lobe for verbal and nonverbal memory encoding. Neuron 20:927–936
Kohler S, Moscovitch M, Winocur G, Houle S, McIntosh AR (1998) Networks of domain-specific and general regions involved in episodic memory for spatial location and object identity. Neuropsychologia 36:129–142
Kojima S, Goldman-Rakic PS (1982) Delay-related activity of prefrontal neurons in rhesus monkeys performing delayed response. Brain Res 248:43–49
Kowalska DM, Bachevalier J, Mishkin M (1991) The role of the inferior prefrontal convexity in performance of delayed nonmatching-to-sample. Neuropsychologia 29:583–600
Kubota K, Niki H (1971) Prefrontal cortical unit activity and delayed cortical unit activity and delayed alternation performance in monkeys. J Neurophysiol 34:337–347
Kuypers HGJM, Szwarcbart MK, Mishkin M, Rosvald HE (1965) Occipitotemporal corticocortical connections in the rhesus monkey. Exp Neurol 11:245–262
Levy R, Goldman-Rakic PS (1999) Association of storage and processing function in the dorsolateral prefrontal cortex of the nonhuman primate. J Neurosci 19:5149–5158
McCarthy G, Puce A, Constable RT, Krystal JH, Gore JC, Goldman-Rakic PS (1996) Activation of human prefrontal cortex during spatial and nonspatial working memory tasks measured by functional MRI. Cereb Cortex 6:600–611
Mesulam MM, Van Hoesen GW, Pandya DN, Geschwind N (1977) Limbic and sensory connections of the inferior parietal lobule (area PG) in the rhesus monkey: a study with a new method for horseradish peroxidase histochemistry. Brain Res 136:393–414
Meunier M, Bachevalier J, Mishkin M (1997) Effects of orbital frontal and anterior cingulate lesions on object and spatial memory in rhesus monkeys. Neuropsychologia 35:999–1015
Miller EK (1999) The prefrontal cortex: complex neural properties for complex behavior. Neuron 22:15–17
Miller EK, Li L, Desimone R (1991) A neural mechanism for working and recognition memory in inferior temporal cortex. Science 254:1377–1379
Miller EK, Li L, Desimone R (1993) Activity of neurons in anterior inferior temporal cortex during a short-term memory task. J Neurosci 13:1460–1478
Mishkin M (1964) Perseverations of central sets after frontal lesions in monkeys. In: Warren JM, Akert K (eds) The frontal granular cortex and behavior. MacGraw-Hill, New York, pp 219–241
Mishkin M, Manning FJ (1978) Non-spatial memory after selective prefrontal lesions in monkeys. Brain Res 143:313–323
Mishkin M, Pribram KH (1955) Analysis of the effects of frontal lesions in object alternation. J Comp Physiol Psychol 48:492–495
Mishkin M, Vest B, Waxler M, Rosvold HE (1969) A re-examination of the effects of frontal lesion on object alternation. Neuropsychologia 7:357–363
O'Scalaidhe SP, Wilson FAW, Goldman-Rakic PS (1997) Areal segregation of face-processing neurons in prefrontal cortex. Science 278:1135–1138
O'Scalaidhe SP, Wilson FAW, Goldman-Rakic PS (1999) Face-selective neurons during passive viewing and working memory performance of rhesus monkeys: evidence for intrinsic specialization of neuronal coding. Cereb Cortex 9:459–475
Owen AM (1997) Tuning in to the temporal dynamics of brain activation using functional magnetic resonance imaging (fMRI). Trends Cogn Sci 1:123–125
Owen AM, Evans AC, Petrides M (1996a) Evidence for a two-stage model of spatial working memory processing within the lateral frontal cortex: a positron emission tomography study. Cereb Cortex 6:31–38
Owen AM, Doyon J, Petrides M, Evans AC (1996b) Planning and spatial working memory: a positron emission tomography study in humans. Eur J Neurosci 8:353–367
Owen AM, Iddon JL, Hodges JR, Summers BA, Robbins TW (1997) Spatial and non-spatial working memory at different stages of Parkinson's disease. Neuropsychologia 35:519–532
Owen AM, Stern CE, Look RB, Tracey I, Rosen BR, Petrides M (1998) Functional organization of spatial and nonspatial working memory processing within the human lateral frontal cortex. Proc Natl Acad Sci USA 95:7721–7726
Owen AM, Herrod NJ, Menon DK, Clark JC, Downey SP, Carpenter TA, Minhas PS, Turkheimer FE, Williams EJ, Robbins TW, Sahakian BJ, Petrides M, Pickard JD (1999) Redefining the functional organization of working memory processes within human lateral prefrontal cortex. Eur J Neurosci 11:567–574
Passingham RE (1975) Delayed matching after selective prefrontal cortex lesions in monkeys (*Macaca mulatta*). Brain Res 92:89–102
Passingham RE (1985) Memory of monkeys (*Macaca mulatta*) with lesions in prefrontal cortex. Behav Neurosci 99:3–21
Perret DI, Rolls ET, Caan W (1982) Visual neurones responsive to faces in the monkey temporal cortex. Exp Brain Res 47:329–342
Petrides M (1995) Impairments on nonspatial self-ordered and externally ordered working memory tasks after lesions of the mid-dorsal part of the lateral frontal cortex in the monkey. J Neurosci 15:359–375
Petrides M, Milner B (1982) Deficits on subject-ordered tasks after frontal- and temporal-lobe lesions in man. Neuropsychologia 20:249–262
Petrides M, Pandya DN (1984) Projection to the frontal cortex from the posterior parietal region in the rhesus monkey. J Comp Neurol 228:105–116
Petrides M, Alivisatos B, Evans AC, Meyer E (1993a) Dissociation of human mid-dorsolateral from posterior dorsolateral frontal cortex in memory processing. Proc Natl Acad Sci USA 90:873–877
Petrides M, Alivisatos B, Meyer E, Evans AC (1993b) Functional activation of the human frontal cortex during the performance of verbal working memory tasks. Proc Natl Acad Sci USA 90:878–882
Pohl W (1973) Dissociation of spatial discrimination deficits following frontal and parietal lesions in monkeys. J Comp Physiol Psychol 82:227–239
Quintana J, Fuster JM (1993) Spatial and temporal factors in the role of prefrontal and parietal cortex in visuomotor integration. Cereb Cortex 3:122–132
Quintana J, Yajeya J, Fuster JM (1988) Prefrontal representation of stimulus attributes during delay tasks. I. Unit activity in cross-temporal integration of sensory and sensory-motor information. Brain Res 474:211–221
Rainer G, Asaad WF, Miller EK (1998) Selective representation of relevant information by neurons in the primate prefrontal cortex. Nature 393:577–579
Rao SC, Rainer G, Miller EK (1997) Integration of what and where in the primate prefrontal cortex. Science 276:821–824
Rodman HR, O'Scalaidhe SP, Gross CG (1993) Response properties of neurons in the temporal cortical visual areas of infant monkeys. J Neurophysiol 70:1115–1136
Romanski LM, Goldman-Rakic PS (1999) Physiological identification of an auditory domain in the prefrontal cortex of the awake behaving monkey. Soc Neurosci Abstr 25:620.1
Romo R, Brody CD, Hernandez A, Lemus L (1999) Neuronal correlates of parametric working memory in the prefrontal cortex. Nature 399:470–473
Rushworth MF, Nixon PD, Eacott MJ, Passingham RE (1997) Ventral prefrontal cortex is not essential for working memory. J Neurosci 17:4829–4838
Selemon LD, Goldman-Rakic PS (1988) Common cortical and subcortical targets of the dorsolateral prefrontal and posterior parietal cortices in the rhesus monkey: evidence for a distributed neural network subserving spatially guided behavior. J Neurosci 8:4049–4068

Seltzer B, Pandya DN (1989) Frontal lobe connections of the superior temporal sulcus in the rhesus monkey. J Comp Neurol 281:97–113

Shallice T (1982) Specific impairments of planning. Philos Trans R Soc Lond B Biol Sci 298:199–209

Shindy WW, Posley KA, Fuster JM (1994) Reversible deficit in haptic delay tasks from cooling prefrontal cortex. Cereb Cortex 4:443–450

Shiwa T (1987) Corticocortical projections to the monkey temporal lobe with particular reference to the visual processing pathway. Arch Ital Biol 125:139–154

Smith EE, Jonides J (1999) Storage and executive processes in the frontal lobes. Science 283:1657–1661

Smith EE, Jonides J, Koeppe RA, Awh E, Schumacher E, Minoshima S (1995) Spatial vs. object working memory: PET investigations. J Cogn Neurosci 7:337–358

Smith EE, Jonides J, Koeppe RA (1996) Dissociating verbal and spatial working memory using PET. Cereb Cortex 6:11–20

Smith EE, Jonides J, Marshuetz C, Koeppe RA (1998) Components of verbal working memory: evidence from neuroimaging. Proc Natl Acad Sci USA 95:876–882

Stamm JS, Rosen SC (1973) The locus and crucial time of implication of prefrontal cortex in delayed response tasks. In: Pibram HK, Luria AR (eds) Psychophysiology of the frontal lobes. Academic Press, New York, pp 139–153

Tanila H, Carlson S, Linnankoski I, Lindroos F, Kahila H (1992) Functional properties of dorsolateral prefrontal cortical neurons in awake monkey. Behav Brain Res 47:169–180

Tanila H, Carlson S, Linnankoski I, Kahila H (1993) Regional distribution of functions in dorsolateral prefrontal cortex of the monkey. Behav Brain Res 53:63–71

Ungerleider LG, Gaffan D, Pelak VS (1989) Projections from inferior temporal cortex to prefrontal cortex via the uncinate fascicle in rhesus monkey. Exp Brain Res 76:473–484

Ungerleider LG, Courtney SM, Haxby JV (1998) A neural system for human visual working memory. Proc Natl Acad Sci USA 95:883–890

Walker AE (1940) A cytoarchitectural study of the prefrontal area of the macaque monkey. J Comp Neurol 73:59–86

Watanabe M (1996) Reward expectancy in primate prefrontal neurons. Nature 382:629–632

Webster MJ, Bachevalier J, Ungerleider LG (1994) Connections of inferior temporal TEO and TE with parietal and frontal cortex in macaque monkeys. Cereb Cortex 5:470–483

Wexler BE, Stevens AA, Bowers AA, Sernyak MJ, Goldman-Rakic PS (1998) Word and tone working memory deficits in schizophrenia. Arch Gen Psychiatry 55:1093–1096

Williams GV, Goldman-Rakic PS (1995) Blockade of dopamine D1 receptors enhances memory fields of prefrontal neurons in primate cerebral cortex. Nature 376:572–575

Wilson FA, O'Scalaidhe SP, Goldman-Rakic PS (1993) Dissociation of object and spatial processing domains in primate prefrontal cortex. Science 260:1955–1958

Adrian M. Owen

The role of the lateral frontal cortex in mnemonic processing: the contribution of functional neuroimaging

Published online: 12 May 2000

Abstract Evidence is now converging which suggests that, at the area level, working-memory processes within the dorsolateral and ventrolateral frontal cortices are organised according to the type of processing required, rather than according to the nature (i.e. domain) of the information being processed, as has been widely assumed. In a recent study using functional magnetic-resonance imaging (fMRI), performance of visual spatial and visual non-spatial working-memory tasks was shown to involve identical regions of the lateral prefrontal cortex when all factors unrelated to the type of stimulus material were appropriately controlled. These results concur fully with recent reviews of the imaging literature, which demonstrate that spatial, visuospatial and verbal working-memory studies have produced distributed patterns of overlapping activation foci within these lateral frontal regions. Moreover, two recent positron-emission tomography studies have demonstrated that either, or both, the ventrolateral and dorsolateral frontal regions can be activated in spatial working-memory tasks, depending on the precise executive processes that are called upon by the task being performed. Similarly, when the executive requirements of a simple verbal working-memory task (e.g. forwards versus backwards digit span) are manipulated, differential activation within these two frontal cortical areas is observed. The results provide further evidence that the mid-dorsolateral and mid-ventrolateral frontal cortical areas make distinct "executive" contributions to memory and correspond with a fractionation of working-memory processes in psychological terms.

Key words Dorsolateral · Ventrolateral · PET · fMRI · Working memory

A.M. Owen
MRC Cognition and Brain Sciences Unit, 15 Chaucer Road, Cambridge CB2 2EF, UK

A.M. Owen
Wolfson Brain Imaging Centre, Box 189, Addenbrooke's Hospital, University of Cambridge, Cambridge, UK

Introduction

While the importance of the prefrontal cortex for "higher-order" cognitive functions is largely undisputed, no consensus has been reached regarding the fractionation of functions within this region. In fact, although some degree of regional specialisation within the frontal lobe seems inevitable, by and large, most attempts to map specific cognitive functions onto neuroanatomical and/or cytoarchitectonic sub-divisions have been disappointing. Perhaps the most widely and passionately debated issue to have emerged in this field in recent years concerns the functional relationship between the dorsal and ventral regions of the lateral frontal cortex and, more specifically, how the "executive" processes assumed to be dependent upon these regions might contribute to aspects of working memory. The concept of working memory has been described and discussed in various ways; as a cognitive system for both the temporary storage and manipulation of remembered information (e.g. Baddeley 1986), as the type of memory that is active and only relevant for a short period of time (e.g. Fuster 1995; Goldman-Rakic 1995) and, most specifically, as the process by which a remembered stimulus is held "on-line" to guide behaviour in the absence of external cues or prompts (Goldman-Rakic 1987, 1996). In part, this descriptive variability reflects the relative interests of those working with different primate species: psychologists working mainly with humans often emphasise the "organisational" or "higher order" aspects of working-memory tasks, whereas those working with non-human primates tend to focus on those aspects of task performance related to the on-line retention or short-term storage of information. The problem of comparison between species is further compounded by Honig's (1978) definition of working memory as applied invariably in rat studies using Olton's radial-arm maze (Olton 1982), which also emphasises the "organisational" or "executive" component of task performance. This description is consistent with the view that working memory should be considered, more generally, in the context of the temporal organisation of action (e.g. Fuster 1997). Nevertheless, in the absence of a precise definition, few disagree that working memory is a fundamental set of processes and an integral component of many cognitive operations, from complex decision making to selective attention (Baddeley 1986).

The prefrontal cortex, which has been the focus of much recent debate regarding the neural basis of working memory processes, is cytoarchitectonically diverse, both in the human brain and in the macaque brain, and comprises a number of specific areas that have distinct patterns of connectivity with other brain regions. Essentially, two divergent positions have emerged which, whilst focusing on a broadly similar distinction between the anatomically and cytoarchitectonically distinct dorsolateral and ventrolateral frontal cortical regions, differ fundamentally in terms of the precise functions ascribed to those regions. On the basis of lesion and electrophysiological-recording studies in the monkey (e.g. Funahashi et al. 1989; Wilson et al. 1993; Levy and Goldman-Rakic 1999), Goldman-Rakic (1987, 1994, 1995) has argued that working-memory processes within the lateral frontal cortex are organised according to the type (e.g. domain) of information being processed, with dorsolateral frontal regions being principally concerned with memory for spatial material, whilst ventrolateral frontal regions subserve memory for non-spatial material. According to this "domain-specific" or "material-specific" model, "informational domain, not process, will be mapped across prefrontal cortex" (Goldman-Rakic 1994, 1995).

Intuitively, this domain-specific theory has some theoretical appeal since, more posteriorly, extrastriate cortical regions are organised, at least in part, into anatomically distinct pathways, functionally specialised for identifying spatial locations (the occipitoparietal pathway or "dorsal stream") or object features (the occipitotemporal pathway or "ventral stream") (Ungerleider and Mishkin 1982). Whilst these posterior association areas project reciprocally to widespread frontal-lobe regions, a certain degree of topographical order appears to be maintained (Barbas 1988; Cavada and Goldman-Rakic 1989; Bates et al. 1994; Rodman 1994; Webster et al. 1994; Carmichael and Price 1995).

An alternative general theoretical framework for understanding the role played by the prefrontal cortex in mnemonic processing and its relationship to more posterior cortical association systems has been proposed by Petrides (1994), based largely on lesion studies in the monkey. According to that model, basic memory functions, including storage and immediate processing of incoming and recalled information, are carried out not within the frontal lobes, but rather within sensory specific and multimodal posterior association areas in the parietal and temporal cortices. The frontal lobes may, however, receive and act upon this information via bi-directional connections between the posterior cortical association areas and the ventrolateral frontal cortex, which, in turn, is closely connected to the mid-dorsolateral frontal cortex, or via direct connections between dorsal regions of the frontal cortex and the medial temporal lobe. Thus, according to this view, the ventrolateral frontal cortex constitutes the first level of interaction between posterior cortical regions and the entire lateral frontal cortex. In this capacity, this region is assumed to be critical for various "second order" memory processes, such as comparisons between, or judgements about the occurrence or non-occurrence of remembered stimuli and the initiation of explicit (i.e. intentional) retrieval of information from long-term memory. In contrast, the mid-dorsolateral frontal cortex is assumed to provide a third level of processing within memory and is recruited when active manipulation or "monitoring" of remembered information is required. According to this view, therefore, working-memory processes within dorsolateral and ventrolateral frontal regions are organised according to the *nature* of the processing required rather than according to the domain of the information to be remembered (Petrides 1994, 1995).

In this article, these two models of lateral-frontal lobe organisation will be evaluated in the light of recent functional neuroimaging studies of spatial, visual and verbal working memory. While focusing, for the most part, on the delineation and neural instantiation of *working memory* processes, it is assumed that the various operations involved are drawn from a single set of "executive" components, which are likely to contribute equally to many other types of tasks that do not necessarily involve, or depend upon, working memory.

Functional neuroimaging studies of spatial and non-spatial (visual) working memory

Until recently, direct investigation of the functional organisation of working-memory processes within the human brain was limited to comparisons between groups of patients with damage to different cortical and/or subcortical regions (e.g. Petrides and Milner 1982; Owen et al. 1990, 1995, 1996b). In patient studies, it is not possible to establish which areas of the frontal cortex are involved in a given cognitive process with any degree of anatomical precision, since the excisions are rarely confined to specific cytoarchitectonic areas. In recent years, however, functional neuroimaging techniques, such as positron emission tomography (PET) and functional magnetic resonance imaging (fMRI), have provided a unique opportunity for assessing the relationship between patterns of cortical and subcortical activation and different aspects of cognitive processing in healthy control volunteers.

Although many recent neuroimaging studies have investigated various components of mnemonic processing, relatively few have attempted to neuroanatomically delineate specific aspects of working-memory processing within the frontal lobe. One approach to this problem is to draw careful comparisons among groups of related studies in order to determine whether consistent patterns of activation occur in association with various types of memory task. Since most functional neuroimaging stud-

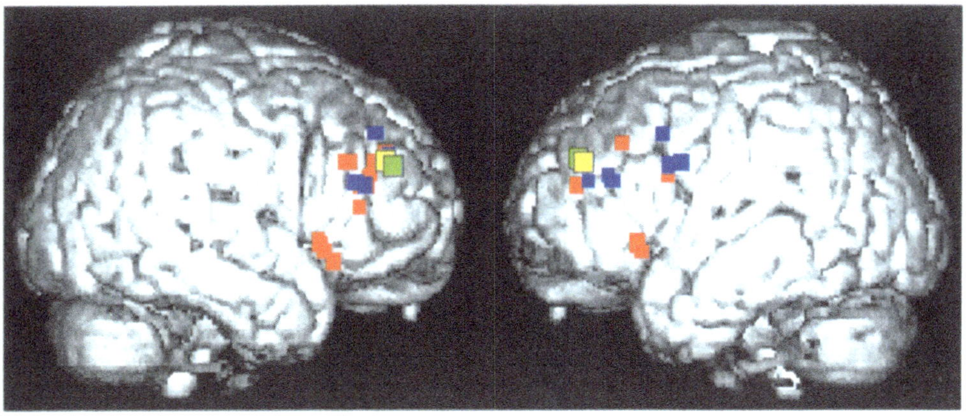

Fig. 1 A schematic diagram illustrating the distribution of activation foci reported in the studies of spatial and non-spatial (visual) working memory (for details, see text). All data have been transformed into standardised sterotaxic space and rendered onto the surface of a three-dimensional magnetic-resonance image. All foci falling within the mid-dorsolateral (areas 9/46, 46, 9) and mid-ventrolateral (44/45, 47) frontal cortices are shown. Activation foci from spatial working-memory tasks are shown in *red*. Activation foci from non-spatial working-memory tasks are shown in *blue*. The *yellow* and *green squares* indicate the precise stereotaxic co-ordinates of the peaks observed during the analogous spatial and visual working-memory tasks, respectively, employed by Owen et al. (1998) (see text)

ies have used the common stereotaxic co-ordinate system based on the three-dimensional atlas of Talairach and Tournoux (1988), direct comparisons across studies are possible. In one recent review of the literature (Owen 1997; Fig. 1), the stereotaxic co-ordinates of activation foci reported within the dorsolateral and ventrolateral frontal cortices during fourteen spatial working-memory tasks (from Jonides et al. 1993; McCarthy et al. 1994, 1996; Smith et al. 1995, 1996; Baker et al. 1996; Goldberg et al. 1996; Owen et al. 1996a, 1998) were compared with those observed during six non-spatial (visual) working-memory tasks (Petrides et al. 1993a; Smith et al. 1995; Baker et al. 1996; Courtney et al. 1996; McCarthy et al. 1996; Owen et al. 1998). The two models of lateral frontal organisation described above make clearly divergent predictions about the likely role in working memory of the dorsolateral and ventrolateral frontal cortical regions. According to the domain-specific model (Goldman-Rakic 1994, 1995), one might expect the results of functional neuroimaging studies to demonstrate that spatial and non-spatial working-memory studies activate distinctly different lateral frontal-lobe regions with a reasonable level of consistency. Examination of the data presented in Fig. 1 suggests that this is not the case. For example, overlapping activation foci within area 9/46 of the mid-dorsolateral frontal cortex have been frequently reported in studies of both spatial and non-spatial (visual) working memory. In fact, across spatial working-memory studies, the mean stereotaxic z-coordinates (inferior-to-superior) for the activation foci falling within areas 9 and 46 are +29 mm (left hemisphere) and +24 mm (right hemisphere). For non-spatial tasks, the corresponding values are +28 mm and +28 mm (for details, see Owen 1997). This simplistic analysis, which takes no account of task-related differences between studies, does demonstrate just how similar the activation foci generated by studies of spatial and non-spatial working memory are; if anything, the trend in the right hemisphere is in the opposite direction of that which would be predicted by the domain-specific hypothesis of lateral frontal organisation.

One logistic problem in comparing the results of unrelated studies is that the tasks used often differ both in terms of their mnemonic (e.g. processing) requirements and in terms of the nature of the material to be remembered (e.g. domain; spatial or non-spatial). In a few cases, however, formally identical spatial and non-spatial working-memory tasks have been used within the same study, and the results of these investigations probably provide the least ambiguous material addressing this issue. For example, we recently used fMRI to compare two experimental tasks that had similar processing requirements (the ability to monitor and manipulate an ongoing series of stimuli within working memory), but differed in the type of stimuli to be remembered (locations versus patterns) (Owen et al. 1998). The first task (spatial working memory) required that subjects continually monitor a sequence of highlighted locations on the screen, responding after each stimulus by selecting the location that was highlighted two steps earlier in the sequence. In a control condition, which required no memory, subjects followed a similar sequence, but responded by touching each location as it was highlighted. In the second task (visual pattern working memory), the same subjects were required to monitor a series of visual patterns presented in one location on the screen, responding after each stimulus by selecting the pattern that was presented one-step earlier in the sequence. In the control condition, which required no memory, each item in a similar series of visual patterns was identical, and subjects responded on each trial by touching the same pattern. Both experimental tasks have the same mnemonic requirements, the only difference being that one required memory for location and the other required memory for abstract patterns with location being irrelevant. Moreover, the two tasks were very closely matched in terms of task difficulty, since within-subject performance measures were statistically indistinguishable. When activity in the spatial working-memory task was compared with that in the spatial control condition, significant increases in signal intensity were observed bilaterally in the mid-dorsolateral frontal cortex in five of the six subjects. In the sixth subject, this change only reached significance in the right hemisphere. The group mean stereotaxic co-ordinates of these activation foci were x=–38, y=42, z=30 (left hemisphere) and x=35, y=44, z=33 (right hemisphere). The pattern of frontal signal-intensity changes observed when the non-spatial working-memory task was compared with the non-spatial control task was almost identical. Thus, significantly increased signal intensity was observed bilaterally in the mid-dorsolateral cortex in five of the six subjects studied and only in the right mid-dorsolateral frontal region in the sixth subject (group mean coordinates; x=–39, y=44, z=32 for the left and x=34, y=45, z=32 for the right). These findings clearly suggest that the mid-dorsolateral frontal region will be activated when subjects have to monitor and manipulate information within working memory, regardless of the domain-specific nature of that information (in this case, spatial or non-spatial). For comparison with the results of previous studies, the group mean stereotaxic co-ordinates reported in that study (Owen et al. 1998) are also plotted in Fig. 1. For both tasks, the peak regional cerebral blood flow (rCBF) changes within the mid-dorsolateral frontal cortex fall within the cluster of activation foci that have been reported in previous studies of spatial and visual working memory. A similar pattern of results has been reported recently by Postle et al. (2000); in that study, equivalent spatial and non-spatial visual working-memory tasks failed to yield dissociable patterns of activation within the prefrontal cortex, although material-specific activation foci were observed in posterior association cortex.

It might be argued that the "visual" working-memory tasks included in the studies described above (Owen et al. 1998; Postle et al. 2000) involve processes that could be considered to be "spatial" in nature and that it is the neural correlates of these processes that emerge as activation foci in the mid-dorsolateral frontal region. However, three observations argue against this hypothesis. First, as in most studies of this type, the non-mnemonic control tasks employed involve the same amount of "spatial information" as the working-memory task of interest; it is reasonable to assume, therefore, that the effects of this variable on CBF would be "subtracted out" when comparisons are made between the two tasks. Second, many working-memory tasks with more explicit spatial components do not activate areas 9/46 of the mid-dorsolateral frontal cortex (Jonides et al. 1993; Smith et al. 1995; Owen et al. 1996a). Third, several recent studies have demonstrated that certain verbal working-memory paradigms also activate similar regions of the mid-dorsolateral frontal cortex (e.g. Cohen et al. 1994; Braver et al. 1997; Smith et al. 1996), even in conditions that involved no visuospatial stimulation at all (e.g. Petrides et al. 1993b).

Functional neuroimaging studies of verbal working memory

Many recent functional neuroimaging studies of working memory have employed verbal stimuli, such as numbers or letters (presented either visually or auditorily), and provide additional material for assessing models of lateral frontal organisation in humans. In one recent review, the stereotaxic co-ordinates of activation foci reported within the dorsolateral and ventrolateral frontal cortices during 27 verbal working-memory studies (Grasby et al. 1993, 1994; Paulesu et al. 1993; Petrides et al. 1993b; Becker et al. 1994; Cohen et al. 1994, 1997; Andreasen et al. 1995; Awh et al. 1996; Coull et al. 1996; Fiez et al.

Fig. 2 A schematic diagram illustrating the distribution of activation foci reported in studies of verbal working memory (for details, see text). All data have been transformed into standardised sterotaxic space and rendered onto the surface of a three-dimensional magnetic-resonance image. All foci falling within the mid-dorsolateral (areas 9/46, 46, 9) and mid-ventrolateral (44/45, 47) frontal cortices are shown. Activation foci from verbal working-memory tasks are shown in *red*. The *yellow* and *blue squares* indicate the precise stereotaxic co-ordinates of the peaks observed during the forwards and backwards digit-span task described in the text, respectively (Owen et al. 2000)

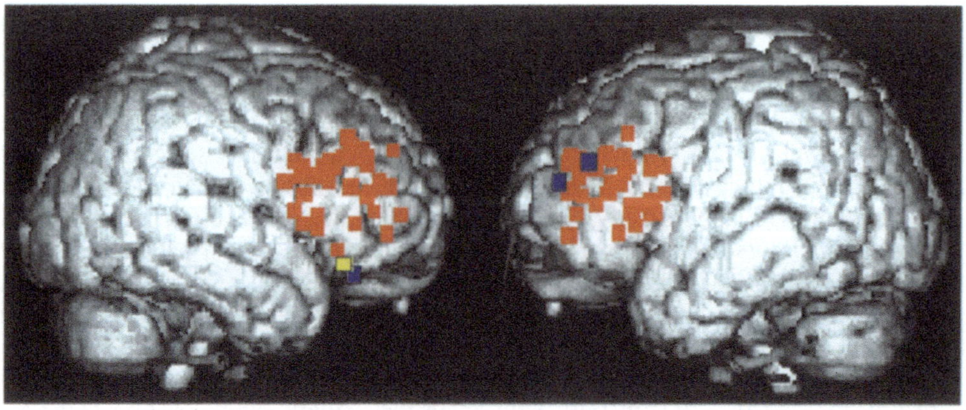

1996; Salmon et al. 1996; Schumacher et al. 1996; Smith et al. 1996; Braver et al. 1997; Jonides et al. 1997, 1998; D'Esposito et al. 1998, 1998; Goldberg et al. 1998; de Zubicaray et al. 1998; Callicot et al. 1999; Collette et al. 1999; Rypma et al. 1999; Barch et al. 1997; Van der Linden et al. 1999) were compared (Owen et al. 2000). Like studies of spatial and visual working memory, a widely distributed pattern of activation foci across both dorsal and ventral frontal areas was observed (Fig. 2). One contributory factor is undoubtedly that the tasks used in different studies vary widely in terms of their specific mnemonic (e.g. processing) requirements. However, it is clear from Fig. 2 that these studies offer no evidence to suggest that, at the area level at least, the lateral frontal cortex is topographically organised according to the nature of the material being processed. In fact, given the considerable overlap between activation foci reported in Fig. 2 and those observed in studies of spatial and non-spatial visual working memory (Fig. 1), it is clear that, in humans, the dorsolateral and ventrolateral frontal regions are broadly polymodal and may each be activated by a variety of tasks involving stimuli of different domains.

Levels of executive processing within the lateral frontal cortex

The "process-specific" model of lateral frontal-lobe organisation rests on the assumption that a functional distinction can be drawn between the mid-dorsolateral and mid-ventrolateral frontal areas, based on the type or nature of the processes that are carried out by those regions (Petrides 1994, 1995). Since this model allows for polymodal representation of information *within* these two frontal regions, its predictions concur fully with the fact that certain spatial, visual and verbal working-memory tasks consistently activate a similar region of the mid-dorsolateral frontal cortex (Figs. 1 and 2). However, one central requirement of this model is that, within a given domain (i.e. spatial or non-spatial), the mid-dorsolateral and mid-ventrolateral prefrontal cortical regions can be shown to play distinct functional roles in working memory. Examination of the studies represented in Fig. 1 offers some, albeit tentative, evidence that this may indeed be the case. Thus, in general, the spatial working-memory tasks that have produced activation foci in mid-ventrolateral area 47 tend to emphasise the active retrieval of one, or a few, pieces of information and the sequencing of responses based directly on that stored information. For example, in the studies by Jonides and colleagues (Jonides et al. 1993; Smith et al. 1995, 1996), the subjects were simply required to remember the location of three simultaneously presented stimuli and then to decide whether or not a probe circle occupied one of those same three locations following a 3-s delay.

In contrast, the spatial working-memory tasks producing increases in rCBF more dorsally, in areas 9 and 46, are often more complex and require additional processing within memory. For example, several studies have used tasks that require the subject to "monitor" or "manipulate" an on-going series of spatial locations within working memory and to make comparisons between each new stimulus and stimuli presented earlier in the sequence (e.g. McCarthy et al. 1994, 1996; Owen et al. 1996a; Smith et al. 1996; for a further description, see Owen 1997). McCarthy et al. (1994, 1996) used functional MRI to measure changes in rCBF while subjects judged whether each of a series of 14 or 15 stimuli was located in a position that had already been occupied earlier in the sequence. The key feature of such tasks appears to be that the response required following each stimulus is invariably not specified directly by that stimulus, but rather has to be computed by comparing that stimulus with information assimilated earlier in the trial (e.g. from previous stimuli).

Similar properties characterise many of the non-spatial working-memory tasks that have been shown to activate the mid-dorsolateral frontal cortex (Fig. 1). In the visual domain, for example, Petrides et al. (1993b) presented subjects with a series of cards, each containing the same eight abstract designs in random positions. The subjects had to select a different design from each card until all eight designs had been selected. Clearly, this type of task requires that the subject constantly monitors an on-going series of visual stimuli within working memory and makes comparisons between each new stimulus and stimuli presented earlier in the sequence. Compared with a control condition, which made minimal demands on working memory, significant increases in rCBF were observed, bilaterally, in the mid-dorsolateral frontal cortex (areas 9/46). Similar findings have been reported in the verbal working-memory literature when conceptually similar tasks are employed. For example, in one parametric fMRI study using letter stimuli, a significant relationship was observed between dorsolateral prefrontal activity and "memory load", which was varied using the widely employed "n-back" paradigm (Braver et al. 1997). This task again requires that subjects maintain and continually update an on-going record of recent stimuli, generating each response by comparing the most recent stimulus with stimuli assimilated earlier in the sequence.

In an attempt to investigate the role of dorsolateral and ventrolateral frontal regions directly, we have recently conducted a series of studies using PET and fMRI, employing spatial, visual and verbal stimuli in tasks that make differing demands on various aspects of executive processing (Owen et al. 1996a, 1999, 2000; Stern et al. 2000). For example, one hypothesis tested was that frontal activation would be confined to the mid-ventrolateral region of the frontal cortex when the experimental task required the subject to hold a sequence of five previously presented spatial locations in memory and, then, to respond directly by touching those same locations following a delay (Owen et al. 1996a, 1999). Thus, the emphasis of the task was on the short-term retention of spatial information; no manipulation of, or computation based

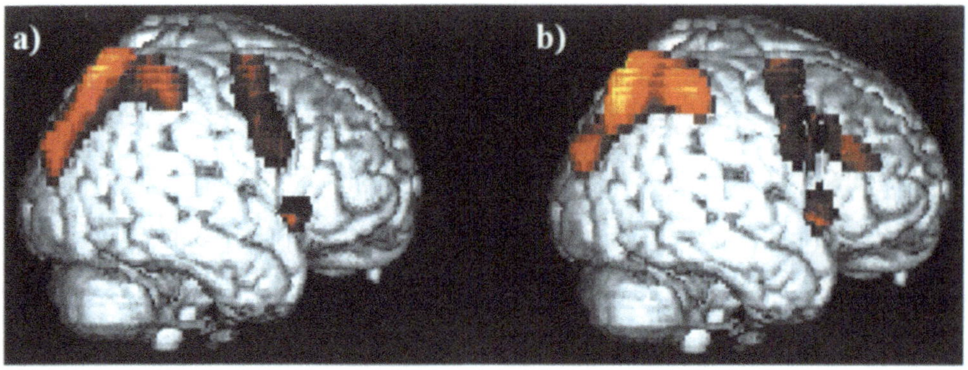

Fig. 3a, b Schematic illustration of the averaged positron-emission-tomography subtraction images rendered onto the surface of a standard three-dimensional magnetic-resonance image. **a** Spatial span minus visuomotor control. Within the prefrontal cortex, a significant regional cerebral-blood-flow (rCBF) change is evident within mid-ventrolateral area 47. **b** Spatial manipulation minus visuomotor control. Within the prefrontal cortex, significant rCBF changes are evident within mid-ventrolateral area 47 and, in addition, within mid-dorsolateral areas 9 and 9/46. The two working-memory conditions differ only with respect to rCBF changes in the mid-dorsolateral frontal cortex (areas 9 and 9/46)

on, this information was necessary. During this variation on the spatial block-tapping test (or "spatial span") of Corsi (see Milner 1971), a significant rCBF increase was observed in ventrolateral area 47 of the right hemisphere at stereotaxic coordinates almost identical to those reported in the studies by Jonides et al. (1993) and Smith et al. (1995, 1996), described above. Similarly, in a second task that required the subjects to execute a fixed sequence of responses to eight previously learned locations, ventrolateral frontal area 47 was significantly activated, bilaterally (Owen et al. 1996a), relative to the same control condition. During both tasks, however, rCBF changes within the dorsolateral frontal region did not approach significance. The second general hypothesis tested was whether there would be significant activation within the mid-dorsolateral frontal cortex (i.e. areas 9 and 46) when the demands of the task were changed to increase the on-going manipulation of information required within working memory. For example, in two tasks, the subject was required to remember which of a set of previously selected locations had been "marked" with a blue circle and to avoid re-selecting those particular locations. Thus, success depended on the ability to maintain, and continually update, an on-line record of which particular locations had been "marked" and, in this sense, the task is conceptually similar to those used by McCarthy et al. (1994) and Petrides et al. (1993b). When the two tasks were compared to a visuomotor control condition, highly significant activation foci were observed in the mid-dorsolateral frontal cortex (area 46/9) of the right hemisphere as well as bilaterally in ventrolateral area 47 (Owen et al. 1996a).

In a follow-up PET study, the five-item spatial span task was used again, but compared with a variation on the widely used spatial "two-back" procedure (Owen et al. 1999). In that task, the subjects were required to monitor a sequence of colour-changing circles on the screen, responding immediately after each stimulus by selecting the circle that changed colour two steps earlier in the sequence. Thus, on each "trial" of the on-going sequence, one of the five red circles was randomly selected by the computer and momentarily changed colour to blue and then back again to red, indicating that it was the next in the series to be remembered. The subject responded immediately not by touching the circle just indicated, but by touching the one two steps earlier in the sequence (i.e. n–2 or "two-back"). Following a fixed delay of 500 ms, the next circle in the sequence changed colour and so on for the entire period of the scan. In the third scanning condition, a matched visuomotor control task, five red circles were again presented in random locations on the screen. On each trial, one of the red circles changed colour to blue and the subject responded immediately by touching that circle and so on. Pilot testing and behavioural results during the scan revealed that, in order to equate the two working-memory tasks for level of difficulty, the parameters should be set to a sequence of five stimuli for the spatial span task and "n–2" for the spatial manipulation task. This provision also ensured that the time between the presentation of a stimulus and the subjects' response *to that stimulus* (e.g. the actual memory time) was identical for the two tasks (for details, see Owen et al. 1999). Moreover, this experimental design ensured that the amount of information that had to be remembered and retrieved during the scan was equivalent for the two working-memory tasks.

As predicted, during the spatial span task, which simply required active (i.e. conscious) retrieval and reproduction of stored information, a significant rCBF increase was observed in the mid-ventrolateral prefrontal cortex at co-ordinates very similar to those reported previous by Owen et al. (1996a) (Fig. 3). In contrast, both the mid-ventrolateral and the mid-dorsolateral prefrontal regions were significantly activated during the two-back task, which required "on-line" manipulation of information within working memory. Moreover, when the spatial span task was subtracted from the spatial manipulation task, the only surviving rCBF difference was located in the mid-dorsolateral prefrontal cortex

Taken together, the results of these two PET studies clearly suggest that, in human subjects, both dorsolateral and ventrolateral frontal cortical areas can be activated by spatial working-memory tasks. Moreover, whether one or both of these regions is recruited appears to depend on the precise cognitive processes that are called upon by the particular task being performed.

In a recent study using fMRI, Courtney et al. (1998) showed that sustained activity during a task that required memory for three locations was observed in the caudal most part of the superior frontal sulcus, immediately anterior to the area defined as the frontal eye field on the basis of activity observed during an occulomotor task. According to a recent cytoarchitectonic analysis of this region (Petrides and Pandya 1994), this peak is located within area 8 [Note that, in both the monkey and in the human brain, the physiologically defined frontal eye field does not correspond to area 8 proper, but rather to the border between area 8 and rostral area 6 (Stanton et al. 1989; Paus 1996)]. A peak in the same location has been reported in previous studies of spatial working memory (e.g. Jonides et al. 1993; Owen et al. 1996a) as well as in studies of spatial attention (e.g. Corbetta et al. 1993; Nobre et al. 1997). A similar peak was also observed in the study described above (Owen et al. 1999) when the visuomotor control task was subtracted from either the spatial span task or the spatial manipulation task. However, as noted in that study, when the spatial span task was subtracted from the spatial manipulation task, there was *no* difference in this region, the only surviving rCBF difference being in the more anteriorly located mid-dorsolateral prefrontal cortex. Given these results, it is now clear that the activation observed in the mid-dorsolateral prefrontal cortex during these tasks is related to the monitoring and manipulation of information within working memory, whereas the peak observed in the posterior dorsolateral cortex (area 8) in this study and in previous studies (e.g. Jonides et al. 1993; Owen et al. 1996a; Courtney et al. 1998) is more likely related to the maintenance of visuospatial attention to the cued locations during the delay period of working memory tasks. Such an interpretation would be entirely consistent with the fact that area 8 is anatomically linked to prestriate visual areas (Barbas and Mesulam 1981). Thus, the mid-ventrolateral, mid-dorsolateral and the posterior dorsolateral prefrontal regions may all be involved in spatial working-memory tasks, but for entirely different reasons.

In a more recent PET study, a direct analogue of the spatial span task was employed to investigate whether these findings could be extended to the verbal domain (Owen et al. 2000). During one experimental task, subjects were required to hold a sequence of five auditorily presented numbers in memory (e.g. 7, 3, 8, 2, 9) and then to respond by (verbally) producing those numbers, in order, following a short delay (e.g. 7, 3, 8, 2, 9). Since the emphasis of this verbal working-memory task was on the active (i.e. conscious) retrieval of remembered information and not on the manipulation of that information, it was predicted that the mid-ventrolateral, but not the mid-dorsolateral prefrontal cortex would be activated. During the second experimental task, the subject was required to listen to similar sequences of numbers, reproducing each sequence *in reverse order* following a short delay (e.g. 9, 2, 8, 3, 7). Since, like the forward digit span task, this task involved the continuous retrieval of information from working memory, it was predicted that the mid-ventrolateral prefrontal cortex would be similarly activated during the two conditions. In addition, however, the backward digit span task places significant demands on the manipulation of the information within working memory; thus, the task requires that the remembered information is re-ordered in order to programme the appropriate sequence of responses. On this basis, the backward digit task was expected to activate, additionally, the mid-dorsolateral prefrontal region. In a third "control" condition, each trial involved an identical digit string, (e.g. 1, 1, 1, 1, 1) and subjects were required to respond by repeating the sequence. In all three conditions, stimuli were presented at a rate of one digit per second with a 6-s intertrial interval (during which time the subject responded). To control for the non-specific effects of task difficulty, each subject underwent a pilot testing session prior to scanning in order to determine their individual forwards and backwards digit spans. During scanning, the number of digits presented in the two experimental conditions was set according to the maximum number of digits that could be recalled accurately in three successive trials.

As predicted, when the forward digits span task was compared to the control, significant activation was observed in right mid-ventrolateral area 47 at co-ordinates slightly anterior to those reported previously in studies of spatial span (Owen et al. 1996a, 1999; see also Jonides et al. 1993). For comparison with previous studies of verbal working memory, the location of this activation focus is represented schematically in Fig. 2. No significant blood-flow changes were observed in the mid-dorsolateral frontal region. In contrast, when the backward digits condition was compared with the control task, significant increases in rCBF were observed in a similar region of the right mid-ventrolateral frontal cortex (area 47) and, in addition, in the left mid-dorsolateral frontal cortex (area 9/46). For comparison with previous studies of verbal working memory, the location of this activation focus is represented schematically in Fig. 2. When the two verbal working-memory tasks were compared directly (backwards minus forwards), only one significant rCBF change emerged, in areas 9 and 9/46 of the mid-dorsolateral frontal cortex (Fig. 2). This focus was located within the left hemisphere, at stereotaxic coordinates almost identical to those observed in the right hemisphere, during tasks which required manipulation of information within *spatial* working memory (Fig. 3; also see Owen et al. 1999). The reverse subtraction yielded no significant rCBF changes within the entire grey-matter volume.

Discussion

It appears, therefore, that the weight of evidence from neuroimaging studies in humans favours the hypothesis that, at the area level at least, the lateral frontal cortex is topographically organised according to the nature of the process being carried out, rather than according to the nature of the material being processed, as previously thought (Wilson et al. 1993; Goldman-Rakic 1995; Courtney et al. 1998; also see Courtney et al. 1996, 1997). However, it is important to emphasise that the findings discussed here do not rule out the possibility that some functional differentiation based on stimulus material might still exist *within* these particular frontal cortical regions. For example, it is plausible that the functional neuroimaging methods used in the studies described in this review have sufficient spatial resolution to detect differences *between*, but not *within* these anatomical regions. Certainly among the mid-dorsolateral activation foci reported in Figs. 1 and 2, there is considerable overlap between studies of spatial, non-spatial and verbal working memory in all three planes (x, y, z). In the ventrolateral cortex, however, there does appear to be some reasonably consistent evidence for differences between those studies that have used spatial stimuli and those that have used non-spatial stimuli in the anterior-posterior (y) plane. Thus, the spatial working-memory tasks used by Jonides et al. (1993), Owen et al. (1996a, 1999) and Smith et al. (1995) all yielded rather posterior ventrolateral activation foci at y co-ordinates of between 14 mm and 24 mm. In two non-spatial studies that employed face stimuli, ventrolateral activation foci were reported rather more anteriorly at y co-ordinates of between 33 mm and 40 mm (Haxby et al. 1995; Courtney et al. 1996). In the verbal working-memory study described in detail above (Owen et al. 2000), ventrolateral activation foci were also observed rather more anteriorly (y=30 and y=34) than those reported in spatial working-memory studies that employed analogous tasks (e.g. Owen et al. 1996a, 1999). Nevertheless, even if such subtle differences in activation were to be confirmed in later studies, they would still not be evidence supporting a functional separation between the anatomically and cytoarchitectonically distinct dorsolateral and ventrolateral frontal-lobe regions that are the focus of this review. Moreover, this general pattern of overlapping activation foci concurs fully with the results of a recent electrophysiological recording study in the monkey designed to investigate where and how information about object-identity is integrated with information about object-location in working memory (Rao et al. 1997). In that study, approximately half of the neurones with delay-related activity were tuned both to visual pattern ("what") and location ("where"). Furthermore, neurones that were tuned only to location or only to visual pattern were equally distributed between the dorsolateral and the ventrolateral prefrontal cortex, neurones tuned to location not being predominant in the dorsolateral prefrontal cortex (Rao et al. 1997; for a further discussion, see Rushworth and Owen 1998).

Finally, recent findings suggest that further insights about the role of human prefrontal cortex in working memory are likely to emerge from comparisons with studies of other types of task assumed to be similarly dependent on the frontal lobe, such as those requiring episodic memory. For example, Fletcher et al. (1998b) reported activation in the mid-ventrolateral frontal cortex during a paired-associates task that required subjects to retrieve previously learned category exemplars in response to a series of category names. In contrast, during a second condition that required subjects to freely recall items from a previously learned list, activation in the mid-dorsolateral frontal cortex was observed (Fletcher et al. 1998b). This dissociation within the frontal-lobes is almost identical to that described above for two types of spatial *working*-memory task (Owen et al. 1999), raising the general issue of developing a theory which is sufficiently comprehensive to incorporate the main findings from ostensibly different types of mnemonic task, but which remains emancipated from a strict localisationalist perspective. In this respect, a fruitful approach may be to assume that the various processes involved in working memory, episodic memory encoding and retrieval, and other "executive" functions not discussed here are drawn from a single set of underlying components, although they may be differentially represented in different tasks. Thus, a general role for the ventrolateral frontal cortex in memory may be to trigger active low-level encoding strategies, such as rehearsal, and to initiate explicit (i.e. intentional) retrieval of information from long-term memory. In the case of working-memory tasks, this would correspond to the relatively straightforward mapping of stimuli to responses, such as that which is assumed to occur in spatial and digit span tasks (e.g. Owen et al. 1996a, 1999) or even simple delayed matching-to-sample paradigms (e.g. Elliott and Dolan 1999). In the case of long-term episodic memory (e.g. verbal paired associate learning), these "active" encoding and retrieval processes might correspond to the active mapping and implementation of a somewhat arbitrary learned response (e.g. a category exemplar) to a specific stimulus (e.g. a category name) (e.g. Fletcher et al. 1998a, 1998b). Indeed, a number of recent episodic-memory tasks that have produced predominantly ventral frontal activation have involved fairly "low-level" mnemonic processes, such as face encoding (Haxby et al. 1996), word-pair encoding (Kapur et al. 1996), short-term word recognition (Andreasen et al. 1995), face recognition (Haxby et al. 1996) and learned picture recognition (Kapur et al. 1995).

In contrast, the mid-dorsolateral frontal cortex may mediate more complex types of processing within memory and will be recruited when active manipulation or "monitoring" of remembered information is required. For example, in the self-ordered spatial working-memory tasks that are sensitive to frontal-lobe damage (Owen et al. 1990, 1996b) and activate both dorsal and ventral frontal-lobe areas (Owen et al. 1996a), an encoding strategy for determining the optimal sequence of choices is required that must be constantly updated or "monitored" during its execution (for a further discussion, see Owen et al. 1996b). Similarly, one key component of the free recall task described by Fletcher et al. (1998b), which activated the dorsolateral frontal cortex, is that each response cannot be made in isolation, but rather can only be made by "monitoring" responses made and information assimilated earlier in each trial. For example, the subject knows, in this case, that there are a specific number of items to be recalled and has to check with each new item produced that it has not been produced before. In general, widespread activation of both ventral and dorsal frontal-lobe areas has been reported during complex episodic memory tasks, such as encoding of temporal order (Cabeza et al. 1997), encoding new associations between nouns and categories (Dolan and Fletcher 1997), word-list encoding with "maximal organisation" (Fletcher et al. 1998a), long-term word recognition (Andreasen 1995), cued recall (Buckner et al. 1995, 1996; Petrides et al. 1995; Cabeza et al. 1997; Fletcher et al. 1998b) and free recall (Petrides et al. 1995).

It would be na, of course, to assume that it will be possible to recast the results of all previous studies of working memory and episodic memory in this light and a systematic re-analysis has not be attempted here. In addition, while this review has focused specifically on the role that various frontal-lobe regions may play in *mnemonic* processing, it is quite clear that a more comprehensive understanding of lateral frontal-lobe organisation will only be achieved by stepping beyond the realm of memory function. For example, similar frontal-lobe regions are widely assumed to contribute to many other aspects of "executive control" that do not directly involve or depend upon working memory; high-level attentional set-shifting behaviour and active inhibition of prepotent responses, being just two examples. Whether such processes can be adequately incorporated within the two-stage conceptual framework suggested by the data reviewed here, will remain a significant challenge for the future.

Acknowledgements I am indebted to Helen Keane for careful assimilation of the verbal working-memory data set described in this review and to Matthew Brett for providing the software for the 3D rendering of spatial, visual and verbal working-memory data sets.

References

Andreasen NC, O'Leary DS, Arndt S, Cizadlo T, Hurtig R, Rezai K, Watkins GL, Boles Ponto LL, Hichwa RD (1995) Short-term and long-term verbal memory: a positron emission tomography study. Proc Natl Acad Sci USA 92:5111–5115

Awh E, Jonides J, Smith EE, Schumacher EH, Koeppe RA, Katz S (1996) Dissociation of storage and rehearsal in verbal working memory: evidence from positron emission tomography. Psychol Sci 7:25–31

Baddeley AD (1986) Working memory. Oxford University Press, New York

Baker SC, Frith CD, Frackowiak RSJ, Dolan RJ (1996) Active representation of shape and location in man. Cereb Cortex 6:612–619

Barbas H (1988) Anatomic organization of basoventral and mediodorsal visual recipient prefrontal regions in the rhesus monkey. J Comp Neurol 276:313–342

Barbas H, Mesulam M-M (1981) Organization of afferent input to subdivision of area 8 in the rhesus monkey. J Comp Neurol 200:407–431

Barch DM, Braver TS, Nystrom LE, Forman SD, Noll DC, Cohen JD (1997) Dissociating working memory from task difficulty in human prefrontal cortex. Neuropsychologia 35:1373–1380

Bates JF, Wilson FAW, O Scalaidhe SP, Goldman-Rakic PS (1994) Area TE connections with inferior prefrontal regions responsive to complex objects and faces. Soc Neurosci Abstr 20: 434.10

Becker JT, Mintun MA, Diehl DJ, Dobkin J, Martidis A, Madoff DC, DeKosky ST (1994) Functional neuroanatomy of verbal free recall: a replication study. Hum Brain Map 1:284–292

Braver TS, Cohen JD, Nystrom LE, Jonides J, Smith EE, Noll DC (1997) A parametric study of prefrontal cortex involvement in human working memory. Neuroimage 5:49–62

Buckner RL, Petersen SE, Ojemann JG, Miezin FM, Squire LR, Raichle ME (1995) Functional anatomical studies of explicit and implicit memory retrieval tasks. J Neurosci 15:12–29

Buckner RL, Raichle ME, Miezin FM, Petersen SE (1996) Functional anatomic studies of memory retrieval for auditory words and visual pictures. J Neurosci 16:6219–6235

Cabeza R, Mangels J, Nyberg L, Habib R, Houle S, Mcintosh AR, Tulving E (1997) Brain regions differentially involved in remembering what and when: a PET study. Neuron 19:863–870

Callicot JH, Mattay VS, Bertolino A, Finn K, Coppola R, Frank JA, Goldberg TE, Weinberger DR (1999) Physiological characteristics of capacity constraints in working memory as revealed by functional MRI. Cereb Cortex 9:20–26

Carmichael ST, Price JL (1995) Sensory and premotor connections of the orbital and medial prefrontal cortex of macaque monkeys. J Comp Neurol 363:642–664

Cavada C, Goldman-Rakic PS (1989) Posterior parietal cortex on rhesus monkey. II. Evidence for segregated corticocortical networks linking sensory and limbic areas with the frontal lobe. J Comp Neurol 287:422–445

Cohen JD, Forman SD, Braver TS, Casey BJ, Servan-Schreiber D, Noll DC (1994) Activation of prefrontal cortex in a non-spatial working memory task with functional MRI. Hum Brain Map 1:293–304

Cohen JD, Perlstein WM, Braver TS, Nystrom LE, Noll DC, Jonides J, Smith, EE (1997) Temporal dynamics of brain activation during a working memory task. Nature 386:604–608

Collette F, Salmon E, Van der Linden M, Chicherio C, Belleville S, Degueldre C, Delfiore G, Franck G (1999) Regional brain activity during tasks devoted to the central executive of working memory. Brain Res Cogn Brain Res 7:411–417

Corbetta M, Miezin FM, Shulman GL, Petersen SE (1993) A PET study of visuospatial attention. J Neurosci 13:1202–1226

Coull JT, Frith CD, Frackowiak RSJ, Grasby PM (1996) A fronto-parietal network for rapid visual information processing: a PET study of sustained attention and working memory. Neuropsychologia 34:1085–1095

Courtney SM, Ungerlieder LG, Keil K, Haxby JV (1996) Object and spatial visual working memory activate separate neural systems in human cortex. Cereb Cortex 6:39–49

Courtney SM, Ungerleider LG, Kell KK, Haxby JV (1997) Transient and sustained activity in a distributed system for human working memory. Nature 386:608–611

Courtney SM, Petit L, Maisog JM, Ungerleider LG, Haxby JV (1998) An area specialized for spatial working memory in human frontal cortex. Science 279:1347–1351

D'Esposito M, Ballard D, Aguirre GK, Zarahn E (1998) Human prefrontal cortex is not specific for working memory: a functional MRI study. Neuroimage 8:274–282

D'Esposito M, Aguirre GK, Zarahn E, Ballard D, Shin RK, Lease J, Tang J (1998) Functional MRI studies of spatial and non-spatial working memory. Brain Res Cogn Brain Res 7:1–13

Dolan RJ, Fletcher PC (1997) Dissociating prefrontal and hippocampal function in episodic memory encoding. Nature 388: 582–585

Elliot R, Dolan RJ (1999) Differential neural responses during performance of matching and nonmatching to sample tasks at two delay intervals. J Neurosci 19:5066–5073

Fiez JA, Raife EA, Balota DA, Schwarz JP, Raichle ME, Petersen SE (1996) A positron emission tomography study of the short-term maintenance of verbal information. J Neurosci 16:808–822

Fletcher P, Shallice T, Dolan RJ (1998a) The functional roles of prefrontal cortex in episodic memory. I. Encoding. Brain 121: 1239–1248

Fletcher P, Shallice T, Frith CD, Frackowiak RSJ, Dolan RJ (1998b) The functional roles of prefrontal cortex in episodic memory. II Retrieval. Brain 121:1249–1256

Funahashi S, Bruce CJ, Goldman-Rakic PS (1989) Mnemonic coding of visual space in the monkey's dorsolateral prefrontal cortex. J Neurophysiol 61:1–19

Fuster JM (1995) Memory in the cerebral cortex: an empirical approach to neural networks in the human and nonhuman primate brain. MIT press, Cambridge

Fuster JM (1997) The prefrontal cortex: anatomy, physiology, and neuropsychology of the frontal lobe, 3rd edn. Lippincott-Raven, Philadelphia

Goldberg TE, Berman KF, Randolph C, Gold JM, Weinberger DR (1996) Isolating the mnemonic component in spatial delayed response: a controlled PET ^{15}O-labeled water regional cerebral blood flow study in normal humans. Neuroimage 3:69–78

Goldberg TE, Berman KF, Fleming K, Ostrem J, Van Horn JD, Esposito G, Mattey VS, Gold JM, Weinberger DR (1998) Uncoupling cognitive workload and prefrontal cortical physiology: A PET rCBF study. Neuroimage 7:296–303

Goldman-Rakic PS (1987) Circuitry of primate prefrontal cortex and the regulation of behavior by representational memory. In: Plum F, Mountcastle V (eds) Handbook of physiology. Section 1, the nervous system, Vol 5. American Physiological Society, Bethesda, pp 373–417

Goldman-Rakic PS (1994) The issue of memory in the study of prefrontal functions. In: Thierry AM, Glowinski J, Goldman-Rakic PS, Christen Y (eds) Motor and cognitive functions of the prefrontal cortex. Springer, Berlin Heidelberg New York, pp 112–122

Goldman-Rakic PS (1995) Architecture of the prefrontal cortex and the central executive. Ann NY Acad Sci 769:71–83

Goldman-Rakic PS (1996) The prefrontal landscape: implications of functional architecture for understanding human mentation and the central executive. Philos Trans R Soc Lond 351:1445–1453

Grasby PM, Frith CD, Friston KJ, Bench C, Frackowiak RSJ, Dolan RJ (1993) Functional mapping of brain areas implicated in auditory-verbal memory function. Brain 116:1–20

Grasby PM, Frith CD, Friston KJ, Simpson J, Fletcher PC, Frackowiak RSJ, Dolan RJ (1994) A graded task approach to the functional mapping of brain areas implicated in auditory-verbal memory. Brain 117:1271–1282

Haxby JV, Ungerleider LG, Horwitz B, Rapoport SI, Grady CL (1995) Hemispheric differences in neural systems for face working memory: a PET-rCBF study. Hum Brain Map 3:68–82

Haxby JV, Ungerleider LG, Horwitz B, Maisog JM, Rapoport SI, Grady CL (1996) Face encoding and recognition in the human brain. Proc Natl Acad Sci USA 93:922–927

Honig WK (1978) Studies of working memory in the pigeon. In: Hulse SH, Fowler H, Honig WK (eds) Cognitive processes in animal behaviour. Lawrence Erlbaum, Hillsdale, pp 211–248

Jonides J, Smith EE, Koeppe RA, Awh E, Minoshima S, Mintun MA (1993) Spatial working memory in humans as revealed by PET. Nature 363:623–625

Jonides J, Schumacher EH, Smith EE, Lauber EJ, Awh E, Minoshima S, Koeppe RA (1997) Verbal working memory load affects regional brain activation as measured by PET. J Cogn Neurosci 9:462–475

Jonides J, Schumacher EH, Smith EE, Koeppe RA, Awh E, Reuter-Lorenz PA, Marshuetz C, Willis CR (1998) The role of parietal cortex in verbal working memory. J Neurosci 18: 5026–5034

Kapur N, Friston KH, Young A, Frith CD, Frackowiak RSJ (1995) Functional role of the prefrontal cortex in memory retrieval: a PET study. Cortex 31:99–108

Kapur S, Tulving E, Cabeza R, Mcintosh AR, Houle S, Craik FIM (1996) The neural correlates of intentional learning of verbal materials: a PET study. Brain Res Cogn Brain Res 4:243–249

Levy R, Goldman-Rakic PS (1999) Association of storage and processing functions in the dorsolateral prefrontal cortex of the non-human primate. J Neurosci 19:5149–5158

McCarthy G, Blamire AM, Puce A, Nobre AC, Bloch G, Hyder F, Goldman-Rakic P, Shulman RG (1994) Functional magnetic resonance imaging of human prefrontal cortex activation during a spatial working memory task. Proc Natl Acad Sci USA 91:8690–8694

McCarthy G, Puce A, Constable RT, Krystal JH, Gore JC, Goldman-Rakic PS (1996) Activation of human prefrontal cortex activation during spatial and non-spatial working memory tasks measured by functional MRI. Cereb Cortex 6:600–611

Milner B (1971) Interhemispheric differences in the localisation of psychological processes in man. Br Med Bull 27:272–277

Nobre AC, Sebestyen GN, Gitelman DR, Mesulam MM, Frackowiak RSJ, Frith CD (1997) Functional localization of the system for visuospatial attention using positron emission tomography. Brain 120:515–533

Olton DS (1982) Spatially organised behaviours of animals: behavioural and neurological studies. In: Potegal M (ed) Spatial abilities. Academic Press, New York, pp 325–360

Owen AM (1997) The functional organization of working memory processes within human lateral frontal cortex: the contribution of functional neuroimaging. Eur J Neurosci 9:1329–1339

Owen AM, Downes JD, Sahakian BJ, Polkey CE, Robbins TW (1990) Planning and spatial working memory following frontal lobe lesions in man. Neuropsychologia 28:1021–1034

Owen AM, Sahakian BJ, Semple J, Polkey CE, Robbins TW (1995) Visuo-spatial short term recognition memory and learning after temporal lobe excisions, frontal lobe excisions or amygdalo-hippocampectomy in man. Neuropsychologia 33:1–24

Owen AM, Evans AC, Petrides M (1996a) Evidence for a two-stage model of spatial working memory processing within the lateral frontal cortex: a positron emission tomography study. Cereb Cortex 6:31–38

Owen AM, Morris RG, Sahakian BJ, Polkey CE, Robbins TW (1996b) Double dissociations of memory and executive functions in working memory tasks following frontal lobe excisions, temporal lobe excisions or amygdalo-hippocampectomy in man. Brain 119:1597–1615

Owen AM, Stern CE, Look RB, Tracey I, Rosen BR, Petrides M (1998) Functional organisation of spatial and non-spatial working memory processes within the human lateral frontal cortex. Proc Natl Acad Sci USA 95:7721–7726

Owen AM, Herrod NJ, Menon DK, Clark JC, Downey SPMJ, Carpenter TA, Minhas PS, Turkheimer FE, Williams EJ, Robbins TW, Sahakian BJ, Petrides M, Pickard JD (1999) Redefining the functional organisation of working memory processes within human lateral prefrontal cortex. Eur J Neurosci 11:567–574

Owen AM, Lee ACH, Williams EJ (2000) Dissociating aspects of verbal working memory within the human frontal lobe: further evidence for a 'process-specific' model of lateral frontal organization. Psychobiology (in press)

Paulesu E, Frith CD, Frackowiak RSJ (1993) The neural correlates of the verbal component of working memory. Nature 362: 342–345

Paus T (1996) Location and function of the human frontal eye-filed: a selective review. Neuropsychologia 34:475–483

Petrides M (1994) Frontal lobes and working memory: evidence from investigations of the effects of cortical excisions in nonhuman primates. In: Boller F, Grafman J (eds) Handbook of neuropsychology, Vol 9. Elsevier, Amsterdam, pp 59–82
Petrides M (1995) Functional organization of the human frontal cortex for mnemonic processing. Ann NY Acad Sci 769: 85–96
Petrides M, Milner B (1982) Deficits on subject-ordered tasks after frontal and temporal lobe lesions in man. Neuropsychologia 20:249–262
Petrides M, Pandya DN (1994) Comparative architectonic analysis of the human and the macaque frontal cortex. In: Boller F, Grafman J (eds) Handbook of neuropsychology, Vol 9. Elsevier, Amsterdam, pp 17–58
Petrides M, Alivisatos B, Evans AC, Meyer E (1993a) Dissociation of human mid-dorsolateral from posterior dorsolateral frontal cortex in memory processing. Proc Natl Acad Sci USA 90:873–877
Petrides M, Alivisatos B, Evans AC, Meyer E (1993b) Functional activation of the human frontal cortex during the performance of verbal working memory tasks. Proc Natl Acad Sci USA 90:878–882
Petrides M, Alivisatos B, Evans AC (1995) Functional activation of the human ventrolateral frontal cortex during mnemonic retrieval of verbal information. Proc Natl Acad Sci USA 92:5803–5807
Postle BR, Stern CE, Rosen BR, Corkin S (2000) An fMRI investigation of cortical contributions to spatial and non-spatial visual working memory. Neuroimage (in press)
Rao SC, Rainer G, Miller EK (1997) Integration of what and where in the primate prefrontal cortex. Science 276:821–824
Rodman HR (1994) Development of inferior temporal cortex in monkey. Cereb Cortex 4:484–498
Rushworth MFS, Owen AM (1998) The functional organization of the lateral frontal cortex: conjecture or conjuncture in the electrophysiology literature. Trends Cogn Sci 2:46–53
Rypma B, Prabhakaran V, Desmond JE, Glover GH, Gabrieli JDE (1999) Load-dependent roles of frontal brain regions in the maintenance of working memory. Neuroimage 9:216–226
Salmon E, Van der Linden M, Collette F, Delfiore G, Maquet P, Degueldre C, Luxen A, Franck G (1996) Regional brain activity during working memory tasks. Brain 119:1617–1625
Schumacher EH, Lauber E, Awh E, Jonides J, Smith E, Koeppe RA (1996) PET evidence for an amodal verbal working memory system. Neuroimage 3:79–88
Smith E, Jonides JJ, Koeppe RA, Awh E, Schumacher EH, Minoshima S (1995) Spatial versus object working memory: PET investigations. J Cogn Neurosci 7:337–356
Smith E, Jonides JJ, Koeppe RA (1996) Dissociating verbal and spatial working memory using PET. Cereb Cortex 6:11–20
Stanton GB, Deng SY, Goldberg ME, McMullen NT (1989) Cytoarchitectonic characteristics of the frontal eye fields in macaque monkeys. J Comp Neurol 282:415–427
Stern CE, Owen AM, Petrides M, Look RB, Tracey I, Rosen BR (2000) Activity in ventrolateral and mid-dorsolateral prefrontal cortex during non-spatial visual working memory processing: evidence from functional magnetic resonance imaging (in press)
Talairach J, Tournoux P (1988) Co-planar stereotactic atlas of the human brain: 3-Dimensional proportional system: an approach to cerebral imaging. Georg Thieme, Stuttgart New York
Ungerleider LG, Mishkin M (1982) Two cortical visual systems. In: Ingle DJ, Goodale MA, Mansfield RJW (eds) Analysis of visual behavior. MIT Press, Cambridge, pp 549–586
Van der Linden M, Collette F, Salmon E, Delfiore G, Degueldre C, Luxen A, Franck G (1999) The neural correlates of updating of information in verbal working memory. Memory 7:549–560
Webster MJ, Bachevalier J, Ungerlieder LG (1994) Connections of inferior temporal areas TEO and TE with parietal and frontal cortx in macaque monkeys. Cereb Cortex 4:470–483
Wilson FAW, Scalaidhe SPO, Goldman-Rakic PS (1993) Dissociations of object and spatial processing domains in primate prefrontal cortex. Science 260:1955–1958
Zubicaray GI de, Williams SCR, Wilson SJ, Rose SE, Brammer MJ, Bullmore ET, Simmons A, Chalk JB, Semple J, Brown AP, Smith GA, Ashton R, Doddrell DM (1998) Prefrontal cortex involvement in selective letter generation: a functional magnetic resonance imaging study. Cortex 34:389–401

Michael Petrides

The role of the mid-dorsolateral prefrontal cortex in working memory

Published online: 20 May 2000

Abstract Recent studies with nonhuman primates have shown that lesions of the mid-dorsolateral prefrontal cortex, which extends from the lip of the dorsal bank of the sulcus principalis to the midline (i.e., dorsal area 46 and 9/46 and area 9), give rise to severe and long-lasting impairments on self-ordered and externally ordered tasks designed to tax executive processing within working memory, rather than short-term memory per se. Lesions limited to area 9 give rise to a mild impairment on these tasks. Thus, the mid-dorsolateral prefrontal region has been shown to be critical for the monitoring of multiple events in working memory. The mid-dorsolateral prefrontal region receives visuospatial input from the posterior dorsolateral region (areas 8 and 6) and from the cortex within the middle part (sulcal area 46) and the caudal part (area 8) of the sulcus principalis. Nonspatial visual input originates from the ventrolateral prefrontal cortex. Thus, lesions focused on the middle to caudal part of the sulcus principalis would affect visuospatial input, but would not affect the flow of nonspatial visual object information that reaches the mid-dorsolateral prefrontal region from the ventrolateral prefrontal cortex. Lesions of the sulcus principalis produce a spatially selective impairment, whereas lesions of the mid-dorsolateral prefrontal region produce a more general impairment of the monitoring and manipulation of information in working memory. The results of recent functional neuroimaging studies with human subjects are consistent with the above findings from work with the monkey.

Introduction

The critical role of the lateral prefrontal cortex in working memory was established by a long line of studies with monkeys, originating in the classic demonstration by Jacobsen (1936) that lesions of the prefrontal cortex impair performance on the delayed-response tasks (e.g., Mishkin 1957; Gross and Weiskrantz 1962; Butters and Pandya 1969; Mishkin et al. 1969; Goldman and Rosvold 1970; Butters et al. 1971; Goldman et al. 1971; Passingham 1975; Mishkin and Manning 1978; Funahashi et al. 1993; Petrides 1991, 1995). Since the 1970s, several studies recording the activity of single neurons in monkeys performing various delayed-response tasks demonstrated that certain neurons in the lateral prefrontal cortex continue to discharge during the delay period, appearing to maintain temporarily the processed information (e.g., Fuster and Alexander 1971; Kubota and Niki 1971; Fuster 1973; Niki 1974a, 1974b; Kojima and Goldman-Rakic 1982; Miller et al. 1996). This work clearly established the existence of sustained neuronal activity during the delay period within the lateral prefrontal cortex and further reinforced the notion that this region of the cortex plays a critical role in working memory.

But what exactly is the role of the prefrontal cortex in working memory? A major puzzle is the fact that patients with damage to the lateral prefrontal-cortical region can perform well on several standard short-term-memory tests. Performance on standard tests of memory, such as simple recognition and story recall, can be adequate even when the lesions are bilateral, as several studies of patients who had undergone frontal lobotomies have clearly demonstrated (see Petrides 1989 for a review). In cases where a severe memory disorder has been reported after frontal lesions, there was involvement of the caudal orbito-medial limbic region of the frontal lobe and the immediately adjacent basal forebrain region (e.g., septal area, nucleus basalis of Meynert, etc.) or there had been significant damage outside the frontal cortex (see Petrides 1989 for a review).

The prefrontal cortex, a large expanse of cortex that reaches its maximum development in the human brain, plays a critical role in various executive processes concerned with the organization (planning) of sequences of

M. Petrides (✉)
Montreal Neurological Institute and Department of Psychology, McGill University, 3801 University Street, Montreal, Quebec, Canada H3A 2B4
e-mail: petrides@ego.psych.mcgill.ca
Tel.: 514-3988375, Fax: 514-3981338

responses and the selection and development of appropriate strategies in complex situations. The contribution of the prefrontal cortex to working memory lies in the application of various executive processes to mnemonic performance. In attempting to characterize one aspect of the essential nature of the specific contribution of the human lateral prefrontal cortex to mnemonic processing, I developed a series of new working-memory tasks, the self-ordered and externally ordered tasks, which could be used both with monkeys and patients. The important aspect of these new tasks was that successful performance could not be based simply on the maintenance of information in short-term memory, but rather taxed the executive requirement that the information in short-term memory be carefully monitored. When we tested patients with lesions involving the lateral prefrontal cortex on these new tasks, we were struck by the severity of the impairments, despite the fact that these same patients could perform well on several other short-term memory tests, such as tests of recognition memory, digit span, and story recall (Petrides and Milner 1982). These early results with patients clearly indicated that a major source of the impairment following lateral prefrontal lesions arose not from the need to maintain the information per se, but rather from the requirement that performance be based on careful monitoring of the information in working memory.

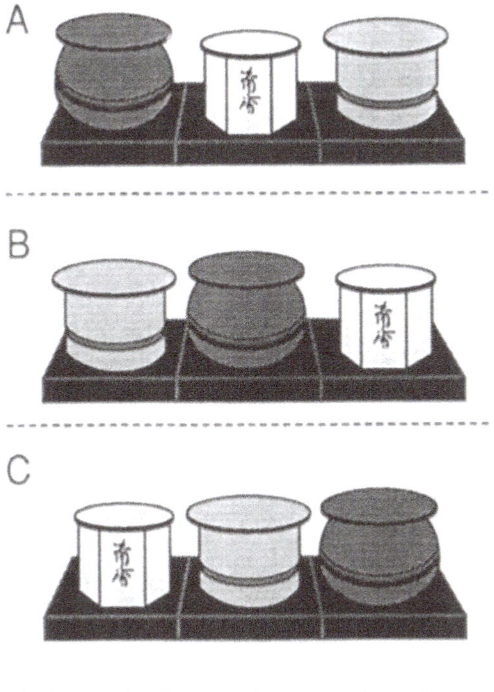

Fig. 1A–C Schematic diagram of the experimental arrangement for the self-ordered task administered to monkeys. On each trial, a set of stimuli (in this case, three objects differing in color and shape) is presented. On the first trial (**A**), selection of any one of the stimuli will lead to reward. After the animal has chosen one of the stimuli and received the reward, the same stimuli (but in a random arrangement) are presented after a short delay period (10 s). The animal must now select any one of the objects not selected on the previous trial in order to receive reward. Testing continues in this manner until all objects are selected once

In the self-ordered working-memory task, the subjects (human or monkey) are presented with different arrangements of the same set of stimuli and, on each trial, they have to select a different stimulus until all have been selected once (Fig. 1) (Petrides 1995). The relative position of the stimuli changes from trial to trial to ensure that the subject is guided by memory of the objects and not their locations. Successful performance, therefore, encourages the subjects to compare carefully those stimuli that they have already selected with those still remaining to be selected. In other words, events in working memory must be closely monitored. In the related externally ordered working-memory tasks, a subset from an expected set of stimuli are presented and the subject is required to monitor which ones from the set of expected stimuli have been presented.

The mid-dorsolateral prefrontal cortex is critical for monitoring of events in working memory

The prefrontal cortex is not a homogeneous region of the cortical mantle, but rather a collection of several distinct architectonic areas (Brodmann 1905, 1908, 1909; Economo and Koskinas 1925; Sarkissov et al. 1955; Sanides 1962; Barbas and Pandya 1989; Petrides and Pandya 1994, 1999). Work in the monkey has indicated that these areas differ in major ways in terms of their cortical and subcortical connections (see Pandya and Yeterian 1985). Undoubtedly, these differences in the local cir-

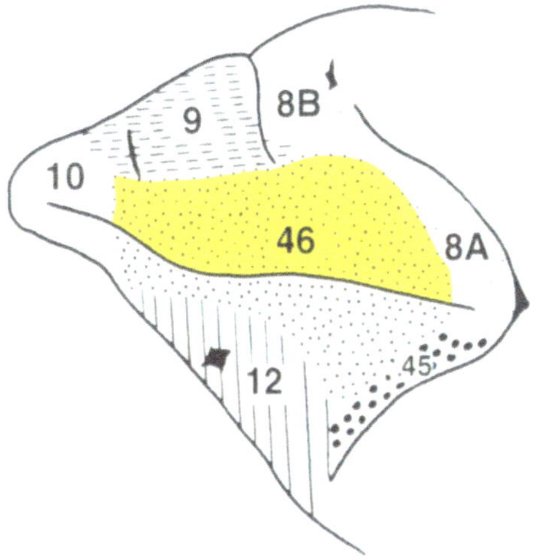

Fig. 2 The classic map of Walker (1940). As can be seen, area 9 occupies approximately the superior half of the mid-dorsolateral prefrontal region. Note that approximately the lower half of the mid-dorsolateral prefrontal region (area marked in *yellow*) is occupied by the dorsal part of area 46, which lies above the sulcus principalis. In a comparative architectonic study of the macaque and the human prefrontal cortex, we noted that Walker's area 9 is comparable with area 9 on the superior frontal gyrus of the human brain, whereas the dorsal part of area 46 of Walker is comparable to dorsal area 46 and 9/46 of the human brain, which occupy the middle frontal gyri (for details, see Petrides and Pandya 1994, 1999). We, therefore, refer to the rostral half of the *yellow region* as 46D and the caudal half as 9/46D (see Fig. 3A)

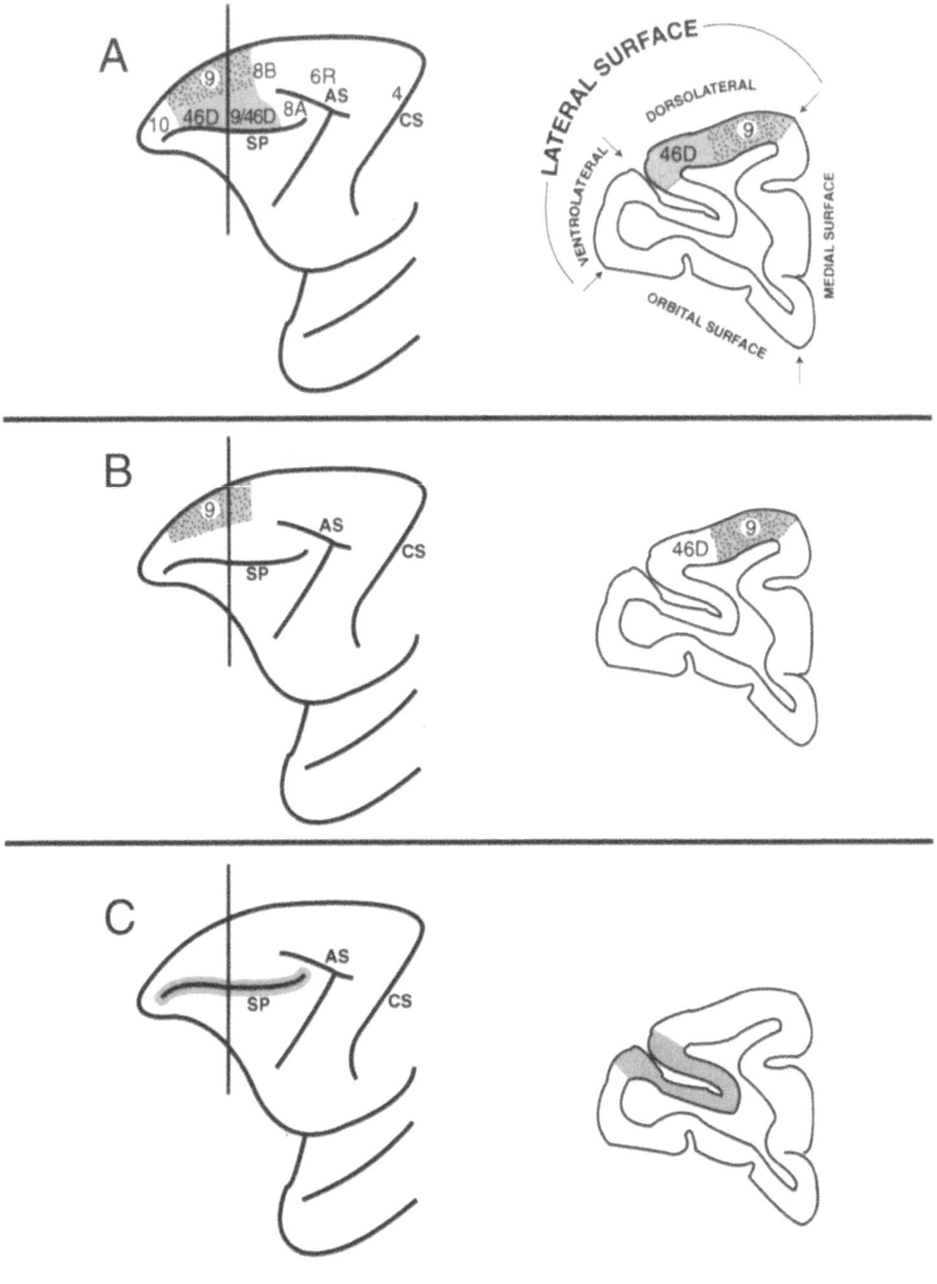

Fig. 3 **A** The mid-dorsolateral prefrontal lesion studied by Petrides (1991, 1995) shown on the lateral surface of the monkey frontal lobe (*left*) and on a coronal section (*right*) taken at the level indicated by the *vertical line*. The mid-dorsolateral prefrontal lesion extends from the lip of the sulcus principalis to the midline, including the granular cortex above the sulcus principalis (dorsal area 46 and dorsal area 9/46) and the dysgranular cortex (area 9) that occupies approximately the upper half of the mid-dorsolateral prefrontal region. **B** The lesion restricted to the superior part (area 9) of the mid-dorsolateral prefrontal region studied by Petrides (1998). **C** The classical sulcus principalis lesion, which is restricted to the cortex lining the banks of the sulcus principalis

cuitry of the various prefrontal areas, which is reflected in their specific cytoarchitectonic pattern, coupled with their distinct inputs and outputs, indicate specialized functional contributions. Thus, one can speak of multiple executive-processing modules within the prefrontal cortex. With regard to the particular issue of whether there is a critical region of the prefrontal cortex that might underlie the monitoring of information in working memory, the work with patients indicated that some part of the dorsolateral prefrontal cortex might be critical, because this region was consistently involved in the patients who were impaired on the self-ordered tasks (Petrides and Milner 1982). The work with the patients, however, could not specify the critical region because the lesions involved multiple areas. Studies with monkeys in which lesions could be restricted with precision within a given region led to the identification of the mid-dorsolateral prefrontal cortex as the critical region for the monitoring of information within working memory (Petrides 1991, 1995).

In the human brain, the dorsolateral prefrontal cortex occupies the gross morphological features of the superior and middle frontal gyri. In the monkey, the dorsolateral prefrontal cortex occupies the cortex extending from the sulcus principalis to the midline. In both the human and the monkey brain, the dorsolateral prefrontal cortex comprises several architectonic areas. The most anterior part of the dorsolateral prefrontal cortex is part of the frontopolar area 10 (Figs. 2 and 3A). Located between this anterior part (i.e. area 10) and the posterior dorsolateral prefrontal cortex (which comprises area 8 and the rostral part of area 6) is the mid-sector of the dorsolateral prefrontal cortex, which is occupied by areas 9 and 46 (Figs. 2 and 3A). We refer to this mid-sector as the mid-dorsolateral prefrontal region to distinguish it from its anterior (area 10) and its posterior part (area 8 and rostral area 6). This mid-dorsolateral prefrontal region can be divided into a superior part, which consists of cortex in which the granular layer IV is not well developed (Walker's area 9) (Fig. 2) and a lower part in which the granular layer IV is well developed. This lower granular half of the mid-dorsolateral prefrontal cortex starts just below area 9, approximately half way in the cortical expanse between the mid-line and the sulcus principalis, and continues within both banks of the sulcus principalis (Figs. 2 and 3). Walker referred to this large granular region as area 46, although both he and subsequent investigators acknowledged that this region is not homogeneous and can be further subdivided (e.g., Barbas and Pandya 1989; Preuss and Goldman-Rakic 1991; Petrides and Pandya 1994, 1999). In a recent comparative architectonic study of the human and the monkey lateral prefrontal cortex, Petrides and Pandya subdivided the granular region extending from the upper bank of the sulcus principalis towards the midline as area 46d and 9/46d (i.e., dorsal area 46 and 9/46) because they are architectonically comparable to certain similarly named areas of the middle frontal gyrus of the human brain (see Petrides and Pandya 1994, 1999 for a discussion). The cortex lining the depths of the sulcus principalis is occupied by sulcal area 46 and, in its caudal portion, by area 8A.

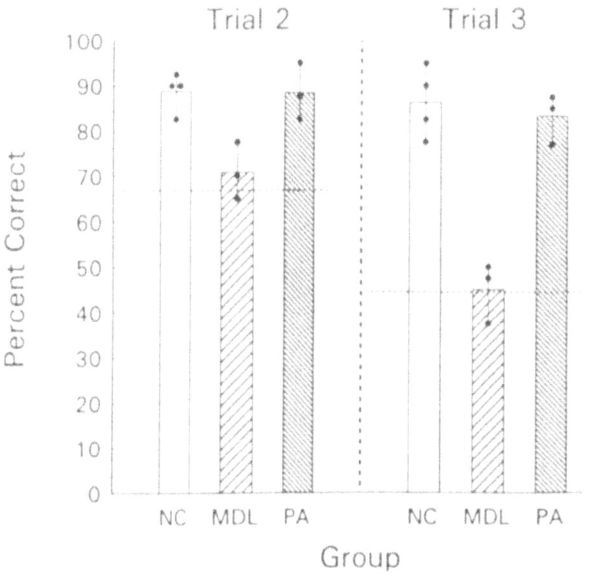

Fig. 4 Mean percentage of correct responses made by normal monkeys (*NC*), monkeys with lesions of the mid-dorsolateral part of the prefrontal cortex (*MDL*), and monkeys with lesions of the periarcuate cortex (*PA*), i.e., the posterior dorsolateral frontal cortex, on trials 2 and 3 of the nonspatial self-ordered task (experiment 1, Petrides 1995). In this experiment, the animals were tested for one set of trials per day for 40 days. Since responses on trial 1 will always be correct, performance measures are only based on trials 2 and 3. The level of chance performance (trial 2=66.6%; trial 3=44.4%) is indicated by the horizontal *dotted line*. *Solid circles* indicate the scores of individual animals in each group

It has been known for a long time that lesions limited to the cortex *within* the sulcus principalis, especially its middle (i.e., sulcal area 46) and caudal (i.e., area 8) portions, which are the focus of major inputs from the parietal cortex (Petrides and Pandya 1984; Schwartz and Goldman-Rakic 1984), produce a rather selective spatial mnemonic impairment that manifests itself on the spatial delayed-response and alternation tasks (Mishkin 1957; Gross and Weiskrantz 1962; Butters and Pandya 1969; Stamm 1969; Goldman and Rosvold 1970; Butters et al. 1971) (Fig. 3C). By contrast, dorsolateral prefrontal lesions that spare the sulcus principalis do not cause an impairment in the classic versions of the spatial delayed-response (Goldman et al. 1971) and delayed-alternation tasks (Mishkin 1957; Goldman and Rosvold 1970). In planning the investigation of the possible role of the dorsolateral prefrontal cortex in the monitoring of information in working memory, the following issues appeared to be critical. Given that the cortex lining the sulcus principalis was known to give rise to a severe spatial delayed-response impairment, it was decided to avoid the cortex within the sulcus principalis in the planned mid-dorsolateral lesion and to extend the lesion from the lip of the sulcus principalis to the midline. Thus, the mid-dorsolateral lesion was to include the granular area (i.e., dorsal area 46 and 9/46), extending from the lip of the dorsal bank of the sulcus principalis to about half of the mid-dorsolateral surface and the dysgranular area 9, which occupies the remaining superior half of this surface (Fig. 3A) (Petrides 1991, 1995). The advantage of such a lesion was that, if any impairments were to be obtained after mid-dorsolateral prefrontal lesions, these could easily be dissociated from the spatial impairment known to follow lesions of the cortex lining the sulcus principalis. Furthermore, since the key question was whether a general problem in monitoring of mnemonic information could be demonstrated after damage to some part of the dorsolateral prefrontal region, the monkeys were to be tested on self-ordered and externally ordered working-memory tasks requiring monitoring of *nonspatial* visual information. Clearly, a demonstration of such an impairment in the nonspatial mode would be particularly indicative of a general problem in the monitoring of mnemonic information rather than a similar deficit on a spatial version of the self-ordered and externally ordered tasks, which might be confused with problems due to a spatial mnemonic impairment.

The mid-dorsolateral prefrontal lesions (i.e., dorsal area 46 and 9/46 and area 9; Fig. 3A) gave rise to severe impairments on the self-ordered and externally ordered working-memory tasks (Petrides 1991, 1995) (Figs. 4 and 5). By contrast, lesions of the posterior dorsolateral region (i.e., the periarcuate region), which result in severe impairments on conditional associative-learning tasks (see Petrides 1987 for a review), did not affect performance on the self-ordered tasks. The deficits on the nonspatial self-ordered tasks after mid-dorsolateral lesions were severe and long-lasting (see experiments 1 and 8, Petrides 1995). Even more important, however, is

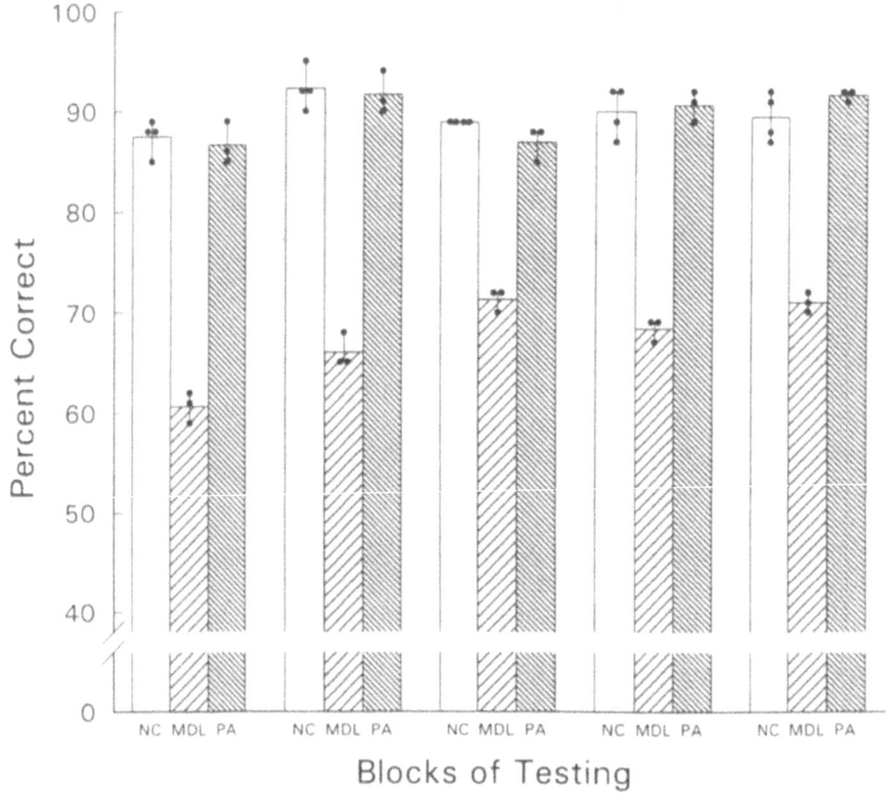

Fig. 5 Mean percentage of correct responses made by normal monkeys (*NC*), monkeys with lesions of the mid-dorsolateral part of the prefrontal cortex (*MDL*), and monkeys with lesions of the periarcuate cortex (*PA*), i.e., the posterior dorsolateral frontal cortex, on a retest on the self-ordered task (experiment 8, Petrides 1995). In this experiment, the animals were tested for five sets of trials per day for 50 days (i.e., a total of 250 sets of trials). The data is presented in blocks of 10 days (i.e., 50 sets of trials). As can be seen, the animals with the mid-dorsolateral prefrontal lesions continue to be severely impaired even on the last block of 10 days of testing. Since responses on trial 1 will always be correct, performance measures are only based on trials 2 and 3. *Solid circles* indicate the scores of individual animals in each group

the fact that it has been possible to analyze the nature of the impairment after lesions of this specific cortical region in isolation from the potentially additive/interactive effects of damage to other prefrontal areas. It is now clear that the impairment on these monitoring working-memory tasks after mid-dorsolateral prefrontal lesions occurs against a background of normal basic mnemonic processing. For instance, monkeys with such lesions (Petrides 1991, 1995), or even larger dorsolateral frontal lesions (Bachevalier and Mishkin 1986), are able to perform normally on basic recognition-memory tasks in which they have to identify novel from familiar stimuli. In addition, monkeys with dorsolateral prefrontal lesions perform well on delayed matching-to-sample tasks in which they have to recognize which one of two constantly recurring stimuli was most recently presented (Passingham 1975) as well as on the delayed object-alternation task in which they have to alternate their response from one stimulus to the other after each delay period (Mishkin et al. 1969; Petrides 1995). In other words, mnemonic judgements based on the relative recency of stimuli and the simple maintenance of information during the delay need not be affected by mid-dorsolateral prefrontal damage. This basic mnemonic processing, however, is inadequate to sustain normal performance on the self-ordered and externally ordered working-memory tasks that are designed to tax monitoring of the information within working memory (Petrides 1991, 1994, 1995).

In summary, the monkeys with mid-dorsolateral prefrontal lesions can perform normally when required to make a choice on the basis of memory of which stimuli were previously seen and which were not (i.e., recognition memory) or on the basis of the relative recency of frequently recurring stimuli. By contrast, these animals are severely impaired when performance cannot be based on these basic memory processes alone (e.g., familiarity, primacy, or recency judgements), but requires that the status of multiple events in working memory be monitored, as in the self-ordered and externally ordered tasks described above.

Manipulation of information in working memory requires precise coding of the current status of an event in memory vis-a-vis the other events so that a transformation in that relative status (i.e., a manipulation) can be effected. I have argued that the capacity to manipulate information in working memory and, therefore, to carry out certain complex plans of action that is so characteristic of primate behavior emerged largely because of the specialized computational capacity of the mid-dorsolateral prefrontal region, which permits marking and monitoring within memory of the relative status of multiple intended acts or expected occurrences (Petrides 1991, 1994). A striking demonstration of the fact that the number of stimuli that must be monitored, and not the maintenance of information per se, is the critical variable affecting the performance of monkeys with mid-dorsolateral prefrontal lesions came from a study that compared the effect of such lesions on visual working memory with the effect of lesions of the rostral part of the inferotemporal cortex (Petrides 1998). The anterior part of the inferotemporal cortex is one of the last stages in the

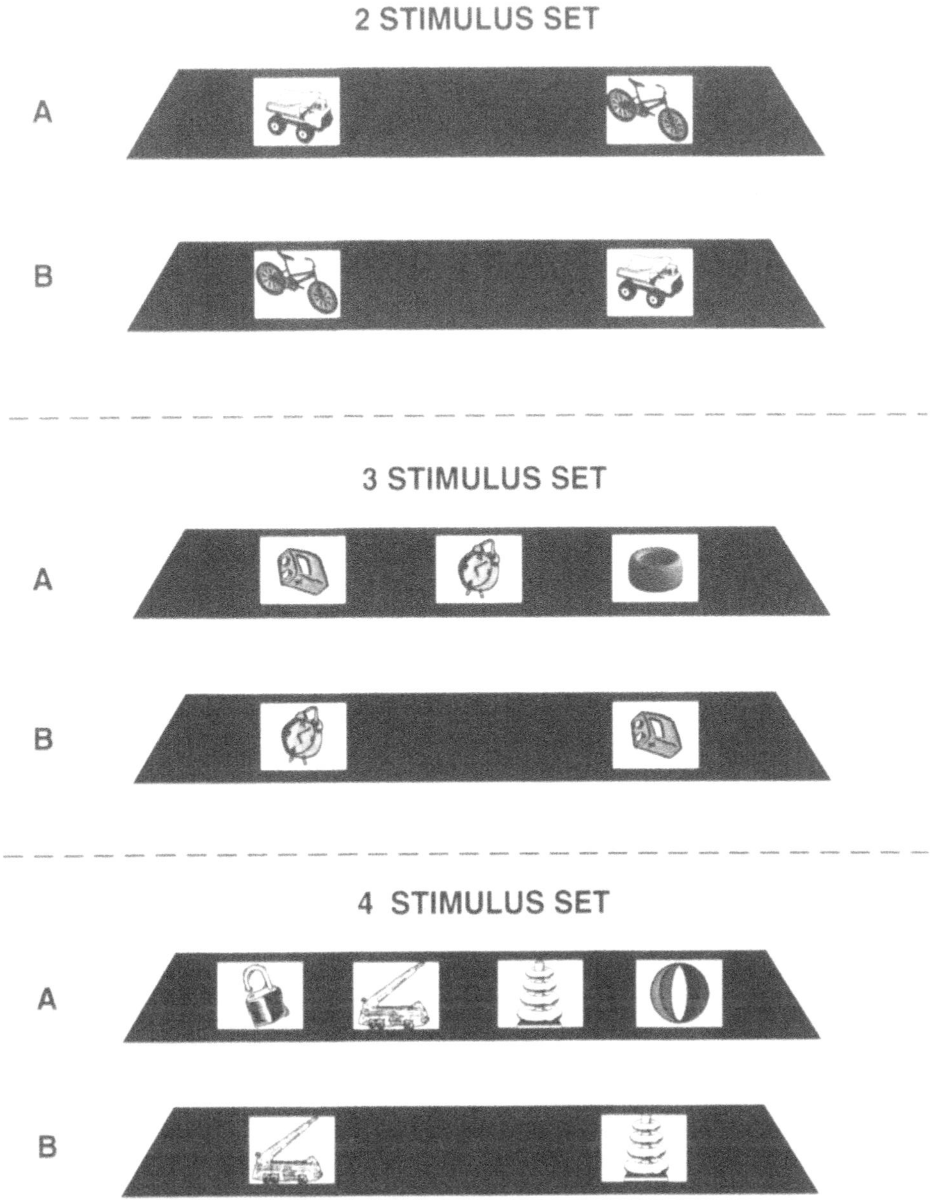

Fig. 6 Schematic diagram of the experimental arrangement in the condition in which the difficulty of monitoring was manipulated. Sets of two, three, four, or five stimuli are presented on the presentation trial (*A*). Once the animal has selected one of the objects, a test trial (*B*) is administered 10 s later, during which the object selected is paired with one of the objects not selected

specialized occipito-temporal system for the processing of visual pattern (object) information (Ungerleider and Mishkin 1982) and has been shown to underlie visual memory operations (Mishkin 1982). We manipulated the load of information within visual working memory in two independent ways: (1) by increasing the length of the delay during which the information had to be maintained (maintenance manipulation), or (2) by increasing the number of stimuli that had to be monitored (monitoring manipulation) (Petrides 1998). This study, in addition to the animals with the complete mid-dorsolateral lesions (Fig. 3A), included a group that had lesions limited to the superior part of the mid-dorsolateral prefrontal cortex, that is area 9 (Fig. 3B) (Petrides 1998). All animals had been highly trained on visual nonspatial self-ordered working-memory tasks. As pointed out above, training on these self-ordered tasks instills the following important principle in the animals: since the same stimuli re-appear on each trial and all the stimuli must be selected only once over the successive trials, successful performance depends on attending to all the stimuli in the set and carefully monitoring successive choices (i.e., noting which stimuli from the set have been selected and which have not yet been selected). This principle was essential for the present experiment, in which monitoring and delay were independently manipulated. As was the case in the self-ordered tasks on which the animals had been trained, the first trial in this experiment was the presentation of an array of objects. This array could consist of a set of 2, 3, 4, or 5 objects (Fig. 6). Once the animal had chosen one of the objects from the array, in the test trial that followed, the animal was faced with a choice between the stimulus it had chosen and one of the stimuli in the previous display that it had not chosen. Given the animal's prior training, the correct (i.e., rewarded) response on this test trial was to select the stim-

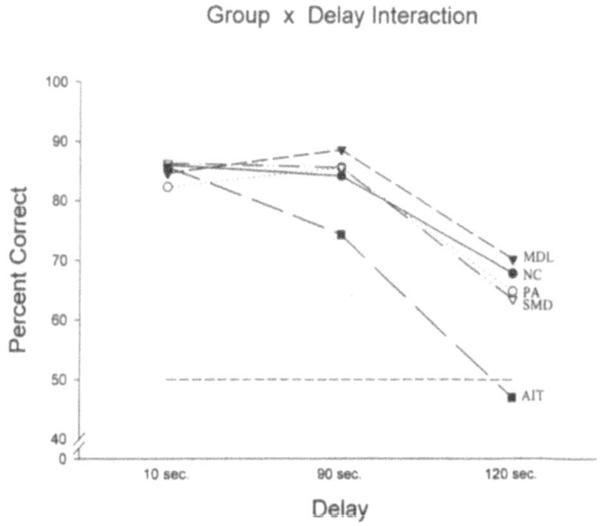

Fig. 7 Graph showing mean performance of the various groups tested across the three delays. The level of chance performance (50%) is indicated by the *horizontal dotted line*. *AIT* group with lesions to the anteroventral inferotemporal region, *MDL* group with damage to both the lower and superior parts of the mid-dorsolateral prefrontal cortex, *NC* normal control group, *PA* group with periarcuate lesions, *SMD* group with damage confined to the superior part of the mid-dorsolateral prefrontal cortex (area 9). In comparison to the control group, the group with anterior inferotemporal lesions (AIT) was significantly impaired at the 90 s and 120 s delays (Petrides 1998)

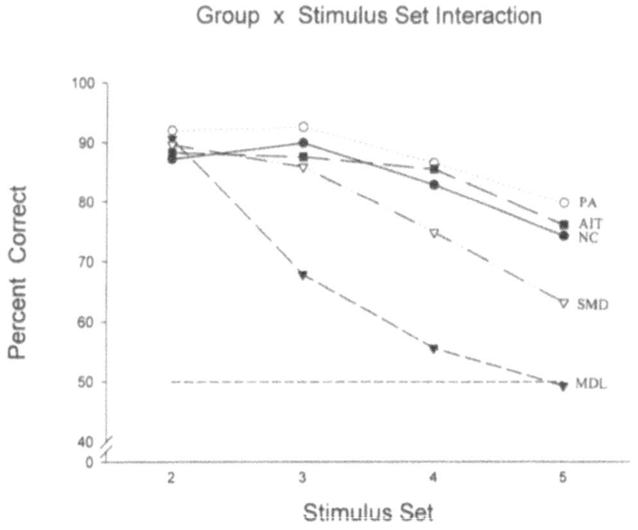

Fig. 8 Graph showing mean performance of each group on the 2, 3, 4, and 5 stimulus sets. The level of chance performance (50%) is indicated by the *horizontal dotted line*. *AIT* group with lesions to the anteroventral inferotemporal region, *MDL* group with damage to both the lower and superior parts of the mid-dorsolateral prefrontal cortex, *NC* normal control group, *PA* group with periarcuate lesions, *SMD* group with damage confined to the superior part of the mid-dorsolateral prefrontal cortex (area 9). As the size of the stimulus set from which the two test stimuli were selected increased, the performance of the two groups with mid-dorsolateral prefrontal lesions deteriorated, whereas that of the animals with anterior inferotemporal lesions and those with posterior dorsolateral prefrontal lesions (i.e., the periarcuate region) was not significantly different from the normal control performance. The animals with the lesions of the complete mid-dorsolateral prefrontal region (MDL group) were more impaired than the animals with the lesions restricted to its upper part (SMD group). The MDL group was impaired at the three-stimulus, the four-stimulus, and the five-stimulus set. The SMD group, on the other hand, was only impaired on the five-stimulus condition

ulus not previously chosen. In one condition, the *size of the stimulus set* was varied during the presentation trials (i.e., 2, 3, 4, or 5 objects), but the delay between the presentation trials and the test trials was held constant at 10 s. The critical manipulation in the present experiment can be summarized as follows. Although the animals would only choose one stimulus (e.g., A) from the display and would have to remember only that stimulus during the 10 s delay, their extensive training on the self-ordered tasks (see above) trained them to attend to the fact that stimulus A, but not B, was selected in the two-object display; stimulus A, but not stimuli B or C, was selected in the three-object display; stimulus A, but not stimuli B, C, or D, was selected in the four-object display; stimulus A, but not B, C, D, or E, was selected in the five-object display. In other words, because of their prior extensive training on the self-ordered task, the animals would be attending not only to the stimulus selected, but also to the other stimuli not selected and which the animals would expect to encounter on the subsequent trials. In the other condition of the experiment, the *length of the delay* between the presentation trials and the test trials was varied (i.e. 10, 90, and 120 s), but the stimulus set during the presentation trials was always two-objects. The order of administration of the two conditions of the experiment (set stimulus-size manipulation versus delay manipulation) was counterbalanced within each group.

The effect of increasing the delay (from 10 to 90 and then to 120 s) whilst keeping the number of stimuli to be monitored low (i.e., two stimuli) can be seen in Fig. 7. The animals with anterior inferotemporal lesions were significantly impaired at the 90 s and 120 s delays; none of the other groups differed from the control group. Thus, both the animals with the complete mid-dorsolateral prefrontal lesions (MDL group) and those with lesions limited to area 9 in the superior part of the mid-dorsolateral region (SMD group) performed as well as the normal control animals and those with the periarcuate lesions. Delay affected differentially only the performance of the animals with lesions to the anterior inferotemporal cortex, these animals performing at chance on the 120 s delay condition.

The effect of increasing the number of stimuli that the animals had to monitor whilst keeping the delay short (i.e., 10 s) is shown in Fig. 8. The animals with the lesions of the complete mid-dorsolateral prefrontal region (MDL group) were more impaired than the animals with the lesions restricted to area 9 in the superior part of this region (SMD group). The MDL group was impaired at the three-stimulus, the four-stimulus, and five-stimulus sets. The SMD group, on the other hand, was only impaired on the five-stimulus condition. Thus, as the size of the stimulus set from which the two test stimuli were drawn increased, the performance of the two groups with mid-dorsolateral prefrontal lesions deteriorated, whereas that of the animals with anterior inferotemporal lesions and of those with posterior dorsolateral prefrontal lesions (i.e,. the periarcuate region) was not significantly different from the normal control performance.

The above results showed that, as the delay during which the information had to be maintained increased, the performance of the animals with the anterior inferotemporal lesions was severely impaired, whereas that of the animals with mid-dorsolateral prefrontal lesions was not different from that of the normal controls. On the other hand, the animals with mid-dorsolateral prefrontal lesions were impaired as the number of the alternative stimuli that they had to monitor increased, a manipulation that did not affect the performance of the animals with inferotemporal lesions. Thus, the number of possible alternative choices that must be considered (i.e., monitored) within working memory, and not the passage of time per se, is the critical factor determining whether or not an impairment will follow mid-dorsolateral prefrontal lesions (Petrides 1995, 1998).

Levy and Goldman-Rakic (1999) have recently examined the effect of lesions limited to the cortex within the sulcus principalis (i.e., sulcal area 46 and area 8) or the superior part of the dorsolateral prefrontal cortex (i.e., area 9 and area 8B) on various delay tasks, including the nonspatial self-ordered task with three stimuli. The results replicated the well-known deficit on spatial delayed-response tasks after lesions limited to the sulcus principalis, which in this study was referred to as the "dorsolateral" lesion. The monkeys with lesions of the sulcus principalis, which spared the mid-dorsolateral region studied by Petrides (1991, 1995), were only transiently impaired on the nonspatial self-ordered task with three stimuli. These results are, therefore, consistent with the widely accepted notion that the deficit after sulcus principalis lesions may be limited to the spatial modality (see Petrides 1994, p. 73). The sulcus principalis lesion, which includes only sulcal area 46 and area 8 in its caudal part (Fig. 3C), differs from the mid-dorsolateral prefrontal lesion studied by Petrides (1991, 1995), which, by contrast, includes dorsal area 46 and 9/46 extending above the sulcus principalis and area 9 (Fig. 3A).

In the Levy and Goldman-Rakic (1999) study, the monkeys with lesions restricted to the superior part of the mid-dorsolateral prefrontal region involving areas 9 and 8B were also transiently impaired on the nonspatial self-ordered task with three stimuli. This lesion, which was referred to as the "dorsomedial" lesion by these authors, was focused on areas 9 and 8B and spared the dorsal area 46 and 9/46, which extends from the lip of the sulcus principalis to the border with areas 9 and 8B. Levy and Goldman-Rakic (1999) discussed this lesion as if it were comparable to the complete mid-dorsolateral lesion of Petrides (1995). This "dorsomedial" lesion, however, differs from the complete mid-dorsolateral lesion studied by Petrides (1991, 1995), which included both area 9 *and dorsal area 46 and 9/46*. The "dorsomedial" lesion in the Levy and Goldman-Rakic (1999) study is comparable to the superior mid-dorsolateral prefrontal lesion studied by Petrides (1998) (Fig. 3B), which spared the lower granular part of the mid-dorsolateral region (dorsal area 46 and 9/46) (see Figs. 2 and 3A). As can be seen in Fig. 8, monkeys with such lesions (SMD group) can perform well on self-ordered trials with a three-stimulus set, although they are impaired with a larger stimulus set (e.g., five stimuli). Thus, both the Petrides (1998) and the Levy and Goldman-Rakic (1999) studies found only a mild impairment after lesions limited to area 9.

The mild impairment after lesions limited to the superior part of the mid-dorsolateral prefrontal cortex (i.e., area 9) contrasts sharply with the severe and long-lasting impairment after complete lesions of the mid-dorsolateral prefrontal region (dorsal area 46 and 9/46 and area 9). Monkeys with complete mid-dorsolateral prefrontal lesions were severely impaired when first tested on the self-ordered task over a 40-day period (Petrides 1995, experiment 1). During this period, they were given only one set of trials per day (Fig. 4). These same animals were then tested for 400 trials on another self-ordered task and continued to perform at chance. This experiment has been published separately (Petrides 1991). The animals then received several hundred trials on various externally ordered tasks that had the same monitoring requirements as the self-ordered tasks, and the animals with mid-dorsolateral prefrontal lesions continued to be severely and consistently impaired (Petrides 1995, experiments 2, 3, 5, and 6). These animals were then re-tested on the self-ordered task for another 250 sets of trials administered over a 50-day period (Petrides 1995, experiment 8), still demonstrating a severe impairment (Fig. 5).

It should be noted here that Levy and Goldman-Rakic (1999) suggested that the deficit after mid-dorsolateral prefrontal lesions in the Petrides (1995) study may have been transient because the monkeys were tested for only 40 sets of trials. These authors were referring to experiment 1 (see Fig. 4) in the Petrides (1995) report and apparently failed to notice the additional 400 trials on which these same animals were tested (reported in Petrides 1991) and the 250 sets of trials administered on the self-ordered task in experiment 8 (see Fig. 5) in Petrides (1995), as well as the hundreds of trials on the externally ordered working-memory tasks (experiments 2, 3, 5, and 6 in Petrides 1995), on all of which the animals with mid-dorsolateral prefrontal lesions exhibited a severe impairment. In summary, complete lesions of the mid-dorsolateral prefrontal cortex (dorsal area 46 and 9/46 as well as area 9) give rise to a severe and long-lasting impairment on the self-ordered and externally ordered tasks requiring monitoring of selections within working memory. By contrast, lesions limited to area 9 (Petrides 1998) give rise to a mild impairment that is evident on longer lists (e.g., set of five stimuli; Fig. 8). This finding is consistent with the report by Levy and Goldman-Rakic (1999) that lesions limited to areas 9 and 8B give rise to only a mild impairment on the self-ordered task with three stimuli.

The findings reported above that the most severe impairment on the self-ordered and externally ordered tasks occur with lesions that involve both the granular (dorsal area 46 and 9/46) and the dysgranular (area 9) parts of the mid-dorsolateral region are particularly interesting because, when comparable self-ordered and externally ordered tasks were used with normal human subjects in functional neuroimaging studies, the observed increases in activity were focused within the mid-dorsolateral prefrontal region on the middle frontal gyrus, where the granular part of the human mid-dorsolateral prefrontal cortex is, and only to a lesser extent on the superior frontal gyrus where the dysgranular area 9 lies (e.g., Petrides et al. 1993).

Inputs of modality-specific information within the mid-dorsolateral monitoring and manipulation system

The data presented above from lesion studies in monkeys provide strong support for the theoretical proposal first made by Petrides in 1991 that the mid-dorsolateral prefrontal cortex (dorsal areas 46 and 9/46 and area 9) constitutes a specialized region for the on-line monitoring and manipulation of multiple cognitive representations within working memory. According to this view, it is a specialized region where stimuli or events that are first interpreted and maintained in posterior association cortical areas can be re-coded so that the on-going relative status of the representations of events that have been planned to occur or are expected to occur can be monitored and manipulated (Petrides 1991, 1994, 1995). Functional neuroimaging data with normal human subjects have provided further strong support to the above theoretical notion in that increases in activity within the human mid-dorsolateral prefrontal region have been consistently demonstrated whenever subjects had to monitor information within working memory regardless of the nature of the stimulus information (visual nonspatial, visual spatial, auditory, etc). These data will not be reviewed here, as they have recently been reviewed by Owen (1997), D'Esposito et al. (1998), and Petrides (2000).

The following question now arises. If the mid-dorsolateral prefrontal region is involved in the monitoring and manipulation of information that is both spatial and nonspatial in nature, how do these inputs reach this region? First, how does visuospatial input reach the mid-dorsolateral region? The middle and caudal parts of the cortex lining the sulcus principalis, which appear to be the critical area for the spatial delayed-response impairment (see Petrides 1994), receive input from visuospatial peristriate and intraparietal regions (Barbas and Mesulam 1985; Petrides and Pandya 1984, 1999; Cavada and Goldman-Rakic 1989; Andersen et al. 1990). Furthermore, the mid-dorsolateral prefrontal region receives input from the posterior dorsolateral prefrontal areas 8A, 8B, and rostral area 6, which have powerful bi-directional connections with the posterior parietal areas, the dorsal prestriate areas, and the medial parieto-occipital regions that are involved in visuospatial processing (e.g., Barbas and Mesulam 1981; Petrides and Pandya 1984, 1999; Huerta et al. 1987; Andersen et al. 1990; Schall et al. 1995) (Fig. 9). The ventral bank of the middle to posterior part of the sulcus principalis also has inputs from somatosensory-related regions of the inferior parietal lobule and insula (Barbas and Mesulam 1985; Petrides and Pandya 1984; Preuss and Goldman-Rakic 1989) that are relevant to the performance of spatial delayed-response tasks. Thus, frontal influences modulating specifically spatial mnemonic information would be expected to occur in these posterior dorsolateral prefrontal areas and in the middle to caudal part of the sulcus principalis. It is interesting to note that the caudal part of the principalis cortex is architectonically part of area 8A (e.g., Brodmann 1905; Walker 1940; Barbas and Pandya 1989; Petrides and Pandya 1994). In contrast to the above mentioned spatial inputs, nonspatial visual input reaches the mid-dorsolateral prefrontal region via connections with the ventrolateral prefrontal region (Petrides and Pandya 1999), the ventrolateral prefrontal region being strongly linked with the inferotemporal region (e.g., Ungerleider et al. 1989), which is primarily involved in the processing on nonspatial visual object information (Ungerleider and Mishkin 1982).

In summary, visuospatial input reaches the mid-dorsolateral prefrontal region involved in the monitoring and manipulation of information via the posterior dorsolateral cortex (areas 8, 6, and middle and caudal principalis), whereas nonspatial visual object input reaches this region via the ventrolateral prefrontal cortex (Fig. 9). The available evidence is consistent with the above view. Lesions focused on the middle to caudal part of the sulcus principalis would affect visuospatial input and, thus, would give rise to a spatially selective impairment since such lesions would not disconnect visual object information that would reach the mid-dorsolateral prefrontal region from the ventrolateral prefrontal areas. The mid-dorsolateral prefrontal region, on the other hand, would be involved whenever monitoring and manipulation is taxed, regardless of whether the information that is being monitored is spatial or nonspatial. The available functional neuroimaging data is also consistent with the above view. Whenever monitoring and manipulation of information were required, increases in activity within the human mid-dorsolateral prefrontal region were observed (for reviews, see Owen 1997; D'Esposito et al. 1998; Petrides 2000). Furthermore, in a recent study by Courtney et al. (1998), in which monitoring and manipulation were minimized, a signal related specifically to the maintenance of an active mnemonic representation of spatial information was observed in a region that was posterior and caudal to the mid-dorsolateral prefrontal region just rostral to an area related to eye movements. Given its location, this signal would be occurring either

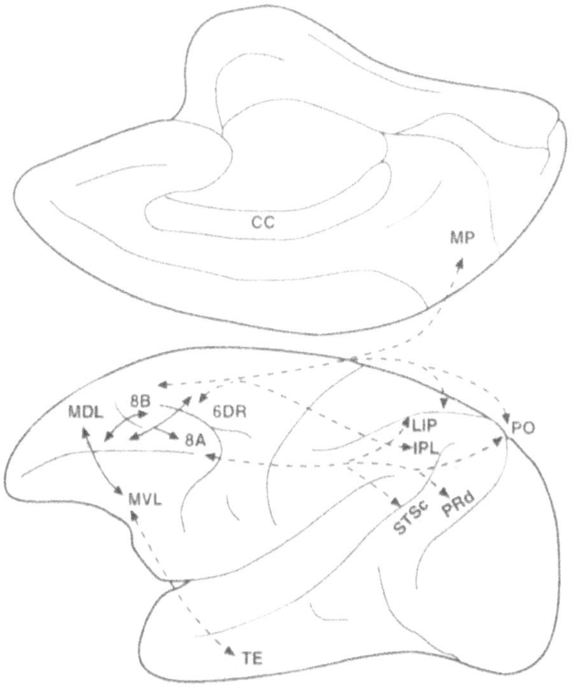

Fig. 9 Schematic diagram of the brain of the macaque monkey to illustrate how two distinct types of visual input enter the mid-dorsolateral prefrontal region (*MDL*), which exercises a higher-order control of mnemonic processing such as monitoring and manipulation of information in working memory. Information from the posterior parietal and adjacent dorsal prestriate region, which is closely involved in the processing of visuospatial information, is strongly linked with the posterior dorsolateral prefrontal cortical region, which includes areas *8A*, *8B*, and the rostral part of dorsal area 6 (*6DR*). Input into this region comes from the lateral bank of the intraparietal sulcus (*LIP*), the caudal part of the inferior parietal lobule (*IPL*), the adjacent area *PO* on the anterior bank of the parieto-occipital sulcus, the medial part of the parieto-occipital region (*MP*), and the motion-related areas in the caudal part of the superior temporal sulcus (*STSc*). Information related to the object features of visual stimuli comes from the anterior part of area *TE* on the inferotemporal surface and interacts, first, with the ventrolateral (*VL*) prefrontal cortex. The *solid arrows* within the frontal lobe show how these posterior dorsolateral and ventrolateral areas interact with the mid-dorsolateral prefrontal region. *CC* Corpus callosum

in rostral area 6, in area 8, or in both. In this respect, it is interesting to note that the posterior part of the sulcus principalis in the monkey is occupied by the rostral extension of area 8A.

Two levels of executive control within the mid-lateral prefrontal cortex

The theoretical position first proposed by Petrides (1991, 1994) argued that, within the lateral prefrontal cortex, a fundamental distinction can be made between the mid-dorsolateral prefrontal region (dorsal areas 46 and 9/46 and area 9), which is primarily involved in the on-line monitoring and manipulation of cognitive representations within working memory, and the mid-ventrolateral prefrontal cortex, which subserves more basic executive processes, such as active selection, comparison, and judgement of stimuli held in short-term and long-term memory (see Petrides 1994 for details). The ventrolateral prefrontal cortex was held to be necessary for active (explicit) encoding and retrieval of information, i.e., processes initiated under conscious effort by the subject and guided by the subject's plans and intentions, but not for automatic stimulus- and context-driven encoding and retrieval of information (Petrides 1996). This theoretical position has sometimes been misinterpreted as denying the existence of modality-specific processing within the prefrontal cortex. However, what has been argued is that the mid-dorsolateral and mid-ventrolateral prefrontal regions subserve different executive processes. As was pointed out above and in the first papers proposing this theoretical model (Petrides, 1991, 1994, p. 73), modality-specific inputs enter particular points of the prefrontal cortex, and lesions there can yield modality-specific impairments. Indeed, it is possible that, within the mid-dorsolateral and mid-ventrolateral prefrontal regions, the application of the particular executive processes subserved by these regions may be partially separable, depending on the way in which inputs from posterior cortical regions enter these regions.

References

Andersen RA, Asanuma C, Essick G, Siegel RM (1990) Corticocortical connections of anatomically and physiologically defined subdivisions within the inferior parietal lobule. J Comp Neurol 296:65–113

Bachevalier J, Mishkin M (1986) Visual recognition impairment follows ventromedial but not dorsolateral prefrontal lesions in monkeys. Behav Brain Res 20:249–261

Barbas H, Mesulam M-M (1981) Organization afferent input to subdivisions of area 8 in the rhesus monkey. J Comp Neurol 200:407–431

Barbas H, Mesulam M-M (1985) Cortical afferent input to the principalis region of the rhesus monkey. Neuroscience 15:619–637

Barbas H, Pandya DN (1989) Architecture and intrinsic connections of the prefrontal cortex in the rhesus monkey. J Comp Neurol 286:353–375

Brodmann K (1905) Beitraege zur histologischen Lokalisation der Grosshirnrinde. III. Mitteilung: Die Rindenfelder der niederen Affen. J Psychol Neurol (Leipzig) 4:177–226

Brodmann K (1908) Beitraege zur histologischen Lokalisation der Grosshirnrinde. VI. Mitteilung: Die Cortexgliederung des Menschen. J Psychol Neurol (Leipzig) 10:231–246

Brodmann K (1909) Vergleichende Localisationslehre der Grosshirnrinde in ihren Prinzipien dargestellt auf Grund des Zellenbaues. Barth, Leipzig

Butters N, Pandya D (1969) Retention of delayed-alternation: effect of selective lesions of sulcus principalis. Science 165: 1271–1273

Butters N, Pandya D, Sanders K, Dye P (1971) Behavioral deficits in monkeys after selective lesions within the middle third of sulcus principalis. J Comp Physiol Psychol 76:8–14

Cavada C, Goldman-Rakic PS (1989) Posterior parietal cortex in rhesus monkey. II. Evidence for segregated corticocortical networks linking sensory and limbic areas with the frontal lobe. J Comp Neurol 287:422–445

Courtney SM, Petit L, Maisog J Ma, Ungerleider LG, Haxby JV (1998) An area specialized for spatial working memory in human frontal cortex. Science 279:1347–1351

D'Esposito M, Aguirre GK, Zarahn E, Ballard D, Shin RK, Lease J (1998) Functional MRI studies of spatial and nonspatial working memory. Cogn Brain Res 7:1–13

Economo C, Koskinas GN (1925) Die Cytoarchitektonik der Hirnrinde des erwachsenen Menschen. Springer, Wien

Funahashi S, Bruce CJ, Goldman-Rakic PS (1993) Dorsolateral prefrontal lesions and oculomotor delayed-response performance: evidence for mnemonic "scotomas". J Neurosci 13: 1479–1497

Fuster JM (1973) Unit activity in prefrontal cortex during delayed-response performance: neuronal correlates of transient memory. J Neurophysiol 36:61–76

Fuster JM, Alexander GE (1971) Neuron activity related to short-term memory. Science 173:652–654

Goldman PS, Rosvold HE (1970) Localization of function within the dorsolateral prefrontal cortex of the rhesus monkey. Exp Neurol 27:291–304

Goldman PS, Rosvold HE, Vest B, Galkin TW (1971) Analysis of the delayed-alternation deficit produced by dorsolateral prefrontal lesions in the rhesus monkey. J Comp Physiol Psychol 77:212–220

Gross CG, Weiskrantz L (1962) Evidence for dissociation of impairment on auditory discrimination and delayed response following lateral frontal lesions in monkeys. Exp Neurol 5:453–476

Huerta MF, Krubitzer LA, Kaas JH (1987) Frontal eye fields as defined by intracortical microstimulation in squirrel monkeys, owl monkeys, and macaque monkeys. II. Cortical connections. J Comp Neurol 271:473–492

Jacobsen CF (1936) Studies of cerebral function in primates. I. The functions of the frontal association areas in monkeys. Comp Psychol Monogr 13:1–60

Kojima S, Goldman-Rakic PS (1982) Delay-related activity of prefrontal neurons in rhesus monkeys performing delayed response. Brain Res 248:43–49

Kubota K, Niki H (1971) Prefrontal cortical unit activity and delayed alternation performance in monkeys. J Neurophysiol 34:337–347

Levy R, Goldman-Rakic PS (1999) Association of storage and processing functions in the dorsolateral prefrontal cortex of the nonhuman primate. J Neurosci 19:5149–5158

Miller EK, Erickson CA, Desimone R (1996) Neural mechanisms of visual working memory in prefrontal cortex of the macaque. J Neurosci 16:5154–5167

Mishkin M (1957) Effects of small frontal lesions on delayed alternation in monkeys. J Neurophysiol 20:615–622

Mishkin M (1982) A memory system in the monkey. Philos Tran R Soc Lond B 298:85–95

Mishkin M, Manning FJ (1978) Non-spatial memory after selective prefrontal lesions in monkeys. Brain Res 143:313–323

Mishkin M, Vest B, Waxler M, Rosvold HE (1969) A re-examination of the effects of frontal lesions on object alternation. Neuropsychologia 7:357–363

Niki H (1974a) Prefrontal unit activity during delayed alternation in the monkey. I. Relation to direction of response. Brain Res 68:185–196

Niki H (1974b) Prefrontal unit activity during delayed alternation in the monkey. II. Relation to absolute versus relative direction of response. Brain Res 68:197–204

Owen AM (1997) The functional organization of working memory processes within the human lateral frontal cortex: the contribution of functional neuroimaging. Eur J Neurosci 9:1329–1339

Pandya DN, Yeterian EH (1985) Architecture and connections of cortical association areas. In: Peters A, Jones EG (eds) Cerebral cortex. Plenum Press, New York, pp 3–61

Passingham RE (1975) Delayed matching after selective prefrontal lesions in monkeys (*Macaca mulatta*). Brain Res 92:89–102

Petrides M (1987) Conditional learning and the primate frontal cortex. In: Perecman E (ed) The frontal lobes revisited. IRBN Press, New York, pp 91–108

Petrides M (1989) Frontal lobes and memory. In: Boller F, Grafman J (eds) Handbook of neuropsychology, Vol 3. Elsevier, Amsterdam, pp 75–90

Petrides M (1991) Monitoring of selections of visual stimuli and the primate frontal cortex. Proc R Soc Lond B Biol Sci 246:293–298

Petrides M (1994) Frontal lobes and working memory: evidence from investigations of the effects of cortical excisions in non-human primates. In: Boller F, Grafman J (eds) Handbook of neuropsychology, Vol 9. Elsevier, Amsterdam, pp 59–82

Petrides M (1995) Impairments on nonspatial self-ordered and externally ordered working memory tasks after lesions of the mid-dorsal part of the lateral frontal cortex in the monkey. J Neurosci 15:359–375

Petrides M (1996) Specialized systems for the processing of mnemonic information within the primate frontal cortex. Philos Trans R Soc Lond B 351:1455–1462

Petrides M (1998) Working memory and the mid-dorsolateral prefrontal cortex. Soc Neurosci Abstr 24:18

Petrides M (2000) Mapping prefrontal cortical systems for the control of cognition. In: Toga A, Mazziotta JC (eds) Brain mapping: the systems. Academic Press, San Diego, pp 157–176

Petrides M, Milner B (1982) Deficits on subject-ordered tasks after frontal- and temporal-lobe lesions in man. Neuropsychologia 20:249–262

Petrides M, Pandya DN (1984) Projections to the frontal cortex from the posterior parietal region in the rhesus monkey. J Comp Neurol 228:105–116

Petrides M, Pandya DN (1994) Comparative architectonic analysis of the human and the macaque frontal cortex. In: Boller F, Grafman J (eds), Handbook of neuropsychology, Vol 9. Elsevier, Amsterdam, pp 17–58

Petrides M, Pandya DN (1999) Dorsolateral prefrontal cortex: comparative cytoarchitectonic analysis in the human and the macaque brain and corticocortical connection patterns. Eur J Neurosci 11:1011–1036

Petrides M, Alivisatos B, Evans AC, Meyer E (1993) Dissociation of human mid-dorsolateral frontal cortex in memory processing. Proc Natl Acad Sci USA 90:873–877

Preuss TM, Goldman-Rakic PS (1989) Connections of the ventral granular frontal cortex of macaques with perisylvian premotor and somatosensory areas: anatomical evidence for somatic representation in primate frontal association cortex. J Comp Neurol 282:293–316

Preuss TM, Goldman-Rakic PS (1991) Myelo- and cytoarchitecture of the granular frontal cortex and surrounding regions in the strepsirhine primate *Galago* and the anthropoid primate *Macaca*. J Comp Neurol 310:429–474

Sanides F (1962) Die Architektonik des menschlichen Stirnhirns. Springer, Berlin

Sarkissov SA, Filimonoff IN, Kononowa EP, Preobraschenskaja IS, Kukuew LA (1955) Atlas of the cytoarchitectonics of the human cerebral cortex. Medgiz, Moscow

Schall JD, Morel A, King DJ, Bullier J (1995) Topography of visual cortex connections with frontal eye field in macaque: convergence and segregation of processing streams. J Neurosci 15:4464–4487

Schwartz ML, Goldman-Rakic PS (1984) Callosal and intrahemispheric connectivity of the prefrontal association cortex in rhesus monkey: relation between intraparietal and principal sulcal cortex. J Comp Neurol 226:403–420

Stamm J (1969) Electrical stimulation of frontal cortex in monkeys during delayed-response performance. J Comp Physiol Psychol 67:535–546

Ungerleider LG, Mishkin M (1982) Two cortical visual systems. In: Ingle DJ, Goodale MA, Mansfield RJW (eds) Analysis of visual behaviour. MIT Press, Cambridge, pp 549–586

Ungerleider LG, Gaffan D, Pelak VS (1989) Projections from inferior temporal cortex to prefrontal cortex via the uncinate fascicle in rhesus monkeys. Exp Brain Res 76:473–484

Walker AE (1940) A cytoarchitectural study of the prefrontal area of the macaque monkey. J Comp Neurol 73:59–86

Lisa Koski · Tomáö Paus

Functional connectivity of the anterior cingulate cortex within the human frontal lobe: a brain-mapping meta-analysis

Published online: 10 May 2000

Abstract A database of positron-emission-tomography studies published between January 1993 and November 1996 was created to address several questions regarding the function and connectivity of the human anterior cingulate cortex (ACC). Using this database, we have previously reported on the relationship between behavioural variables and the probability of blood-flow response in distinct subdivisions of the ACC. The goal of the current analysis was to discover which areas of the frontal cortex show increased blood-flow co-occurring consistently with increased blood-flow in the ACC. Analyses of the frequency distributions of peaks in the ACC and the remaining frontal cortex (FC) yielded several important findings. First, FC peaks in the precentral gyrus, superior frontal gyrus, middle frontal gyrus, inferior frontal gyrus, medial frontal gyrus and orbitomedial frontal gyri were more frequent in subtractions that also yielded a peak in the ACC than in those that did not yield an ACC peak. Second, regional differences in the frequency distribution of these FC peaks were observed when the ACC peaks were subdivided into the rostral versus caudal ACC and supracallosal versus subcallosal ACC. Peaks in the precentral gyrus and in the vicinity of the supplementary motor area were more prevalent in subtractions with co-occurring peaks in the caudal than with the rostral ACC. Peaks in the middle frontal gyrus were more frequent in subtractions with co-occurring peaks in the paralimbic part of the supracallosal ACC, relative to the subcallosal or limbic supracallosal ACC. These observations are consistent with known differences in the anatomic connectivity in these cortical regions, as defined in non-human primates. Further analyses of the influence of behavioural variables on the relationships between the ACC and other regions of the frontal cortex suggested that this type of meta-analysis may provide testable hypotheses about functional and effective connectivity within the human frontal lobe.

Key words Anterior cingulate · Positron emission tomography · Meta-analysis · Frontal cortex

L. Koski · T. Paus (✉)
Montreal Neurological Institute, 3801 rue University, Montreal, Quebec H3A 2B4, Canada
e-mail: tomas@bic.mni.mcgill.ca
Tel.: 514-398-8504, Fax: 514-398–1338

Introduction

The anterior cingulate cortex (ACC) is a heterogeneous region in terms of its cytoarchitecture, connectivity and function. Since Brodmann's initial classification of areas 24, 25 and 32, evidence has emerged for the further subdivision of the ACC into limbic and paralimbic regions (Sanides 1964). Anatomists working in both the human and monkey brain have identified several cytoarchitecturally distinct regions within area 24, denoted as 24a, 24b and 24c (human: Petrides and Pandya 1994; Vogt et al. 1995; Zilles et al. 1995; monkey: Barbas and Pandya 1989; Matelli et al. 1991; Petrides and Pandya 1994; Vogt and Pandya 1987; Vogt et al. 1987). Different cortical zones can also be distinguished along the rostral-caudal plane of the human ACC. The most obvious of these is the gigantopyramidal field located in the caudalmost portion of area 24c, in the dorsal bank of the cingulate sulcus (Braak 1976). Subtle variations in cytoarchitecture define further subdivisions of area 24 as it curves around rostral to the genu of the corpus callosum (Vogt et al. 1995). Cytoarchitectural differences along the rostral-caudal plane are also seen in area 32, a transitional cortex that shares many features of its neighbouring neocortical areas. Sarkissov's brain map (Sarkissov et al. 1955) emphasises the resulting gradations from caudal to rostral to subcallosal area 32 in the use of the labels 32/8, 32/9, 32/10 and 32/12 (see Fig. 1).

The anatomic and functional specificity of these subdivisions is illustrated by the presence of one or more cingulate motor areas in the caudal portion of area 24 (Luppino et al. 1991; Shima et al. 1991) that contain direct topographic connections to the spinal cord (Dum and Strick 1991; He et al. 1995). Functional neuroimag-

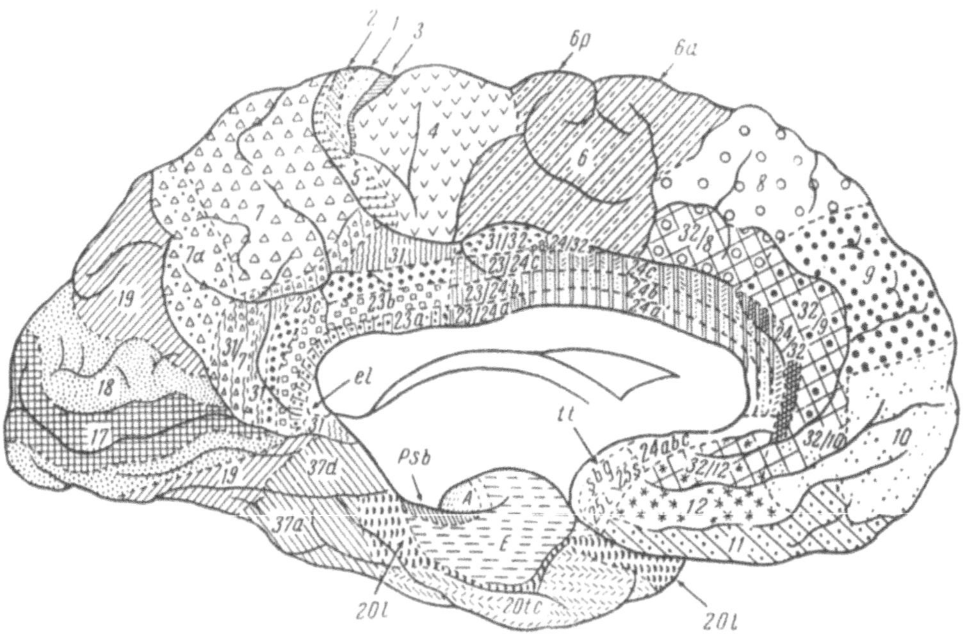

Fig. 1 Cytoarchitectonic divisions of the frontal cortex according to Sarkissov et al. (1955). Note the ventral to dorsal differentiation of parts a, b, and c within area 24. Also note that the paralimbic anterior cingulate area 32 is labelled as a transitional cortex that shares some of the features of medial areas 8, 9, 10 and 12

ing studies in humans support the existence of regions within the ACC that are differentially involved in manual, oculomotor and vocal responses (Paus et al. 1993; Picard and Strick 1996).

Although the empirical evidence is less striking, a distinction has also been made between the functions of the supracallosal, or "cognitive", and the subcallosal, or "visceral", parts of the ACC (Mayberg 1997; Vogt et al. 1995). In the monkey, these regions show somewhat distinct patterns of connectivity. Areas 24 and 32 are predominantly supracallosal and are interconnected with dorsolateral frontal areas (Barbas and Pandya 1989; Morecraft et al. 1993), which have been implicated in cognitive functions such as attention (Mesulam 1981; Posner and Petersen 1990) and working memory (Goldman-Rakic 1987; Petrides 1996). Subcallosal area 25 is interconnected with posterior orbitofrontal area 13 (Barbas and Pandya 1989) and has been implicated in the control of respiration, blood pressure and other autonomic functions (see Kaada 1960 for a review).

Our knowledge of the connections between the ACC and other parts of the frontal cortex has been restricted to non-human primates (Barbas and Pandya 1989; Bates and Goldman-Rakic 1993; Luppino et al. 1993; Morecraft and Van Hoesen 1992, 1993; Vogt and Pandya 1987), as the invasiveness of anatomical tracing techniques precludes their use in humans. Research into the connectivity of the human brain relies on the recent development of new techniques using functional neuroimaging. First, statistical methods such as principal components analysis (Friston et al. 1993), structural equation modelling (Horwitz et al. 1995; McIntosh et al. 1994) and multivariate partial least squares (McIntosh et al. 1996, 1999) have been used to evaluate co-activations of brain regions during the performance of cognitive tasks. Depending on the approach, different aspects of inter-regional interactions are emphasised: the term "functional" connectivity is often used when referring to simple inter-regional correlations, whereas "effective" connectivity refers to a more causal relationship between two systems such that one neural system exerts direct influence over the other (Friston et al. 1996). Second, new experimental methods that combine transcranial magnetic stimulation with positron emission tomography (Paus et al. 1997), functional magnetic resonance imaging (Bohning et al. 1998) or electroencephalography (Ilmoniemi et al. 1997) promise to demonstrate effective connectivity, without the behavioural confound inherent in traditional imaging approaches. Finally, with the growing body of PET experiments, it is now possible to analyse large sets of data in which multiple brain regions may show activation peaks within the same subtraction. The present study demonstrates how these data may be used to establish which areas of the brain show changes in activity that co-occur in a consistent manner with changes in a particular region of interest, i.e. across studies and across various behavioural manipulations.

We recently compiled a database of 107 published PET studies and were able to demonstrate a quantitative relationship between increases in the rate of behavioural response across tasks and increases in activation specific to the caudal part of the ACC (Paus et al. 1998). We also found that increases in task difficulty affected cingulate blood-flow in a regionally differentiated way, with the greatest increases seen in the paralimbic part of the supracallosal section of the ACC, smaller increases seen in the limbic part of the this section, and negligible changes seen in the subcallosal portion of the ACC.

For the present study, we looked for evidence of functional connectivity between the ACC and other parts of the frontal cortex by returning to our database and assessing which areas of the frontal cortex contained activation peaks in the same subtractions that produced peaks in subregions of the ACC. This approach was validated by the confirmation of strong predictions of functional connectivity between the caudal ACC and the primary and supplementary motor areas. Our approach also suggested connections between supracallosal cingulate and the middle frontal gyrus. Finally, we investigated whether these relationships between subregions were dependent on the behavioural requirements of tasks.

Materials and methods

Database

Only a short description of the original database is provided here, as full details have been reported elsewhere (Paus et al. 1998). In brief, we reviewed 107 PET studies published between January 1993 and November 1996. These studies had reported their findings as peaks of significant difference in cerebral blood flow (CBF) between two scans/tasks and had located the peaks in standardised stereotaxic space (Talairach and Tournoux 1988). Each task was coded along several behavioural dimensions, including type of input (e.g. visual) and output (e.g. hand movement), involvement of perceptual judgements (e.g. direction of motion), linguistic operations (e.g. detection of a phoneme), recent and remote memory, selective attention and relative task difficulty (Paus et al. 1998). A difference score was calculated for each subtraction. For subtractions yielding ACC peaks, the coordinates were entered. These peaks were classified into the following subdivisions: rostral versus caudal, supracallosal versus subcallosal or limbic versus paralimbic part of the supracallosal ACC (Fig. 2A).

Classification of peaks in the frontal cortex

The first author returned to the papers included in the database to record the x,y,z coordinates of all activation peaks obtained in the frontal lobe. Using a probabilistic atlas of the human frontal lobe (Kabani et al. 1997), each peak was classified automatically as located in one of the following frontal gyri in either the left or right hemisphere: precentral gyrus, superior frontal gyrus, middle frontal gyrus, inferior frontal gyrus, lateral orbitofrontal gyrus, medial orbitofrontal gyrus or medial frontal gyrus (Fig. 2B). Peaks outside the frontal cortex, including those classified as white matter, were excluded from further analyses. From this point on, for ease of communication, we will use the term "frontal cortex" (FC) to refer to peaks in the frontal cortex, but outside the ACC.

Statistical analyses

All tests were based on frequency distributions of categorical data. The number of subtractions yielding a peak in a particular frontal subdivision was compared for subtractions with an ACC-peak versus no ACC-peak. Further comparisons were conducted between subdivisions of the ACC (rostral versus caudal, supra- versus subcallosal, limbic versus paralimbic part of the supracallosal subdivision) to determine which ones were associated with peaks in a particular region of the FC. The frequencies were evaluated with a X^2, with the level of statistical significance set at P=0.01.

Further analyses were conducted to determine whether the observed relationships between subdivisions of the ACC and other regions of the frontal cortex could be attributed to the presence of a confounding behavioural variable. The behavioural variables selected were those that had been identified in our earlier review (Paus et al. 1998) as task parameters associated with particular subregions of the ACC. These parameters were: presence of a Hand/Arm Response, Output Rate and Visual Judgement for the caudal, rather than rostral, ACC; Auditory Input, Hand/Arm Response, Oculomotor Response, Recent Memory and Difficulty Level for the supracallosal, rather than subcallosal, cingulate; and Difficulty Level for the paralimbic, rather than limbic, portions of the supracallosal cingulate.

Only those subtractions containing at least one peak in the ACC and one peak elsewhere in the frontal cortex were included in the dataset for the present study. Therefore, the first step of this analysis was to conduct a set of tests to determine whether the relationships between the ACC subdivisions and the behavioural variables observed in the earlier study remained significant. Once again, the frequency distributions were evaluated with a X^2, with the level of statistical significance set at P=0.01.

In the second step, we compared the distribution of ACC and frontal cortex peaks in subtractions with positive values on a behavioural variable (i.e. >0) with their distribution in subtractions where the behavioural variable was subtracted out (i.e. =0). A series of analyses assessed the influence of each behavioural variable on the distribution of peaks within the ACC and frontal cortex. For example, the distribution of peaks to the ACC (rostral vs. caudal) and the prefrontal gyrus (yes vs. no) in subtractions with an Output Rate of zero was used to predict the expected distribution of peaks in subtractions with an Output Rate of greater than zero. The observed and expected frequencies for the four cells were compared using a goodness-of-fit X^2 test based on the sum of the squared differences, with a critical value based on three degrees of freedom and a P=0.01 level of significance. An assessment of the contribution of each cell was made following a significant result.

Results

The resulting database consisted of 413 subtractions, of which 174 yielded at least one ACC peak. Of these 174 subtractions, 114 yielded at least one FC peak. The total number of cingulate peaks was 227, of which 157 were from subtractions that also produced at least one peak elsewhere in the frontal cortex. The number of FC peaks obtained and their classifications are detailed in Table 1.

Comparison of ACC with no-ACC subtractions

The occurrence of a FC peak was significantly more likely in subtractions that also yielded an ACC peak (69%) than in those that did not (52%; X^2=20.4, P<0.0001). Table 1 shows the number of peaks in each FC classification for subtractions with and without a concomitant ACC peak. All subdivisions of the frontal cortex appeared to contribute equally to this finding. An exception was seen for peaks in the lateral orbitofrontal cortex, which showed the reverse pattern. Lateral orbito-

Table 1 Number of subtractions with one or more peaks in a particular region of the frontal cortex. *ACC* Anterior cingulate cortex

	ACC peak	
	Yes	No
Precentral gyrus	43	23
Superior frontal gyrus	29	15
Middle frontal gyrus	83	52
Inferior frontal gyrus	41	36
Lateral orbitofrontal gyri	7	22
Medial orbitofrontal gyri	16	6
Medial frontal gyrus	54	28

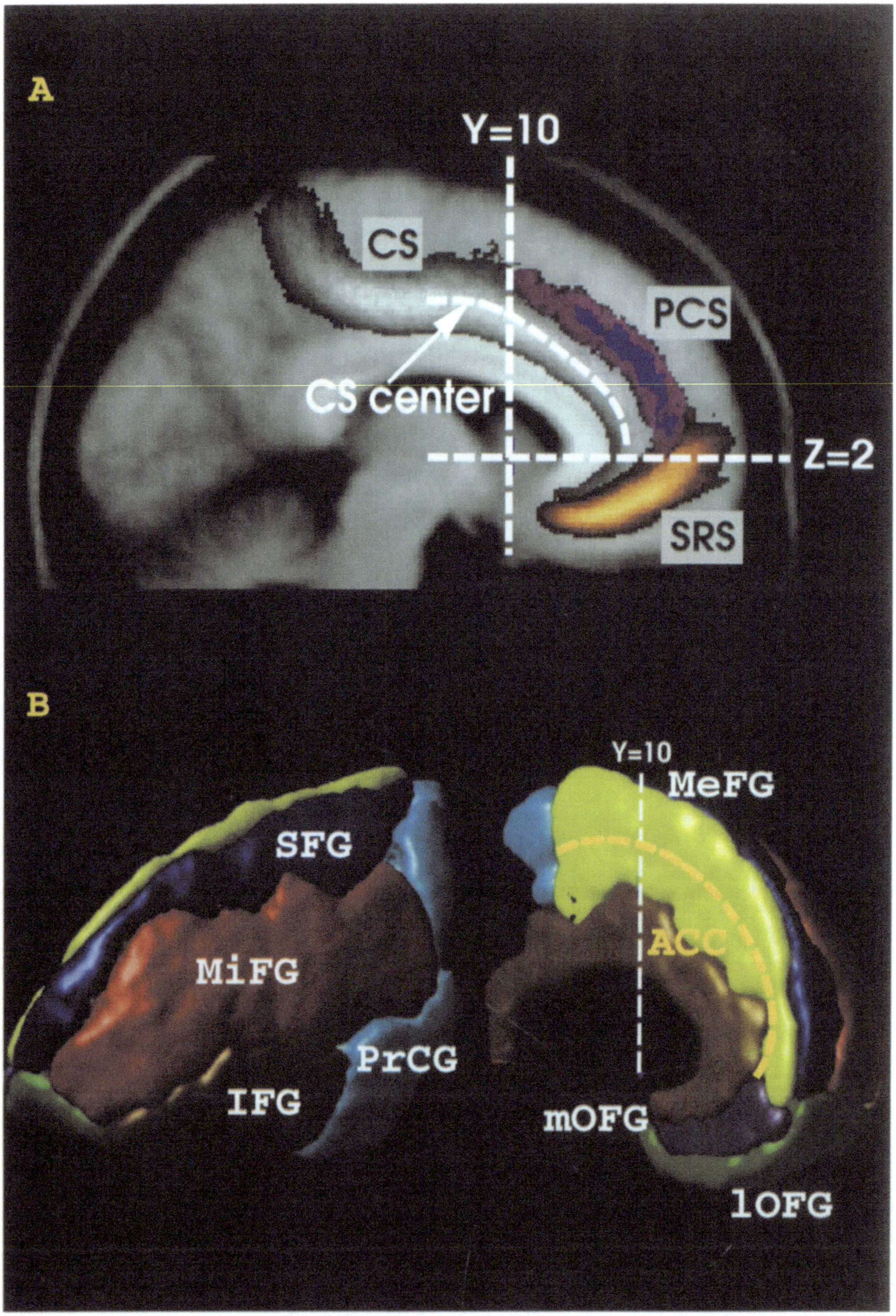
A
Y=10
CS
PCS
CS center
Z=2
SRS
B
Y=10
MeFG
SFG
MiFG
ACC
PrCG
IFG
mOFG
lOFG

frontal peaks occurred more frequently in the absence of a concurrent ACC peak (X^2=14.8, *P*=0.0001).

Rostral versus caudal ACC

Table 2 presents the frequency of FC peaks in each region with respect to the rostral and caudal subdivisions of the ACC. The co-occurrence of a frontal peak in the precentral gyrus was more likely in the caudal part than in the rostral part of the ACC (X^2=12.8, *P*=0.0004). A similar pattern was seen for frontal peaks in the medial frontal gyrus (X^2=9.1, *P*=0.003). By splitting the peaks into two groups, we tested the prediction that this pattern was driven by peaks occurring in the posterior part of the medial frontal gyrus, which contains the supplementary motor area (SMA). Peaks whose y-coordinate was ≤10 were considered as having a high probability of falling in the SMA. Note that, within this database, the border between the SMA and the ventrally located cingulate motor areas was defined on the basis of a coordinate in the dorsoventral plane: z=50 (Paus et al. 1996). The remaining peaks were called non-SMA. The frequency of a SMA peak did in fact discriminate between the rostral and caudal ACC in the expected direction (X^2=12.4, *P*<0.0004). The differences between subtractions with rostral or caudal ACC peaks were not significant for any other region of the FC.

◀ **Fig. 2** **A** Subdivisions of the anterior cingulate cortex (ACC). Probabilistic maps (Paus et al. 1996) of the cingulate sulcus (*CS*), paracingulate sulcus (PCS) and superior rostral sulcus (SRS) are superimposed on a magnetic-resonance image of the human brain; the maps and the brain are co-registered within standardised stereotaxic space (Talairach and Tournoux 1988). The border between the caudal and rostral ACC runs along the vertical plane located 10 mm anterior (Y=10) to the anterior commissure; this plane was chosen so that the caudal section includes the gigantopyramidal field of Braak (1976) as well as the cingulate hand/arm representations localised in our previous blood-flow-activation studies (Paus et al. 1993). The border between the supracallosal and subcallosal ACC runs along the horizontal plane located 2 mm above the anterior commissure (Z=2); this plane is located at the ventro-rostral tip of the CS and PCS probabilistic maps. This border thus approximates the split between the supracallosal areas 24 and 32 (in and around the CS and PCS) and the subcallosal areas 25 and 12 (in the SRS and below). The border between the paralimbic and limbic portions of the supracallosal ACC was chosen to coincide with the centre of gravity of the CS probabilistic map: the paralimbic areas 24c and 32 and the limbic areas 24a and 24b should lie, on average, above and below the CS centre, respectively. **B** Subdivisions of the frontal cortex. The divisions are based on the application of an automatic segmentation method to the magnetic resonance volumes of 33 normal, right-handed adults (Kabani et al. 1997). The frontal cortical volumes were divided into superior (*SFG*), middle (*MiFG*) and inferior frontal gyri (*IFG*), medial frontal (*MeFG*) and cingulate gyri on the medial wall, medial (*mOFG*) and lateral orbitofrontal gyri (*lOFG*), and the precentral gyri (*PrCG*). For consistency with our definition of anterior cingulate cortex, peaks in those portions of paralimbic ACC lying outside the cingulate sulcus (i.e. area 32, inside *dotted yellow boundary*) were reclassified as *ACC*, rather than as part of the medial frontal gyrus (as classified by the automatic segmentation method)

Table 2 Frequency of co-occurring rostral versus caudal anterior-cingulate-cortex (ACC) peaks in each frontal cortex region. *P*-values associated with significant differences in frequency distributions are in *italics*

	Rostral		Caudal		*P*
	Yes	No	Yes	No	
Precentral gyrus	23	93	20	21	*0.0004*
Superior frontal gyrus	21	95	8	33	842
Middle frontal gyrus	64	52	19	22	330
Inferior frontal gyrus	36	80	5	36	018
Lateral orbitofrontal gyri	6	110	1	40	465
Medial orbitofrontal gyri	15	101	1	40	0.056
Medial frontal gyrus	32	84	22	19	*0.003*
Supplementary motor area Y≤10	12	20	21	4	*<0.001*

Table 3 Frequency of co-occurring supracallosal versus subcallosal anterior-cingulate-cortex (ACC) peaks in each frontal cortex region. *P*-values associated with significant differences in frequency distributions are in *italics*

	Supra-callosal		Sub-callosal		*P*
	Yes	No	Yes	No	
Precentral gyrus	37	84	6	30	0.100
Superior frontal gyrus	24	97	5	31	0.420
Middle frontal gyrus	71	50	12	24	*0.007*
Inferior frontal gyrus	31	90	10	26	0.796
Lateral orbitofrontal gyri	6	115	1	35	0.578
Medial orbitofrontal gyri	4	117	12	24	*<0.001*
Medial frontal gyrus	41	80	13	23	0.805

Supracallosal versus subcallosal ACC

The frequency of co-occurrence of FC peaks in each region with respect to the supra- and subcallosal ACC is shown in Table 3. Only two comparisons were significant for these contrasts. A co-occurring peak in the middle frontal gyrus was more frequent for the supracallosal than for the subcallosal portion of the ACC (X^2=7.2, *P*=0.007). In contrast, a peak in the medial orbitofrontal gyri was more likely in subtractions that yielded a peak in the subcallosal than in the supracallosal ACC (X^2=27.3, *P*<0.0001).[1]

Paralimbic versus limbic ACC

The supracallosal portion of the ACC was further divided into a paralimbic and a limbic part. Despite this relatively small number of peaks in the limbic ACC (see Table 4), one FC region emerged as discriminating the

[1] For subtractions with more than one ACC peak, each peak was represented as a separate subtraction with all associated FC peaks, to ensure that all ACC peaks received equal weight. Since peaks in the medial orbitofrontal gyrus were relatively rare, this procedure resulted in a biased distribution of peaks co-occurring in the subcallosal cingulate and the medial orbitofrontal gyrus on the basis of a single experiment. Thus, we did not interpret the significant co-activation of these regions.

limbic from paralimbic ACC. Peaks in the middle frontal gyrus co-occurred more often with peaks in the paralimbic than in the limbic ACC (X^2=6.4, *P*=0.01).

Behavioural variables and the ACC subdivisions

The subtraction scores for behavioural-task parameters Hand/Arm Response and Output Rate were differently distributed for subtractions with significant CBF peaks in the rostral and caudal parts of the anterior cingulate region (see Table 5). In the caudal ACC, compared with the rostral ACC, peaks occurred more often in subtractions in which Task A had a higher Hand/Arm Response value than Task B (X^2=25.7, *P*<0.001). The same pattern was found for Output Rate (X^2=15.7, *P*<0.001). The difference between the rostral and caudal ACC in terms of Visual Judgement was not significant in this data set (X^2=1.5, *P*<0.48).

Higher scores on the Hand/Arm-Response, Oculomotor-Response, Recent-Memory and Difficulty-Level parameters were associated with subtractions that yielded significant peaks in the supracallosal, rather than the subcallosal, part of the anterior cingulate region (X^2=8.6, X^2=11.1, X^2=18.2 and X^2=49.7, respectively; *P*≤0.01). On the distribution of the Auditory-Input scores, the difference between the supracallosal and subcallosal ACC was not significant in this data set (X^2=3.6, *P*=0.06). The difference between the paralimbic and limbic portions of the supracallosal ACC in terms of Difficulty Level was not statistically significant in this data set (X^2=5.3, *P*=0.07).

Table 4 Frequency of co-occurring paralimbic versus limbic anterior-cingulate-cortex (ACC) peaks in each frontal cortex region. *P*-values associated with significant differences in frequency distributions are in *italics*

	Para-limbic		Limbic		*P*
	Yes	No	Yes	No	
Precentral gyrus	18	54	19	30	0.106
Superior frontal gyrus	17	55	10	42	0.560
Middle frontal gyrus	49	23	22	27	*0.011*
Inferior frontal gyrus	21	51	10	39	0.279
Lateral orbitofrontal gyri	4	68	2	47	0.714
Medial orbitofrontal gyri	3	69	1	48	0.521
Medial frontal gyrus	19	53	22	27	0.035

Behavioural contributions to the relationships between frontal cortex and ACC

Rostral versus caudal ACC

As demonstrated in Table 6, the pattern of occurrence of peaks in the precentral gyrus (yes/no) and in the ACC (rostral/caudal) was different for those subtractions in which a Hand/Arm Response was present rather than subtracted out (X^2=47, *P*<0.001). However, the change in distribution pattern across the four cells was *not* due to an increase in the frequency of co-occurring precentral gyrus and caudal ACC peaks when a Hand/Arm Response was present (X^2=2.0, *P*=0.2). In fact, a significant increase in the number of co-activations of caudal ACC

Table 5 Test of the relationships between subdivisions of the anterior cingulate region that showed cerebral blood-flow (CBF) peaks and relevant task-difference scores. *ACC* Anterior cingulate cortex. *P*-values associated with significant differences in frequency distributions are in *italics*

Task parameter	ACC subdivision	Subtraction score for behavioural parameter			*P*
		0	1	–1	
Hand/arm response	Rostral	109	4	3	*<0.001*
Caudal		28	13	0	
Output rate	Rostral	65	19	11	*<0.001*
Caudal		17	19	0	
Visual judgement	Rostral	107	4	5	0.481
Caudal		39	0	2	
Auditory input	Supracallosal	109	11	0	0.06
Subcallosal		36	0	0	
Hand/arm response	Supracallosal	103	17	1	*0.014*
Subcallosal		34	0	2	
Eye response	Supracallosal	114	6	1	*0.004*
Subcallosal		32	0	4	
Recent memory	Supracallosal	86	29	6	*<0.001*
Subcallosal		26	1	9	

Task parameter	ACC subdivision	Subtraction score for behavioural parameter					*P*
		–2	–1	0	1	2	
Difficulty level	Supracallosal	3	9	11	54	30	*<0.001*
Subcallosal		9	14	7	3	3	
Difficulty level	Paralimbic	3	4	5	31	21	0.071
Limbic		0	5	6	23	9	

Table 6 Test of the influence of behavioural variables on the distribution of co-activations in rostral versus caudal anterior cingulate cortex with different frontal cortex regions. *Y* Yes, *N* no, *SMA* supplementary motor area. *P*-values associated with significant differences in frequency distributions are in *italics*

Behavioural variable	Frontal region		Behaviour absent		Expected distribution		Observed distribution		*P*[a]		*P*-sum[b]
			rostral	caudal	rostral	caudal	rostral	caudal	rostral	caudal	
Hand	PreCentral	Y	23	16	2.9	2.0	0	4	0.09	0.15	*<0.001*
		N	86	12	10.7	1.5	4	9	0.04	*<0.001*	
Output	PreCentral	Y	16	10	7.4	4.6	2	7	0.05	0.27	*<0.001*
		N	49	7	22.7	3.2	17	12	0.23	*<0.001*	
Hand	Medial	Y	26	12	3.2	1.5	3	10	0.90	*<0.001*	*<0.001*
		N	83	16	10.3	2.0	1	3	*<0.01*	0.47	
Output	Medial	Y	4	7	3.2	5.6	18	12	*<0.001*	*<0.01*	*<0.001*
		N	47	10	37.3	7.9	17	7	*<0.001*	0.74	
Hand	SMA	Y	9	11	3.8	4.6	3	10	0.69	*0.01*	*<0.001*
		N	17	1	7.2	0.4	0	3	*<0.01*	*<0.001*	
Output	SMA	Y	7	6	4.8	4.1	0	12	0.03	*<0.001*	*<0.001*
		N	11	1	7.5	0.7	2	3	0.05	*<0.01*	
Hand	PreCentral	Y	23	16	1.5	1.0	0	4	0.23	*<0.01*	*<0.001*
	Nonmedial	N	65	6	4.1	0.4	1	2	0.12	*<0.01*	

[a] Probability estimate based on the comparison of the squared differences between observed and expected frequencies against a X^2 distribution with one degree of freedom

[b] Probability estimate based on a comparison of the sum of squared differences against a X^w distribution with three degrees of freedom

Table 7 Test of the influence of behavioural variables on the distribution of co-activations in supracallosal (Supra) versus subcallosal (Sub) anterior cingulate cortex with the middle frontal gyrus region. *Y* Yes, *N* no. *P*-values associated with significant differences in frequency distributions are in *italics*

Behavioural variable	Middle gyrus	Behaviour absent		Expected distribution		Observed distribution		*P*		*P*-sum
	Y/N	Supra	Sub	Supra	Sub	Supra	Sub	Supra	Sub	
Hand	Y	62	12	7.7	1.5	9	0	0.64	0.22	0.11
	N	41	22	5.1	2.7	8	0	0.20	0.10	
Eye	Y	67	11	2.8	0.5	4	0	0.45	0.50	0.60
	N	47	21	1.9	0.9	2	0	0.96	0.35	
Recent memory	Y	54	9	14.5	2.4	17	1	0.51	0.36	0.07
	N	32	17	8.6	4.6	12	0	0.21	0.03	
Difficulty	Y	7	5	35	25	57	1	*<0.001*	*<0.001*	*<0.001*
	N	4	2	20	10	27	5	0.12	0.11	

peaks with *non*-precentral gyrus peaks was the main contributor to the change in distribution (X^2=37.9, P<0.001). Similar results were obtained from the analysis of the influence of Output Rate on the distribution of these peaks (see Table 6).

The relationship between peaks in the medial frontal gyrus and ACC peaks (rostral vs. caudal) was significantly altered by the presence of either a Hand/Arm Response (X^2=57.6, P<0.001) or an Output Rate greater than zero (X^2=87.8, P<0.001; see Table 6). However, the relationship was influenced differently for the two behavioural variables. For the presence of Hand/Arm Response, the change in distribution was due to an increase in the frequency of caudal ACC and medial frontal cortex co-activations (X^2=48.7, P<0.001). This increase was significant whether the co-activated medial frontal peak was in the SMA or rostral to it. For Output Rates greater than zero, both caudal and rostral ACC showed increased co-activations with the medial frontal gyrus.

Based on the observed relationship between peaks in the medial frontal gyrus and the caudal ACC, a further analysis of the peaks in the precentral gyrus was carried out. We tested the hypothesis that the medial frontal peaks accounted for the increased association, noted above, between *non*-precentral gyrus peaks and caudal ACC in the presence of a Hand/Arm Response. A comparison was made between subtractions with peaks within the precentral gyrus and subtractions with peaks outside the precentral gyrus *excluding the medial frontal gyrus*. Using this contrast, the presence of a Hand/Arm Response led to increased association of caudal ACC peaks with either precentral (X^2=8.7, P=0.003) or non-precentral/non-medial peaks (X^2=6.9, P=0.008).

Supracallosal versus subcallosal ACC

Table 7 shows the results of the analyses of the influence of Hand/Arm Response, Oculomotor Response, Recent Memory demands and Difficulty Level on the relationship between the middle frontal gyrus and the supracallosal ACC. The presence of a Hand/Arm Response (X^2=6.1, *P*=0.1), Oculomotor Response (X^2=1.9, *P*=0.17) or Recent Memory requirement (X^2=7.2, *P*=0.06) did not significantly alter the pattern of distribution of co-activations in the ACC and middle frontal cortex. In contrast, greater Difficulty Level was associated with a different pattern of co-activations relative to those subtractions in which Difficulty Level was equal (X^2=41.8, *P*<0.001). Both an increase in the co-activation of supracallosal ACC with middle frontal gyrus (X^2=13.8, *P*<0.001) and a concomitant decrease in the co-activation of subcallosal ACC with middle frontal gyrus (X^2=23.0, *P*<0.001) contributed to this change.

Discussion

This analysis of the peaks obtained from PET-study subtractions demonstrated that several frontal-lobe gyri were consistently linked with changes in activity in the anterior cingulate cortex. First, blood-flow changes in most subdivisions of the frontal cortex occurred more often in subtractions that also showed changes in the anterior cingulate. These results confirm our previous observations of a tendency toward concomitant activation within these areas during functional neuroimaging studies. We have suggested that such co-activation may reflect the transmission of information computed in the prefrontal cortex to the ACC, where it is modulated by non-specific arousal systems as it is forwarded to motor channels (Paus et al. 1993). Neuroanatomic studies in the monkey indicate that these regions are richly interconnected, in that the ACC projects to, or receives projections from, virtually all areas of the frontal cortex (see Barbas 1995 for a review). Indeed, Barbas (1995, 1997) has noted that dysgranular, or "limbic", cortex (including areas 24, 25 and 32) tends to have more widespread connections relative to eulaminate (6-layer) cortical regions.

Interestingly, the pattern of association between ACC and frontal cortex was reversed for changes in the lateral orbitofrontal cortex, a subdivision that probably includes at least Brodmann's area 12 and the lateral portions of 11 and 13 as well. Two separate architectonic trends have been described within the prefrontal cortex, following relatively separate courses along the basoventral and mediodorsal cortices (Barbas and Pandya 1989). The basoventral trend begins in the periallocortex of the caudal orbitofrontal region, continues to area 13 and then through areas 11, 12 and 14, coursing up to area 10, lateral area 12 and ventral areas 46 and 8. The mediodorsal trend begins in the periallocortex at the rostral tip of the corpus callosum, spreads to areas 25, 24 and 32, and then on through medial areas 9, 10 and 14 to lateral areas 10 and 9 and dorsal areas 8 and 46. Although areas 11, 12 and 13 do send a few projections to the anterior cingulate (Barbas and Pandya 1989; Vogt and Pandya 1987), for the most part, the interconnections between the two trends occur between cortical areas of similar stages of architectonic differentiation (Barbas and Pandya 1989). This may account for our observation that peaks in the lateral orbitofrontal cortex did not co-occur with peaks in the ACC.

The patterns of association between the anterior cingulate cortex and the rest of the frontal cortex were dissected to explore contrasts between several subdivisions of the anterior cingulate. Further analyses were conducted to assess the degree to which the "co-activation" of specific regions could be attributed to behavioural components of the tasks performed during scanning.

Caudal ACC and other motor areas

The first important observation was that peaks in the precentral gyrus region co-occurred significantly more often in subtractions that also yielded a peak in the caudal, as compared with the rostral, ACC. This relationship was not influenced by the presence of manual responses and greater response rates in the subtractions that yielded caudal ACC peaks. Therefore, the hypothesis that the association between caudal ACC and the precentral gyrus is based on these behavioural confounds in the data set may be rejected.

A second finding concerned the relationship between the caudal ACC and the medial frontal gyrus, particularly in the region of the supplementary motor area. Output rate did not have a selective influence on the association between caudal ACC and the medial frontal gyrus. On the other hand, an increase co-activation of caudal ACC and medial frontal gyrus was seen for tasks with a manual response. The latter finding raises the possibility that the tendency of peaks in these regions to occur in the same subtractions was to some degree a function of the task demands in these functional-imaging studies. However, the observed relationship between caudal ACC and the supplementary motor area portion of the medial frontal gyrus was *not* influenced by manual response or output rate.

The consistent co-activation of these specific regions of the ACC and frontal cortex across studies using vastly different behavioural tasks is quite remarkable, particularly when it can be demonstrated that these relationships were not influenced by the behavioural components common to the tasks. We propose, therefore, that these results may reflect underlying anatomic connectivity between these cortical areas. This interpretation is supported by the results of several studies in the monkey. By injecting neuronal tracers, it has been demonstrated that both the primary (Morecraft and Van Hoesen 1992, 1993) and supplementary (Bates and Goldman-Rakic 1993; Luppino et al. 1993) motor areas are densely interconnected with the caudal ACC. This pattern of connectivity, along with the presence of direct corticospinal projections from the caudal ACC (Dum and Strick 1991; He et al. 1995) has resulted in the term cingulate motor area to describe a particular portion of caudal ACC located in the depths of the cingulate sulcus. The definition of the caudal ACC used in this meta-analysis was based on our original observations of significant peaks during simple finger movements (Paus et al. 1993) and includes all peaks associated with simple hand or arm movement tasks in Picard and Strick's (1996) review of 29 PET studies.

Supracallosal ACC and the middle frontal gyrus

Peaks in the middle frontal gyrus occurred more frequently in subtractions with a peak in the supracallosal ACC than in subtractions with a peak in the subcallosal ACC. Within the supracallosal part of the anterior cingulate, middle frontal gyrus peaks were seen more often in subtractions yielding a peak in paralimbic regions than in limbic regions of the ACC. That more dorsally located regions of the anterior cingulate cortex are concomitantly activated with dorsolateral regions of the prefrontal cortex suggests their preferential involvement in the computations underlying complex cognitive tasks, such as those requiring conditional associative learning or working memory (Goldman-Rakic 1988; Petrides 1989).

The relationship between the supracallosal cingulate and the middle frontal gyrus was not influenced by the greater presence of manual and oculomotor responses in these subtractions, nor did the greater recent-memory requirements prove consistent in their contributions to the pattern. In contrast, increased difficulty of the task appears to have strongly determined the co-activation of these regions. The association of the supracallosal cingulate and the middle frontal gyrus was significantly greater in those subtractions that yielded positive differences in task-difficulty levels. Furthermore, co-activation of the middle frontal gyrus and the subcallosal cingulate was significantly less frequent in subtractions with greater difficulty levels. The potential contribution of difficulty level to the specific relationship between middle frontal gyrus and paralimbic ACC was not assessed, as the relationship between difficulty level and paralimbic ACC was not significant in this study.

A distinction has appeared in the literature between the functions of the supracallosal, rostral and subcallosal regions of the anterior cingulate cortex (Devinsky et al. 1995; Mayberg 1997; Vogt et al. 1995). Devinsky and colleagues (Devinsky et al. 1995) proposed that dorsal regions of the ACC are involved in cognition while rostral and subcallosal portions of the ACC are engaged in emotional behaviour. Based on early stimulation work in the rat (Neafsey 1990), the cat, the monkey and in humans undergoing psychosurgery (see Kaada 1960 for a review), the importance of the perigenual and subcallosal regions for modulating autonomic or visceral aspects of emotion has been emphasised. For example, electrical stimulation of these regions produces changes in respiration, blood pressure and vocalisation. Evidence from other methodologies has tended to support this view of the functions of the subcallosal anterior cingulate cortex. In the human, for example, skin-conductance response in anticipation of rewards and penalties is absent in patients with bilateral lesions centred within the ventromedial prefrontal lobe (Bechara et al. 1996), and abnormalities in the cortical volume of and the blood flow to subcallosal cingulate areas have been observed in patients with mood disorders (Drevets et al. 1997). The precise location of the cingulate areas that participate in autonomic functions in the human remains unclear, however, due to differences in the anatomy and physiology of the monkey and the human. Kaada's early work in the macaque monkey pointed to the existence of functionally distinct areas within the ACC. Electrical stimulation in the perigenual cingulate area yielded respiratory inhibition, decreased arterial pressure, inhibition of reflexes and inhibition of movements induced by cortical stimulation (Kaada 1960). This region was considered to influence "visceral" functions. In contrast, stimulation of the cortex outside this area, in more caudal parts of the supracallosal and subcallosal anterior cingulate, elicited "arousal" effects, including increased respiration rate, facilitation of movements induced by cortical stimulation, dilation of pupils and increased cortical arousal on electroencephalogram. A recent comparative study of the architectonic structure of the macaque monkey and the human shows that the monkey area 32 is located in the perigenual and subcallosal portions of the cingulate, whereas in the human the greater portion of area 32 is located supracallosally (Petrides and Pandya 1994). Thus, it is likely that the region associated with visceral functions in the monkey was comprised largely of area 32. Yet, in the human, these effects appear to have been restricted to stimulation of rostral area 24, and not rostral area 32 (Kaada and Jasper 1952; Pool and Ransohoff 1949). More recent histological studies in the monkey support the subdivision of the monkey ACC into supracallosal and subcallosal regions, and into paralimbic and limbic regions, based on their differential connectivity with the hypothalamus (Ongur et al. 1998), striatum (Kunishio and Haber 1994) and periaqueductal grey (An et al. 1998). Whether these connections are also present in the human brain is unknown. However, the differential patterns of co-activation observed here between supracallosal and subcallosal ACC and between paralimbic and limbic portions of the supracallosal ACC suggest that the distinctions may also be valid for the human.

The results of the present study extend our previous findings of functional heterogeneity within the anterior cingulate cortex (Paus et al. 1998) by demonstrating that increases in activity within a particular subdivision of the cingulate occur most often along with increases in activity in specific regions of the frontal cortex. Equally importantly, we have been able to conduct analyses of the impact of certain behavioural demands of the tasks on the observed patterns of co-activations. First, the relationship between supracallosal cingulate and the middle frontal gyrus was significantly stronger in subtractions associated with a greater difficulty level. Thus, more difficult tasks may demand the joint efforts of both supracallosal cingulate and middle frontal cortex areas or include several cognitive components that independently engage the two regions. Second, it was demonstrated that the presence of movement does not underlie the relationship between caudal ACC and other motor areas of the frontal cortex. Having ruled out the most obvious explanation for the relationship, i.e. that the two regions were activated independently due to their role in motor control, we propose that these findings suggest effective connectivity between the caudal ACC and the primary and supplementary motor areas.

Our conclusions as to the potential of statistical analyses of large data sets to yield evidence by which we may infer anatomic connectivity in the human remain tentative at present. In demonstrating relationships between cortical areas that are independent of potential behavioural confounds, we have drawn closer to our goal. However, several limitations of the current approach must be considered. First, the selection of behavioural parameters that were most likely to account for some portion of the co-activations observed was based on our earlier experience with this database. Other task parameters were not analysed, including behavioural confounds of a more subtle nature that proved too difficult to code objectively in the original study. Furthermore, the analysis of a large and heterogeneous data set precludes the evaluation of several important task variables that have been associated with anterior cingulate activation (e.g. response competition), as these were common to only a handful of studies in the set. Indeed, our most "cognitive" variable, Difficulty Level, encompassed a deliberately broad range of task comparisons. Second, relationships involving interactions among task parameters were too complex for the current methods of analysis. Typically, a log linear analysis would be appropriate for testing the size of the behavioural contribution to the co-activation patterns as well as the potential influence of behavioural interactions; however, the presence of zero or near-zero values in some cells precluded the use of this statistic (Tabachnick and Fidell 1989). A larger database might permit the use of more sophisticated statistical approaches for evaluating the relationships between behavioural variables and activation peaks.

Nevertheless, the results of the present study could prove valuable in terms of generating hypotheses about functional and effective connectivity within the frontal cortex that may then be tested by combining, for example, PET with transcranial magnetic stimulation (TMS). Once a cortical target for stimulation has been selected, TMS and PET can be used to examine the effective connectivity between a particular region on the lateral convexity of the frontal cortex and deeper structures, including the anterior cingulate. In this instance, one might stimulate at several sites over the cortex of the middle frontal gyrus and look for evidence of increased blood flow in the paralimbic ACC.

A recent review by Fox (Fox et al. 1998) highlighted the importance of combining data obtained from different studies and in different laboratories for generating new hypotheses. The present meta-analysis is among the first to use quantitative statistical methods to test the consistency of the patterns of activation observed across multiple experiments. We anticipate that the emergence of statistical methods that use the standardised coordinate system as their unit of measurement will contribute in an important way to the use of the information contained in larger databases such as that developed by Fox and his colleagues (Fox and Lancaster 1996).

Acknowledgements We gratefully acknowledge the help of Dr. Rhonda Amsel in the form of statistical advice. This work was funded in part by the Canadian Medical Research Council (MT-14505).

References

An X, Bandler R, Ongur D, Price J (1998) Prefrontal cortical projections to longitudinal columns in the midbrain periaqueductal grey in macaque monkeys. J Comp Neurol 401:455–479

Barbas H (1995) Anatomic basis of cognitive-emotional interactions in the primate prefrontal cortex. Neurosci Biobehav Rev 19:499–510

Barbas H (1997) Two prefrontal limbic systems: their common and unique features. In: Sakata H, Mikami A, Fuster J (eds) The association cortex: structure and function. Harwood Academic Publishers, Amsterdam, pp 99–116

Barbas H, Pandya DN (1989) Architecture and intrinsic connections of the prefrontal cortex in the rhesus monkey. J Comp Neurol 286:353–375

Bates JF, Goldman-Rakic PS (1993) Prefrontal connections of medial motor areas in the rhesus monkey. J Comp Neurol 336:211–228

Bechara A, Tranel D, Damasio H, Damasio A (1996) Failure to respond autonomically to anticipated future outcomes following damage to prefrontal cortex. Cereb Cortex 6:215–225

Bohning D, Shastri A, Nahas Z, Lorberbaum J, Andersen S, Dannels W, Haxthausen E, Vincent D, George M (1998) Echoplanar BOLD fMRI of the brain activation induced by concurrent transcranial magnetic stimulation. Invest Radiol 33:336–340

Braak H (1976) A primitive gigantopyramidal field buried in the depth of the cingulate sulcus of the human brain. Brain Res 109:219–233

Devinsky O, Morrell MJ, Vogt BA (1995) Contributions of anterior cingulate cortex to behaviour. Brain 118:279–306

Drevets W, Price J, Simpson J, Todd R, Reich T, Vannier M, Raichle M (1997) Subgenual prefrontal cortex abnormalities in mood disorders. Nature 386:824–827

Dum RP, Strick PL (1991) The origin of corticospinal projections from the premotor areas in the frontal lobe. J Neurosci 11: 667–689

Fox P, Lancaster JL (1996) Neuroscience on the net. Science 226:994–996

Fox P, Parsons LM, Lancaster JL (1998) Beyond the single study: function/location metaanalysis in cognitive neuroimaging. Curr Opin Neurobiol 8:178–187

Friston KJ, Frith CD, Liddle PF, Frackowiak RS (1993) Functional connectivity: the principal-component analysis of large (PET) data sets. J Cereb Blood Flow Metab 13:5–14

Friston KJ, Frith CD, Fletcher P (1996) Functional topography: multidimensional scaling and functional connectivity in the brain. Cereb Cortex 6:156–164

Goldman-Rakic PS (1987) Circuitry of primate prefrontal cortex and regulation of behavior by representational memory. In: Plum F (ed) Handbook of physiology. The nervous system, Vol 5. American Physiological Society, Bethesda, pp 373–417

Goldman-Rakic P (1988) Topography of cognition: parallel distributed networks in primate association cortex. Annu Rev Neurosci 11:137–156

He SQ, Dum RP, Strick PL (1995) Topographic organization of corticospinal projections from the frontal lobe: motor areas on the medial surface of the hemisphere. J Neurosci 15:3284–3306

Horwitz B, McIntosh AR, Haxby JV, Grady CL (1995) Network analysis of brain cognitive function using metabolic and blood flow data. Behav Brain Res 66:187–193

Ilmoniemi R, Virtanen J, Ruohonen J, Karhu J, Aronen H, Naatanen R, Katila T (1997) Neuronal responses to magnetic stimulation reveal cortical reactivity and connectivity. Neuroreport 8:3537–3540

Kaada B (1960) Cingulate, posterior orbital, anterior insular and temporal pole cortex. In: Field J, Magoun H, Hall V (eds) Neurophysiology, Vol II. American Physiological Society, Washington DC, pp 1345–1372

Kaada B, Jasper H (1952) Respiratory responses to stimulation of temporal pole, insula, and hippocampal and limbic gyri in man. Arch Neurol Psychiatry 68:609–619

Kabani N, Collins L, Evans A (1997) Hemispheric differences in gray matter volume of adult human brain (abstract). Annual Meeting of the Society for Neuroscience, Poster Presentation

Kunishio K, Haber S (1994) Primate cingulostriatal projection: Limbic striatal versus sensorimotor striatal input. J Comp Neurol 350:337–356

Luppino G, Matelli M, Camarda RM, Gallese V, Rizzolatti G (1991) Multiple representations of body movements in mesial area 6 and the adjacent cingulate cortex: an intracortical microstimulation study in the macaque monkey. J Comp Neurol 311:463–482

Luppino G, Matelli M, Camarda R, Rizzolatti G (1993) Corticocortical connections of area F3 (SMA-proper) and area F6 (pre-SMA) in the macaque monkey. J Comp Neurol 338:114–140

Matelli M, Luppino G, Rizzolatti G (1991) Architecture of superior and mesial area 6 and the adjacent cingulate cortex in the macaque monkey. J Comp Neurol 311:445–462

Mayberg H (1997) Limbic-cortical dysregulation: a proposed model of depression. J Neuropsychiat 9:471–481

McIntosh AR, Grady CL, Ungerleider LG, Haxby JV, Rapoport SI, Horwitz B (1994) Network analysis of cortical visual pathways mapped with PET. J Neurosci 14:655–666

McIntosh AR, Bookstein FL, Haxby JV, Grady CL (1996) Spatial pattern analysis of functional brain images using partial least squares. Neuroimage 3:143–57

McIntosh AR, Rajah MN, Lobaugh NJ (1999) Interactions of prefrontal cortex in relation to awareness in sensory learning. Science 284:1531–1533

Mesulam MM (1981) A cortical network for directed attention and unilateral neglect. Ann Neurol 10:309–325

Morecraft RJ, Van Hoesen GW (1992) Cingulate input to the primary and supplementary motor cortices in the rhesus monkey: evidence for somatotopy in areas 24c and 23c. J Comp Neurol 322:471–489

Morecraft RJ, Van Hoesen GW (1993) Frontal granular cortex input to the cingulate (M3), supplementary (M2) and primary (M1) motor cortices in the rhesus monkey. J Comp Neurol 337:669–689

Morecraft RJ, Geula C, Mesulam MM (1993) Architecture of connectivity within a cingulo-fronto-parietal neurocognitive network for directed attention. Arch Neurol 50:279–284

Neafsey E (1990) Prefrontal cortical control of the autonomic nervous system: anatomical and physiological observations. In: Uylings H, VanEden C, DeBruin J, Corner J, Feenstra M (eds) Progress in brain research, Vol 85. Elsevier Science, New York, pp 147–166

Ongur D, An X, Price J (1998) Prefrontal cortical projections to the hypothalamus in macaque monkeys. J Comp Neurol 401:480–505

Paus T, Petrides M, Evans AC, Meyer E (1993) Role of the human anterior cingulate cortex in the control of oculomotor, manual, and speech responses: a positron emission tomography study. J Neurophysiol 70:453–469

Paus T, Tomaiuolo F, Otaky N, MacDonald D, Petrides M, Atlas J, Morris R, Evans A (1996) Human cingulate and paracingulate suci: pattern, variability, asymmetry, and probabilistic map. Cereb Cortex 6:207–214

Paus T, Jech R, Thompson CJ, Comeau R, Peters T, Evans AC (1997) Transcranial magnetic stimulation during positron emission tomography: a new method for studying connectivity of the human cerebral cortex. J Neurosci 17:3178–3184

Paus T, Koski L, Caramanos Z, Westbury C (1998) Regional differences in the effects of task difficulty and motor output on blood flow response in the human anterior cingulate cortex: a review of 107 PET activation studies. Neuroreport 9:R37–R47

Petrides M (1989) Frontal lobes and memory. In: Boller F, Grafman J (eds) Handbook of neuropsychology, Vol 3. Elsevier Science, Amsterdam New York, pp 75–90

Petrides M (1996) Specialized systems for the processing of mnemonic information within the primate frontal cortex. Philos Trans R Soc Lond B Biol Sci 351:1455–1462

Petrides M, Pandya DN (1994) Comparative architectonic analysis of the human and the macaque frontal cortex. In: Boller F, Grafman J (eds) Handbook of neuropsychology, Vol 3. Elsevier Science, Amsterdam New York, pp 17–58

Picard N, Strick PL (1996) Motor areas of the medial wall: a review of their location and functional activation. Cereb Cortex 6:342–353

Pool J, Ransohoff J (1949) Autonomic effects on stimulating rostral portion of cingulate gyri in man. J Neurophysiol 12:385–392

Posner MI, Petersen SE (1990) The attention system of the human brain. Annu Rev Neurosci 13:25–42

Sanides F (1964) Structure and function of the human frontal lobe. Neuropsychologia 2:209–219

Sarkissov S, Filimonoff J, Kononova E, Preobraschenskaja I, Kukuew L (1955) Atlas of the cytoarchitectonics of the human cerebral cortex. Medzig, Moscow

Shima K, Aya K, Mushiake H, Inase M, Aizawa H, Tanji J (1991) Two movement-related foci in the primate cingulate cortex observed in signal-triggered and self-paced forelimb movements. J Neurophysiol 65:188–202

Tabachnick B, Fidell L (1989) Using multivariate statistics. Harper and Row, New York

Talairach J, Tournoux P (1988) Co-planar stereotaxic atlas of the human brain. Thieme Medical, New York

Vogt BA, Pandya DN (1987) Cingulate cortex of the rhesus monkey. II. Cortical afferents. J Comp Neurol 262:271–289

Vogt BA, Pandya DN, Rosene DL (1987) Cingulate cortex of the rhesus monkey. I. Cytoarchitecture and thalamic afferents. J Comp Neurol 262:256–270

Vogt BA, Nimchinsky EA, Vogt LJ, Hof PR (1995) Human cingulate cortex: surface features, flat maps, and cytoarchitecture. J Comp Neurol 359:490–506

Zilles K, Schlaug G, Matelli M, Luppino G, Schleicher A, Qu M, Dabringhaus A, Seitz R, Roland PE (1995) Mapping of human and macaque sensorimotor areas by integrating architectonic, transmitter receptor, MRI and PET data. J Anat 187:515–537

Joaquín M. Fuster

Executive frontal functions

Published online: 10 May 2000

Abstract This chapter presents a conceptual model of the representational and executive functions of the cortex of the frontal lobe derived from empirical evidence obtained principally in the monkey. According to this model, the neuronal networks of the frontal lobe that represent motor or executive memories are probably the same networks that cooperate with other cerebral structures in the temporal organization of behavior. The prefrontal cortex, at the top of the perception-action cycle, plays a critical role in the mediation of contingencies of action across time, an essential aspect of the temporal organization of behavior. That role of cross-temporal mediation is based on the interplay of two short-term cognitive functions: one retrospective, of short-term memory or sensory working memory, and the other prospective, of attentive set (or motor working memory). Both appear represented in the neuronal populations of dorsolateral prefrontal cortex. At least one of the mechanisms for the retention of working memory of either kind seems to be the reentry of excitability through recurrent cortical circuits. With those two complementary and temporally symmetrical cognitive functions of active memory for the sensory past and for the motor future, the prefrontal cortex secures the temporal closure at the top of the perception-action cycle.

Key words Prefrontal cortex · Cross-temporal contingencies · Short-term memory · Motor attention · Perception-action cycle

Introduction

The entire cortex of the primate's frontal lobe seems dedicated to organismic action. It can, thus, be considered, as a whole, "motor" or "executive" cortex in the broadest sense. The frontal cortex participates in all aspects of active adaptation of the organism to the environment: skeletal and ocular movement, reasoning, and the spoken language. Visceral actions and emotional behavior are modulated to some extent by orbital and medial areas of the frontal cortex. In this chapter, the focus is on the role of the dorsolateral prefrontal cortex in the cognitive aspects of the temporal organization of action, in other words, in the cognitive aspects of executive function. In the present model, there is no need for a "central executive". Such a hypothetical entity would be distributed here in dorsolateral prefrontal cortex.

It is a reasonable assumption that the cognitive functions of the prefrontal cortex, as those of any other part of the neocortex, consist of the activation and processing within and between distributed networks of neurons representing the environment and the organism within it; in other words, within and between memory networks (review in Fuster 1997b). These networks are organized hierarchically and are highly specific, defined by their connectivity. The memory code, in this sense, is a relational code, and all memory is associative. Memory networks extend across cortical modules and areas, overlapping and extensively interconnected with one another. One neuron or group of neurons anywhere in the cortex can be a part of many memory networks and, therefore, many memories.

In the cortex of the frontal lobe, executive networks are hierarchically organized like the perceptual networks of posterior, post-rolandic, cortex. The primary motor cortex is the lowest level of the cortical motor hierarchy; it represents and executes elementary muscular movements. Above it, the premotor cortex is the substrate for more complex movements, defined by goal and trajectory. At the top is the prefrontal cortex. On the basis of neuropsychological data, it appears that this cortical region represents the broad schemas of action in skeletal and speech domains. Furthermore, it seems crucially involved in the executions of those schemas. One of the most consistent components of the prefrontal-lesion syndrome is the difficulty in formulating and enacting plans of behavioral, linguistic, or cognitive action.

J.M. Fuster (✉)
UCLA Neuropsychiatric Institute, 760 Westwood Plaza,
Los Angeles, CA 90024, USA
e-mail: joaquinf@ucla.edu
Tel.: +1-310-8250247, Fax: +1-310-8256792

Temporal organization

It follows from these general concepts and assumptions that the cognitive functions of the prefrontal cortex cannot be isolated from those of the rest of the neocortex and the subjacent stages of the executive hierarchy. It is erroneous to localize in the prefrontal cortex cognitive functions that are not localizable. This is true for working memory, for the so-called "central executive," for spatial memory, and for various forms or aspects of attention. All these cognitive functions are subserved by the frontal lobe, but none of them is localized in it. Only parts of the networks of executive memory are localized there. By neural processing within and between those networks, and between those networks and others elsewhere in the neocortex, the prefrontal cortex plays its role in the temporal organization of behavior, speech, and logical reasoning.

An outline follows of physiological processes behind the postulated role of the prefrontal cortex in temporal structures of action. At the root of that role is a set of cognitive operations that mediate *cross-temporal contingencies*. The dorsolateral prefrontal cortex plays a critical role in that mediation, as is now substantiated in the human and non-human primate. Behaviorally, the best way to study the mediation of cross-temporal contingencies is by use of the delay-task paradigm. In delay tasks, motor acts are contingent on sensory cues that the animal must retain for a period (delay) of seconds or minutes. A single trial in one such task is an example of temporal structure or "gestalt." Since each trial temporally separates events that are mutually contingent, and since those events are novel – inasmuch as they change randomly between trials – the task is based on the mediation of cross-temporal contingencies.

What follows is a brief summary of some of our evidence for: (1) the crucial importance of the dorsolateral prefrontal cortex for the mediation of cross-temporal contingencies; (2) the role of prefrontal networks in active short-term memory, or working memory, the retrospective aspect of cross-temporal contingencies; (3) the role of prefrontal networks in short-term attentive set, the prospective aspect of cross-temporal contingencies; and (4) the mechanisms of short-term active memory.

Cooling dorsolateral prefrontal cortex – parts of areas 9 and 46 – in the monkey induces reversible deficits in visual, auditory, and tactile delay tasks (Fuster 1997a). It appears that the animal with functionally depressed prefrontal cortex cannot mediate across time the contingency between a stimulus and the consequent behavioral response to it, especially if the time between the two is long (>5 s). If the task is visual (delayed matching to sample), a similar deficit can be obtained by bilaterally cooling the inferotemporal cortex. There is considerable anatomical and physiological evidence for areal specificity within the dorsolateral prefrontal cortex, with regard to stimuli as well as contingency tasks (Fuster et al. 1982; Petrides et al. 1993a; Petrides and Pandya 1994; Goldman-Rakic 1995). Imaging studies corroborate that evidence (Paulesu et al. 1993; Petrides et al. 1993b; Courtney et al. 1996; Owen et al. 1996; Smith et al. 1996; Aguirre et al. 1998; Gabrieli et al. 1998). These studies demonstrate that several prefrontal areas are activated during working memory. We contributed to this evidence with a positron emission-tomography (PET) deoxyglucose in human subjects performing a visual delayed matching-to-sample task (Swartz et al. 1995).

The mechanisms of cortical activation in short-term memory can best be investigated in real time at the cellular level. Neuronal phenomena show that the mediation of cross-temporal contingencies depends on two temporally symmetrical functions: (1) active short-term (working) memory and (2) short-term attentive set or motor memory.

Active short-term memory

The results from numerous studies clearly indicate that the dorsolateral prefrontal cortex is critically involved in all forms of working memory toward a goal, whether in behavior, reasoning, or speech (Fuster 1997a). Frontal memory in the active state is defined by its teleological quality. All the physiological attributes of single areas and cell groups in the dorsolateral frontal cortex seem to be related to that teleological quality of frontal memory. In that cortex, sensory-cell groupings and memory maps may be simply the pathways of access to executive action. Sensory working memory is one of the cognitive functions at the service of that executive action. It assists in organizing behavior in the temporal domain. Some areas of ventral or orbital cortex receive information related to reward or emotion. That too may have teleological significance, for that information may serve the fulfillment of drives. Those areas have important inputs from the limbic system, notably the amygdala.

The involvement of prefrontal neurons in short-term active memory is amply documented by descriptions of single units that respond by activation of firing frequency to the presence of a sensory memorandum for prospective action (e.g., Fuster 1973; Niki 1974; Funahashi et al. 1989). Such units have two characteristics that define them as so-called "memory cells": (1) specific response to one or more memoranda, and (2) temporal decay of their firing during memorization (delay); this phenomenon is most evident in manual memory tasks with long delays (over 5 s). Those cells are apparently constituents of motor memory networks that are activated by stimuli that need to be retained toward a goal. Their firing frequency is related not only to those stimuli or memoranda, but to the level of correctness of performance of the task. Different sensory memoranda have different prefrontal distributions.

In a task with varying probability of association between a visual stimulus and a later manual act, we studied the temporal characteristics of sensory and motor memory cells in dorsolateral prefrontal cortex (Quintana and Fuster 1999). The task is a combination of delayed matching to sample and delayed conditioned discrimination. Each trial begins with the presentation of a color, the initial cue. Following a delay of 12 s, a second visual cue is given, and the animal is required to perform a manual choice that depends on both the first and the second cue; therefore, on the combination of two visual stimuli separated by time. Since each combination of the two stimuli – double contingency – determines whether the response after the delay will be to the left or to the right, the trial-initiating color (red, green, blue, or yellow) predicts with a given degree of probability (100% or 75%) the response direction.

In the prefrontal cortex, during performance of that double-contingency task, two broad categories of "memory cells" can be observed, that is, of cells with elevated discharge during the memory period (delay). The first respond with a different level of activation depending on the color of the initial cue; their discharge descends toward baseline level in the course of the delay. They seem to distinguish and remember the colors, and their discharge during that period seems to reflect the decay of working memory.

The second type of cells behave in the opposite way. Their firing during the delay is related to the direction of the approaching manual response, before it is prompted by the second cue. These cells appear to anticipate the response. They accelerate their firing as the delay advances. Moreover, the degree of acceleration varies in proportion to the certainty with which the animal can predict the direction of the response. Both types of cells, sensory-coupled and motor-coupled cells, are intermixed, and, therefore, it is not possible to identify a separate cortical topography for each of them. Thus, it seems that, during the delay, there is a transfer of information from sensory-memory cells to motor-set cells. More precisely, there appears to be a temporal transfer from one prefrontal network to another, both connected to the visual networks of posterior cortex (inferotemporal) and the motor networks downstream.

Attentive set

The other category of prefrontal units, those that seem to anticipate the action (Quintana and Fuster 1999), may be the substrate for the short-term activation of motor memory, that is, the converse of sensory working memory. Consequently, there seems to be a sensory and a motor short-term memory, one retrospective and the other prospective, the two complementing each other at the service of the frontal executive in the mediation of cross-temporal contingencies.

Active prospective memory is also the motor equivalent of sensory attention; it may be called "motor attention." It would be a function in some way related to, if not the same as, what has been termed the "memory of the future" (Ingvar 1985). The cellular manifestations of motor set acquire special significance in view of the neuropsychological evidence that the dorsolateral prefrontal cortex is profoundly implicated in the formulation and execution of plans of action. The motor-set cells would be the support for the frontal planning functions in the short-term.

The sustained activations of prefrontal cells in delay tasks are related to the field potentials observable in the human frontal cortex between mutually contingent and temporally separate events, especially the "contingent negative variation" or CNV. The accelerating cell activations of "set cells" are undoubtedly related to the "Bereitschaftspotential," or "readiness potential," which is another negative potential that takes place after the CNV, immediately preceding a pre-instructed motor act. These surface negative potentials, which appear over frontal cortex after a sensory stimulus and before an action that is contingent on it, probably reflect the activation of large neuronal populations involved in working memory and motor set.

To summarize, the ramping-up cells and the surface negative field potentials, in particular the "readiness potential," appear to be electrophysiological manifestations of attentive set, or motor attention, the prospective function of the dorsolateral prefrontal cortex. This would be attention focused on the action in preparation, in other words, focused in the representations of the actions about to take place. It is attention directed to the components of long-term motor memory that are activated successively for the execution of the behavior in progress. Those cells apparently predicting future actions indicate the presence of mechanisms in the dorsolateral prefrontal cortex preparing the motor apparatus for those actions. It is possible that such mechanisms result in the priming of lower motor structures (e.g., premotor cortex, basal ganglia, pyramidal system) for those actions.

The perception-action cycle

Finally, to conclude this chapter, a few considerations are in order regarding the mechanisms of functional coordination of working memory and attentive set, the two prefrontal functions mentioned above, in the temporal organization of behavior. What are the mechanisms by which the prefrontal cortex mediates the transfer of information from the past to the future and from the perception to the action? Undoubtedly, these mechanisms involve local transactions, as the two functional types of neighboring cells suggest, and also remote or transcortical processes, as some of our other cellular evidence suggests. Reentry or reverberation through recurrent circuits may play a role in both these kinds of processes, local and remote.

Several methods have been used with the purpose of testing the reentry hypothesis. First, an artificial network model was developed with an architecture that was profusely recurrent. We trained that model to "sample" an external input, to retain it in memory, and to elicit

Fig. 1 The cortical stages of the perception-action cycle. The *arrows* represent connections demonstrated anatomically in the non-human primate. (Schematic diagram of the human brain with color-coded representation of the sensory- and motor-processing hierarchies)

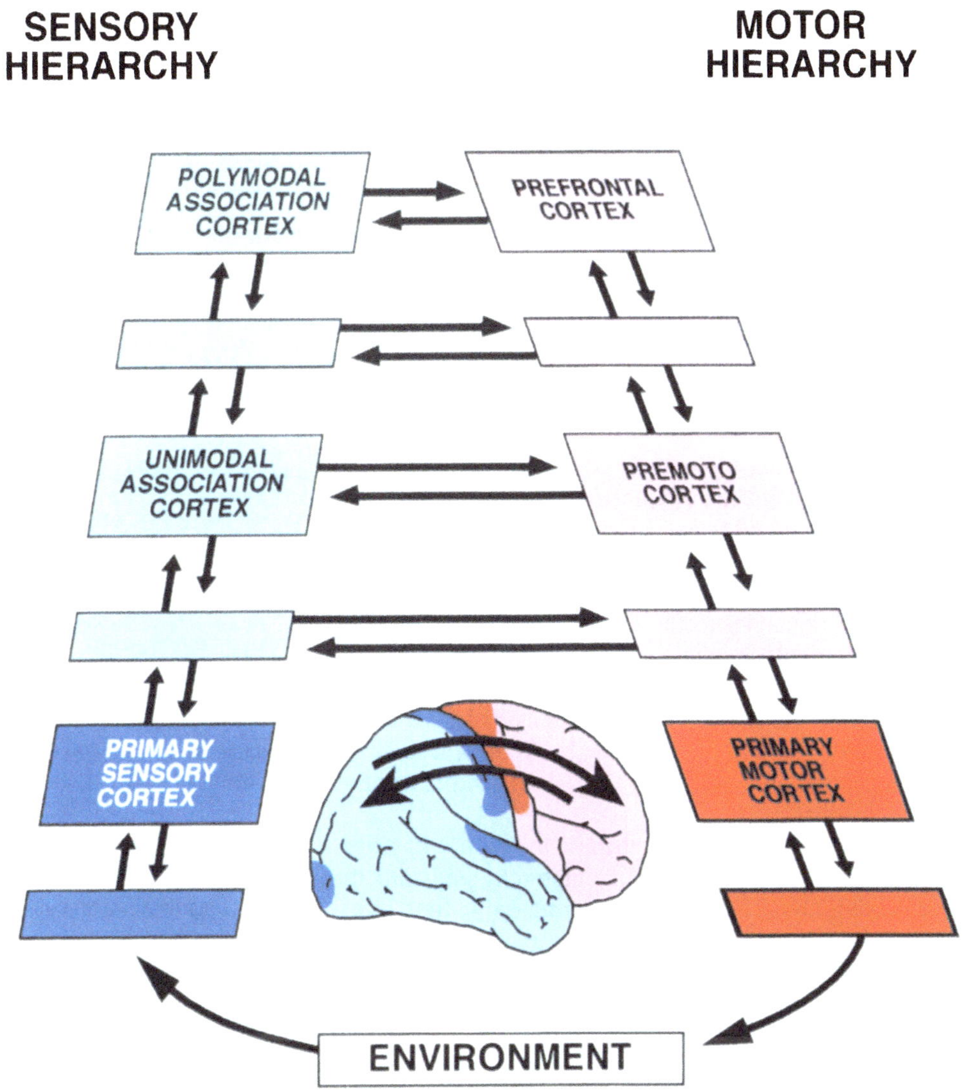

an output that was a specified function of the input (Zipser et al. 1993). To train the model, we used the back-propagation method. This is an error-reducing method allowing the network, through multiple iterations, to adjust synaptic weights to keep a stable relationship between input and output, despite fluctuations in the input. The weights stay fixed after the training has been completed, after the network has "learned."

In the fully trained network, a memory trial is simulated by loading an input, that is, the memorandum, and by holding a gate open through a memory period or delay until the recall, when another load signal closes the gate and emits the output. The output cells behave predictably and unremarkably, because they only reflect the input-output function specified by the modeler. Exceptionally remarkable, however, is the discharge of the internal or "hidden units" of the network. With appropriate scaling, these cells appear to behave like real cells in a delay-memory task. It can be concluded from this finding that the firing patterns of cortical cells are consistent with the sustained activation of fully trained recurrent networks with fixed and pre-established synaptic weights. Thus, the model supports the concept of reentry as a mechanism in the cortical dynamics of short-term memory.

The reentry mechanism in short-term memory is also supported by experiments with reversible cortical depression by cooling (Fuster et al. 1985). Monkeys were trained to perform a delayed matching task with colors. After the animals were trained, cooling probes and microelectrode carriers were implanted, bilaterally, on two cortical areas known to participate in the performance of that task, the dorsolateral prefrontal cortex and the inferotemporal cortex. While the animal performed the task, prefrontal or temporal cortex was cooled bilaterally, and units were concomitantly recorded from the noncooled cortex.

By cooling either inferotemporal or parietal cortex to 20°C, a reversible impairment is induced in the monkey's performance of the task. The procedure also modifies the spontaneous and memory – delay period – discharge of the cells in the other (non-cooled) cortex. Under normal conditions, some prefrontal and inferotemporal cells are differentially activated during the memorization of the color sample: they seem to prefer one color in short-term memory over the other colors in the same condition. Under cooling of the other, distant cortex, these cells show lesser differences in their color-related memory discharge; they differentiate less the colors in memory than when that cortex is at normal temperature. Therefore, it appears that, in the absence of input from the remote cortex (under cooling), neurons in both prefrontal and inferotemporal cortex are less active in the memorization of their preferred color. At the same time, the monkey is less able to retain the colors in short-term memory. This leads to the inference that short-term visual memory is maintained active by reentrant, reverberating, neuronal influences between inferotemporal and prefrontal cortices.

In broader neurobiological terms, the apparent recurrent excitation between the prefrontal cortex and the sensory association cortex can be viewed as a mechanism of temporal closure at the summit of the perception-action cycle. This cycle is the circular flow of neural processing linking the organism to the environment. Anatomically, the cycle basically consists of two parallel hierarchies of neural structures, one sensory and the other motor, which extend along the nerve axis from the spinal cord to the highest cortex of association (Fig. 1). At all levels, structures are interconnected reciprocally: by feedforward as well as feedback.

In new or recently learned behavior, sensory impulses are processed along the sensory hierarchy and into the motor hierarchy. That sensory information is thus translated into action, processed down the motor hierarchy to produce changes in the environment. Such changes elicit new sensory impulses, which are processed in the sensory hierarchy and then modulate further action, and so on. The posterior cortex of association and the dorsolateral prefrontal cortex are part of the processing cycle, if the behavior contains novelty or uncertainty, and has to bridge temporal gaps with short-term memory and attentive set; in other words, if it has to mediate cross-temporal contingencies. As the behavior becomes automatic (e.g., walking, skilled routines), the action is integrated in lower structures (e.g., premotor cortex, basal ganglia), and the processing is shunted at lower levels. This is probably why, with the over-learning of tasks that do not require working memory, metabolic activations disappear from the highest cortical levels of the perception-action cycle (Grafton et al. 1992; Raichle et al. 1994). At the top of the perception-action cycle, the dorsolateral prefrontal cortex integrates actions with perceptions, especially in situations marked by novelty, ambiguity, and complexity. In order to do it, the prefrontal cortex works in close cooperation with other areas of the neocortex and with subcortical structures in lower stages of the executive hierarchy.

References

Aguirre GK, Zarahn E, D'Esposito M (1998) Neural components of topographical representation. Proc Natl Acad Sci USA 95:839–846

Courtney SM, Ungerleider LG, Keil K, Haxby JV (1996) Object and spatial visual working memory activate separate neural systems in human cortex. Cereb Cortex 6:39–49

Funahashi S, Bruce CJ, Goldman-Rakic PS (1989) Mnemonic coding of visual space in the monkey's dorsolateral prefrontal cortex. J Neurophysiology 61:331–349

Fuster JM (1973) Unit activity in prefrontal cortex during delayed-response performance: neuronal correlates of transient memory. J Neurophysiol 36:61–78

Fuster JM (1997a) The prefrontal cortex anatomy: physiology and neuropsychology of the frontal lobe. Lippincott-Raven, Philadelphia

Fuster JM (1997b) Network memory. Trends Neurosci 20:451–459

Fuster JM, Bauer RH, Jervey JP (1982) Cellular discharge in the dorsolateral pefrontal cortes of the monkey in cognitive tasks. Exp Neurol 77:679–694

Fuster JM, Bauer RH, Jervey JP (1985) Functional interactions between inferotemporal and prefrontal cortex in a cognitive task. Brain Res 330:299–307

Gabrieli JDE, Poldrack RA, Desmond JE (1998) The role of left prefrontal cortex in language and memory. Proc Natl Acad Sci USA 95:906–913

Goldman-Rakic PS (1995) Architecture of the prefrontal and the central executive. Proc Natl Acad Sci USA 769:71–83

Grafton ST, Mazziotta JC, Woods RP, Phelps ME (1992) Human functional anatomy of visually guided finger movements. Brain 115:565–587

Ingvar DH (1985) "Memory of the future": an essay on the temporal organization of conscious awareness. Human Neurobiol 4:127–136

Niki H (1974) Differential activity of prefrontal units during right and left delayed response trials. Brain Res 70:346–349

Owen AM, Evans AC, Petrides M (1996) Evidence for a two-stage model of spatial working memory processing within the lateral frontal cortex: a positron emission tomography study. Cereb Cortex 6:31–38

Paulesu E, Frith CD, Frackowiak RSJ (1993) The neural correlates of the verbal component of working memory. Nature 362: 342–344

Petrides M, Pandya DN (1994) Comparative architectonic analysis of the human and the macaque frontal cortex. In: Boller F, Grafman J (eds) Handbook of neuropsychology. Elsevier, Amsterdam, pp 17–58

Petrides M, Alivisatos B, Evans AC, Meyer E (1993a) Dissociation of human mid-dorsolateral from posterior dorsolateral frontal cortex in memory processing. Proc Natl Acad Sci USA 90:873–877

Petrides M, Alivisatos B, Meyer E, Evans AC (1993b) Functional activation of the human frontal cortex during the performance of verbal working memory tasks. Proc Natl Acad Sci USA 90:878–882

Quintana J, Fuster J (1999) From perception to action: temporal integrative functions of prefrontal and parietal neurons. Cereb Cortex 9:213–221

Raichle ME, Fiez JA, Videen TO, MacLeod A-MK, Pardo JV, Fox PT, Petersen SE (1994) Practice-related changes in human brain functional anatomy during nonmotor learning. Cereb Cortex 4:8–26

Smith EE, Jonides J, Koeppe RA (1996) Dissociating verbal and spatial working memory using PET. Cereb Cortex 6:11–20

Swartz BE, Halgren E, Fuster JM, Simpkins F, Gee M, Mandelkern M (1995) Cortical metabolic activation in humans during a visual memory task. Cereb Cortex 3:205–214

Zipser D, Kehoe B, Littlewort G, Fuster J (1993) A spiking network model of short-term active memory. J Neurosci 13:3406–3420

Rüdiger J. Seitz · Klaus Martin Stephan
Ferdinand Binkofski

Control of action as mediated by the human frontal lobe

Published online: 16 May 2000

Abstract Conscious control of action involves the voluntary initiation and the continuous adjustment of motor activity. Neuroimaging data provide evidence that the plan for a movement is developed with respect to the behavioral context in prefrontal cortex, while the synergies of a motor program are coded by premotor cortex and the specific movement parameters by the motor cortex. It is suggested that the initiational aspects of conscious motor activity are implemented in a medial system of information flow and the integrative aspects in a lateral system of the human frontal lobe.

Key words Voluntary movement · Prefrontal cortex · Premotor cortex · Motor cortex · Functional neuroimaging

Introduction

The frontal lobe comprises the motor cortex, the premotor cortex, and the prefrontal cortex, which all contribute to executive functions. The executive functions can be conceptualized as a hierarchical system of action control comprising volition, planning, selection, programming, and performance of movement. An intentional system allows movements to be voluntarily selected and initiated. The intended movement has to be imbedded in the behavioral context and planned accordingly. Further, movement synergies have to be programmed to generate a desired action. Finally, movement parameters have to be specified in relation to the physical state of the subject to allow for automatic performance.

Neuroimaging methods open avenues to disentangle the cerebral structures involved in the different aspects underlying executive functions. Here, we were interested in three different processes of movement control. Using simple finger movements of both hands, we wished to identify the brain structures controlling bimanual actions. Specifically, subjects were required to adjust simultaneous or alternating movements with both hands in a self-paced manner to each other. In a second experiment, we were interested in mapping the cortical representations of movements in space. A third study aimed at identifying the cortical areas involved in temporal control of movements. We will describe that these motor-control tasks share common, but also involve different subareas of the premotor and prefrontal cortex in the human frontal lobe. These findings will be supplemented by studies in patients showing the critical importance of some of these subareas both for movement performance and recovery.

R.J. Seitz (✉) · K.M. Stephan · F. Binkofski
Department of Neurology, Heinrich-Heine-University Düsseldorf, Moorenstrasse 5, 40225 Düsseldorf, Germany
e-mail: seitz@neurologie.uni-duesseldorf.de
Tel.: +49-211-8118974, Fax: +49-211-8118485

Materials and methods

Subjects

Three groups of right-handed male volunteers (age range: 25–40 years), with no history of neurological illness, participated in functional magnetic resonance imaging (fMRI) studies. In addition, patients (age range: 39–66 years), with either a focal lesion of the mediofrontal wall area or after recovery from hemiplegic infarction in the middle cerebral-artery territory, were investigated. In the patients, cerebral activations were studied with measurements of the regional cerebral blood flow (rCBF) with positron emission tomography (PET). All of them gave an informed consent. The studies were approved by the Ethics Committee of the Heinrich-Heine-University, Düsseldorf. Right handedness was assessed by the Edinburgh Inventory (Oldfield 1971).

Behavioral tasks

In the first task, six healthy subjects and two patients with ventral frontomedial-wall lesions were required to perform tapping movements of their index fingers on the thumb. Movements were performed with both hands either simultaneously (in-phase) and alternating (anti-phase), respectively. The control condition was rest. Eyes were closed in all conditions. Details of the kinematic behavior and of imaging data are given by Stephan et al. (1999a).

In a second task, six subjects had to perform four different motor-imagery conditions. In one condition, they were asked to imagine moving their outstretched right index finger at a rate of 0.5 Hz, while having their hands and arms relaxed and their eyes closed. In this movement, the tip of the index finger described a spatial trajectory of a double circle. In a second condition, the subjects imagined the same movement of the right index finger, but were required to imagine that it followed a visual target while having their eyes closed. During the scan, no target was presented; however, before the scan, the subjects had become acquainted with pursuing the bicircular path of the target with their right index finger. In the third condition, the subjects were asked to imagine themselves, with their eyes closed, from a third person's perspective lying in the fMRI scanner and moving the right index finger following the target. In the final condition, the subjects had to imagine the light point moving on the screen with their eyes closed. They were asked to imagine the path of the moving target, but not to imagine themselves to perform any movement. During the control period, they were asked to avoid any imagery while having their eyes closed.

In a third task, eight healthy subjects were required to tap with their right index finger on an electrical switch to acoustic tones. The pacing metronome tones were generated using a sine-wave generator at a frequency of 1000 Hz with a plateau time of 50 ms and presented through a loudspeaker. In the isochronous condition, the tones were presented every 1250 ms. In two further conditions, the intervals of the pacing tones were modulated following a cosine-wave pattern with a period of four samples and a time span of 30 ms and 200 ms, respectively. The tapping movements were recorded via the switch at a sampling rate of 1000 Hz and stored on a computed for off-line analysis.

Finally, seven patients who had recovered from their first hemiparetic stroke were required to perform sequential finger movements with their recovered hand while being blindfolded. The clinical, electrophysiological, and imaging data of the patients have been detailed elsewhere (Seitz et al. 1998). Here, the cortical areas related to motor control compared with rest shall be addressed. The finger-movement sequence consisted of successive tapping of the thumb on the second to fifth finger and backwards with one hand.

Functional imaging

Functional magnetic resonance imaging (fMRI) of cerebral blood oxygen-level dependent signal changes was performed on a Siemens 1.5T scanner with a gradient booster and standard rf coil, as described in detail elsewhere (Binkofski et al. 1999; Stephan et al. 1999a). Contiguous horizontal slices parallel to the intercommissural line with a thickness of 4.4 mm were acquired every 3 s using echoplanar imaging sequences (TE=66 ms, α=90°). The field of view was 200×200 pixels in a 64×64 matrix. In-plane resolution of the image slices was 3.12×3.12 mm. The image slices covered the dorsal part of the brain above the internal capsule. Each experiment consisted of 50 images representing five alternating control-active pairs allowing ten images for each epoch. In addition, anatomical imaging was performed using volumetric three-dimensional T1-weighted high contrast sequences.

Measurements of the rCBF using PET were performed on a SIEMENS ECAT+ and an eight-ring GE/SCANDITRONIX PC4096 plus PET camera, respectively. PET scanning was performed as described in detail elsewhere following intravenous bolus injection of [^{15}O]-butanol (Herzog et al. 1996; Seitz et al. 1998; Stephan et al. 1999a). A transmission scan using a rotating ^{68}Ge pin source was obtained prior to the emission scans to correct for attenuation. The PET images were reconstructed with a Hanning filter to an effective image resolution (FWHM) of 8 mm. Quantitation of the rCBF was performed with a combined dynamic-autoradiographic approach (Herzog et al. 1996).

The fMRI data were analyzed off-line using SPM96 software of the Leopold Müller Functional Imaging Laboratory, London. After correction for head movements and signal-intensity variation, images were normalized spatially into stereotactic space and smoothed with an 8 mm isotropic Gaussian kernel. Thereafter, group analysis of the data was performed. Significance was assessed using the delayed box-car reference function of the SPM96 software. Pixels were considered significant when they had a correlation of their time series with the reference function exceeding a Z-score of 2.66 (corresponding to $P<0.01$). In addition, activated areas were required to reach a cluster threshold of 0.05 (corrected for resolution elements). The PET image data of the patients were analyzed with SPM96 and the computerized brain atlas, respectively. In the latter approach, all brain lesions were reoriented to the left side during the spatial standardization procedure, as detailed elsewhere (Seitz et al. 1998). Thereafter, t-maps were thresholded corresponding to $P<0.01$ and a cluster criterion to correct for autocorrelation of adjacent pixels corresponding to $P<0.05$, corrected for image resolution (Wunderlich et al. 1997). For visualization, the loci of the peak activations were superimposed onto the lateral brain template of the atlas of Talairach and Tournoux (1988).

Results

Control of bilateral movements

Sequential index-finger-to-thumb opposition movements can be performed easily by healthy subjects and have been shown to activate the motor cortex and the supplementary motor area (Seitz and Roland 1992a; Shibasaki et al. 1993). Bilateral finger movements can also be performed easily when they are being performed simultaneously (in-phase) in a mirror-like fashion. The task becomes far more complicated when the same movements have to be performed alternatively with both hands (anti-phase). The comparison of anti-phase to in-phase movements showed that co-ordination of bilateral index-to-thumb tapping movements is especially dependent on ventral and dorsal medial-wall areas, including the supplementary motor area and the cingulate motor area, as well as on the dorsolateral premotor cortex (Stephan et al. 1999b). The stereotactic coordinates of these areas are given in Table 1. A similar activation pattern was found when parallel performance of sequential finger movements of both hands was compared with mirrored performance (Sadato et al. 1997). Figure 1 demonstrates the cortical network involved in phase control of bimanual movements. In this figure, the hypothetical anatomic connections among these areas are depicted. As became evident by the patients, lesions in the ventromedial wall area around the cingulate sulcus interfere with bimanual synchrony and induce a pathological facilitation of associated movements (Stephan et al. 1999a). This area probably corresponds to the cingulate motor area, which was shown to be activated in signal-triggered and self-paced movements in the monkey (Shima et al. 1991). In contrast, the patients with lesions in this part of the ventromedial cingulate had no problems with the early stages of motor planning, including selecting the appropriate action in response to sensory cues which is characteristic for patients with lesions of the more dorsally located supplementary motor area (Halsband and Freund 1990). The impaired bimanual phase control induced by a cingulate lesion appeared to be due to its strategic location, which probably interfered with the transcallosal connections of the homologue cingulate areas (Fig. 1). Thus, it

Table 1 Activation loci in frontal lobe related to movement control. Coordinates in stereotactic space (x, y, z in mm) of Talairach and Tournoux (1988). *PMC* Premotor cortex, *SMA* supplementary motor area, *CMA* cingulate motor area

PMC	SMA	CMA	Anterior cingulate	Prefrontal
Bimanual finger movements:				
Bilateral (Dorsal) 39, –9, 50	Bilateral 2, –4, 60	Bilateral 8, –8, 38		
Imagery of spatial movements of right index finger:				
Bilateral (Dorsal) 39, –10, 50	Bilateral 5, –2, 50	Left 5, –8, 38	Right 8, 12, 36	
(Ventral) 57, 3, 31				
(Opercular) 56, 8, 11				
Irregularly paced right index-finger tapping:				
Left (Dorsal) 33, –3, 47			Right 3, 18, 42	Bilateral 42, 30, 33
Bilateral (Opercular) 51, 16, 3				
Finger movement sequences with recovered hand:				
Bilateral (Dorsal) 29, –1, 47	Left 8, 1, 47		Left 9, 16, 33	Left 24, 50, 11

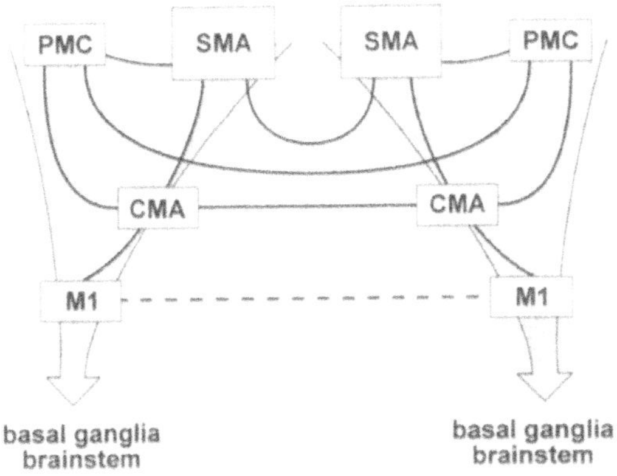

Fig. 1 Scheme of the bihemispheric cortical network related to control of bimanual anti-phase compared with in-phase index-finger-to-thumb tapping movements in healthy subjects. *CMA* Cingulate motor area, *M1* primary motor area, *PMC* premotor cortex, *SMA* supplementary motor area

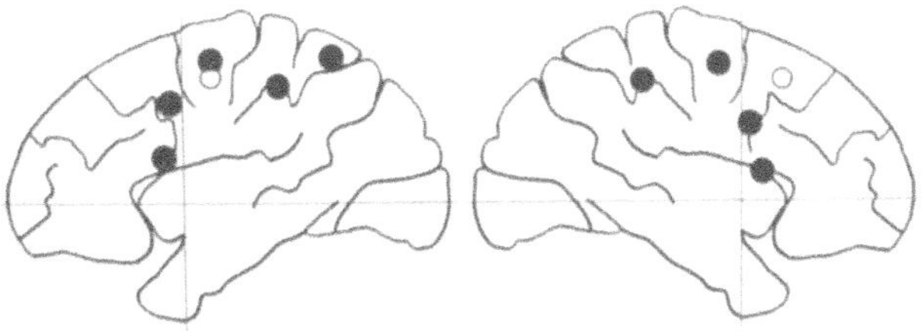

Fig. 2 Cortical activations (*filled circles*) related to imagery of motion trajectories on the lateral prospect of the human brain, as compared with rest in healthy volunteers. Activations are plotted into Talairach and Tournoux (1988) space. *Open circles* Activations of right anterior cingulate and left supplementary motor area

can be speculated that the greater activation related to anti-phase movements in premotor cortex than that related to in-phase movements (Table 1) assisted the interhemispheric coordination of the movements, which crucially depended on the integrity of the cingulate and ventral supplementary motor area.

These results are augmented by recent findings by Fink et al. (1999), who studied out-of-phase movements of the two hands during incongruent proprioceptive and visual feedback compared with in-phase movements of the two hands. The authors observed a specific activation of the caudal dorsolateral prefrontal cortex with a clear right-sided predominance during anti-phase movements of both hands (Fink et al. 1999). This activation was ascribed to the subjects' intention to cope with the conflict of their senses during task performance. In contrast to our observations, the activations of the medial wall areas and of the dorsolateral premotor cortex were canceled out in the study design by Fink et al. (1999).

Control of spatial movements

During imagery and performance of trajectorial finger movements as compared with rest, the lateral premotor cortex became activated in a topographically differential manner. The stereotactic locations of the activation areas are summarized in Table 1 and illustrated on the lateral aspect of the brain (Fig. 2). During imagery of index-finger movements that followed an eight-shaped trajectory, two different sub-fields of premotor cortex were activated in association with anterior and posterior parietal cortical areas lining the intraparietal sulcus (Fig. 2). The frontal activations were localized bilaterally in a dorsal and ventral location of the lateral premotor cortex, the supplementary motor area, and the left cingulate motor area. In addition, there was an activation in the right anterior cingulate gyrus (Table 1). These activations corresponded to similar findings by Kawashima et al. (1994), Grafton et al. (1996), and Seitz et al. (1997) during actual execution of graphomotor trajectories as well as during pointing and reaching movements. During imagery of motion from an observer's perspective, there were additional activation areas bilaterally in the opercular part of the premotor cortex (Table 1). Imagery of target motion activated the right opercular premotor cortex, an area also activated during recognition of gestures and finger-movement sequence learning (Seitz and Roland 1992a; Bonda et al. 1993; Parsons et al. 1995; Rauch et al. 1995). On the contrary, imagery of a third-party finger motion activated the left opercular premotor cortex, as did recognition of tactually explored objects (Binkofski et al. 1999). The lateralization of these opercular activations was also significant in direct comparison of these two imagery tasks. Interestingly, all imagery conditions related to imagery of one's own movements engaged the left supplementary motor area and the right cingulate cortex, whereas imagery of target motion which did not involve movements of one's own fingers did not engage these medial wall areas. Notably, there were no activations in the visual motion area (Watson et al. 1993; Tootell et al. 1995; Goebel et al. 1998). The lack of activation of the visual motion area in this group study was due to the limited field of view, which did not cover this part of the brain in all subjects.

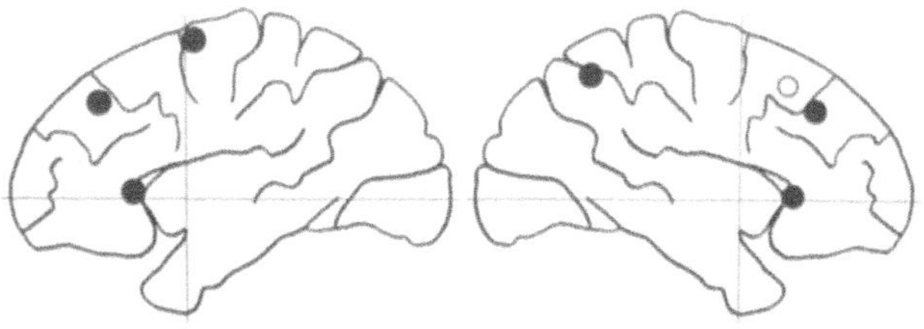

Fig. 3 Cortical activation areas (*filled circles*) related to conscious, metronome-paced finger tapping in healthy volunteers. Metronome pacing was modulated at a time span of 200 ms, while, in the control condition, the pacing of the finger movements was modulated at a time span of 30 ms, which meant that the subjects were not aware of the metronome modulation. *Open circle* Activation of the right anterior cingulate. Not shown are the activation areas in the left cerebellum. Activations are plotted into Talairach and Tournoux (1988) space

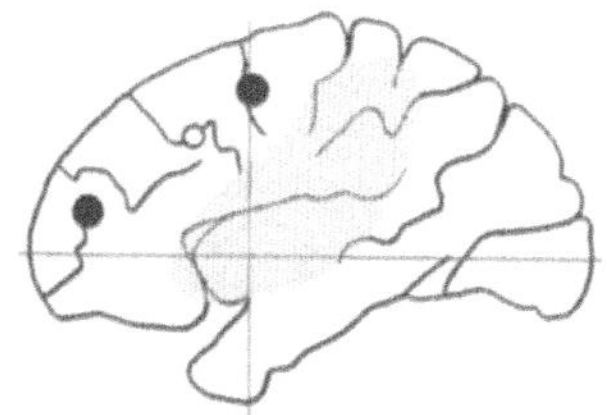

Fig. 4 Prefrontal and premotor activations during sequential finger movements of the recovered hand compared with rest in patients after hemiparetic stroke. The activation of the supplementary motor area and of the contralesional premotor cortex project behind the ipsilesional premotor activation. The common stroke lesion involving the pre- and postcentral gyrus and the periinsular cortex is indicated by the *stippled area*. Activations are plotted into Talairach and Tournoux (1988) space

Temporal control of movements

The cortical-activation patterns related to acoustically cued finger movements are shown in Fig. 3. They were critically affected by the awareness of the subjects regarding the temporal characteristics of the pacing tone. The subjects were required to tap to a metronome, while – unknown to the subjects – the metronome beat was modulated. When the deviation from isochrony was in the range of 30 ms, the subjects were not aware of this modulation, but their tapping behavior became more irregular. At a modulation of the beat in the range of 200 ms, all subjects were aware of the kind of modulation and changed their behavior consciously. Specifically, they switched their anticipatory tapping observed during isochrony to a fully aware stimulus-response pattern. During the modulation of 200 ms compared with the 30 ms modulation, the activations involved the dorsolateral prefrontal cortex, the dorsolateral premotor cortex, as well as the inferior parietal cortex close to the intraparietal sulcus, and left cerebellum. The cortical activation pattern was clearly different from the other conditions, as can be seen in Table 1. At the medial cerebral surface, an activation area in the right anterior cingulate was evident, which corresponded to the right cingulate activation during imagery of movement trajectories. The prefrontal activations corresponded to activation areas of similar location during awareness of sensory-information processing (Fink et al. 1999; McIntosh et al. 1999). Clearly, these activations coincided with the peak activations in a number of studies focusing on response conflict, on an incompatible stimulus response situation, on the response to task novelty, and on monitoring tasks manipulating working memory (Duncan and Owen 2000). In this meta-analysis, also anterior cingulate activations were found, showing the importance of the anterior cingulate for conscious behavior. Remarkably, in our study, there was a clear right hemispheric predominance of the prefrontal and premotor activations, which corresponded to the observation by Fink et al. (1999). This receptive right-hemispheric dominance seems to have its counterpart in the left-hemispheric activation during associative conscious syntactic processing (McIntosh et al. 1999).

Figure 4 shows that the prefrontal cortex also plays an important role during movement execution after recovery from hemiparetic stroke. This figure shows activations in the patients performing a simple finger-movement sequence with their recovered hand compared with rest. The activations occurred adjacent to the stroke lesions, which extended from the dorsolateral part of the precentral and postcentral gyrus down to the peri-insular cortex, but spared the internal capsule and the thalamus. The activations were observed bilaterally in the dorsal premotor cortex, the supplementary motor area, the anterior cingulate, and the prefrontal cortex on the left (Table 1). The activations of the dorsolateral premotor cortex and the supplementary motor area occurred in typical locations similar to other movement tasks. However, the prefrontal activation was more ventral and rostral than in the healthy subjects during tapping to a frequency-modulated metronome (Table 1, Fig. 3). The greater activation of the ipsilesional prefrontal cortex in the stroke patients than in the healthy subjects during performance of unilateral finger-movement sequences can be interpreted in the light of conscious monitoring of the action performed. Since the patients needed to focus on their performance, which remained slightly abnormal compared with healthy volunteers (Seitz et al. 1999), they engaged prefrontal cortex. The interesting aspect of this observation is that patients with a circumscribed brain lesion affecting the sensorimotor system engage for a simple task a comparable control strategy as normal people do under enhanced task difficulty.

Discussion

Our studies aimed at exploring the role of premotor and prefrontal cortex for conscious control of action. As summarized in Table 1, we showed that the dorsal premotor cortex became engaged in relation to all types of finger movements studied, while the opercular part appeared to code more complex spatial and temporal movement characteristics. The ventral premotor cortex was only activated in spatial movement control. The supplementary motor area and the cingulate motor area appeared to be co-activated in relation to intentional and imagined movement generation. Prefrontal cortex and the anterior cingulate were engaged in situations when subjects had to bring their movement activity in register with additional constraints. These data will be discussed according to the established parcellation of the motor areas in the human frontal lobe.

Parcellation of the frontal lobe

Motor cortex

The human motor cortex is physiologically characterized by a low threshold for electrical stimulation, by which twitching of single or groups of muscles can be elicited with a gross somatotopic organization of head, trunk, and limb muscles (Foerster 1936). Recent evidence in non-human primates substantiates earlier observations by Penfield and Boldrey (1937) showing that, within topographic areas, there is a considerable spatial overlap of neuronal populations projecting to different muscles as, for example, to intrinsic hand muscles of different fingers (Schieber and Hibbard 1993; Stepniewska et al. 1993). In correspondence, recent neuroimaging observations suggest that this intermingled organization of finger-movement representations is also present in human motor cortex (Sanes et al. 1995; Kleinschmidt et al. 1997). Thus, motor cortex appears to effect movement by driving groups of muscles with different synergistic and kinematic specifications (Georgopoulos et al. 1982, 1992, 1993). The phylogenetic increase of corticospinal neurons projecting from motor cortex to the intermediate part and the ventral horn of the spinal cord represents the substrate for the unprecedented individualization of digit movements in humans (Bortoff and Strick 1993; He et al. 1993). Conversely, damage to the corticospinal neurons and the cortical spinal tract impair or even abolish fractionated finger movements as well as grip-force production in a related fashion (Binkofski et al. 1996; Pendlebury et al. 1999).

In the studied presented in this report, movement activity was present both in the specific activation and in the control conditions. Thus, activations related to basic motor control were canceled out in the direct comparisons between both conditions.

Premotor cortex

The cortical area bordering the motor cortex rostrally on the precentral gyrus and in the depth of the precentral sulcus along the entire medio-dorsal dimension of the precentral gyrus is composed by a number of subareas, which can be differentiated on the basis of their cytoarchitectonic and electrophysiological characteristics as well as by their afferent and efferent connections (Wise 1991). As was shown in non-human primates, the premotor cortical areas comprise area F3 (supplementary motor area) and area F6 (pre-supplementary motor area) on the medial hemispheric surface (Luppino et al. 1991; Matelli et al. 1991; Tanji 1994). Areas F2, F4, and F5 are located on the cerebral convexity (Gentilluci et al. 1988), while area F7, which probably includes the location for the supplementary eye field (Schlag and Schlag-Rey 1987), is located in the dorsolateral aspect frontally adjacent to area F2 (Rizzolatti et al. 1998). From these areas, electrical stimulation can evoke movements at higher thresholds than from motor cortex, and the elicited movements have a complex appearance such as, for instance, the fighter posturing upon stimulation of the medial brain surface (Foerster 1936). Subareas F2–F5 receive intensive input from the parietal cortex in a topographically highly organized fashion related to spatial characteristics of movement (Godschalk et al. 1984; Hummelsheim et al. 1988; Fogassi et al. 1992; di Pelligrino and Wise 1993). In the dorsolateral premotor cortical areas F2 and F4, purposeful synergies are coded, with the more dorsal parts conveying proximal movements and the more ventral lateral cortical portions conveying more distal movements (Weinrich et al. 1984; Rizzolatti et al. 1988, 1990; Jeannerod et al. 1995). In our experiment on imagery of movement trajectories, we found activations of three different portions of the lateral aspect of the premotor cortex as well as anterior parietal activations along the intraparietal sulcus (Fig. 2). These data show that the mental representation of movement is sufficient to engage the cortical areas engaged for coding motor acts, even in absence of movement. Area F5 appears to be particular, since it comprises so-called mirror neurons (Gallese et al. 1996). These neurons exhibit reactivity towards movement-related sensory stimuli when the monkey observes a particular movement and also in an identical fashion when the monkey performs this movement himself. The activations of the posterior portion of the inferior frontal cortex related to imagery of motion from an oberserver's perspective or of a target suggests that the opercular premotor cortex codes abstract movement concepts, which are also relevant for motor learning and recognition of gestures (Seitz and Roland 1992a; Bonda et al. 1993; Parsons et al. 1995).

The supplementary motor area (F3), which has a prominent corticospinal projection (Dum and Strick 1991; Galea and Darian-Smith 1994) and is the origin of the corticoreticulospinal tract in non-human primates (Keizer and Kuypers 1989), appears to play a significant role for movement sequencing (Gaymard et al. 1993) and for limb posturing during an intended act involving bilateral limbs (Brinkmann 1984; Massion et al. 1989; Luppino et al. 1991; Kozennikov et al. 1994). In the studies presented here, we observed activations of the supplementary motor area during motor imagery, acoustically cued right index-finger apping, and performance of sequential finger movements in patients who had recovered from hemiparetic stroke (Table 1). These data accord with a large number of studies showing activation of the supplementary motor area, particularly under enhanced task difficulty (Shibasaki et al. 1993; Jahanshahi et al. 1995; Seitz et al. 1997). Furthermore, we found that the more ventral aspects of the supplementary motor area were active during bimanual, anti-phase finger tapping, reflecting the impact of this area of the control of bilateral limb movements (Lang et al. 1990). From the supplementary motor area, there are intense projections to the basal ganglia, linking the basal ganglia to neuronal processes underlying limb- and eye-movement initation (Alexander et al. 1986; Mink and Thach 1993; Petit et al. 1993). In Parkinson's disease, the supplementary motor area has been shown to be less active than in healthy controls, reflecting the problem of movement initiation in this condition (Jahanshahi et al. 1995). The more rostral subareas F6 and F7 do not receive afference from parietal cortex, but rather massive input from the prefrontal areas (Luppino et al. 1990). Therefore, they do no appear to be related to sensory-guided movement control, but to a higher aspect of action control. Deiber et al. (1991) reported that selection of movement specifically activates the fronto-mesial cortex anterior to the frontal plane through the anterior commissure, probably including the pre-supplementary motor area. Since in none of our tasks was selection of movement required, we did not observe pre-SMA activations.

Prefrontal cortex

The prefrontal cortex is engaged in controlling executive functions (Fuster 1993). It is well-established that neurons in the dorsolateral prefrontal cortex around the principle sulcus mediate cue-directed actions, such as spatially directed saccades in delay-response paradigms (Funahashi et al. 1989). Recent evidence was obtained showing that object-related information and spatial-related information of visual stimuli, which are processed along different routes in the occipital-temporal and occipital-parietal pathways, respectively, are integrated in area 9 in the prefrontal cortex (Rao et al. 1997a). These data suggest that, in the dorsolateral prefrontal cortex, pre-processed contents of present perception and of previous experience about the external world become relevant for behavior. In correspondence to this suggestion, we found a strong prefrontal activation in healthy subjects when they consciously adjusted their motor behavior to a temporally modulated acoustic stimulus (Fig. 3). Similarly, prefrontal activation occurred in neurological patients, who performed a sequential motor task that required conscious monitoring of performance (Fig. 4). Specifically, behavior-related actions were made possible by prefrontal cortex, such that knowledge about the external targets or events was being kept online until the adequate action was performed. As evident from human lesion studies, patients with lesions of prefrontal cortex have difficulties in planning actions in a complex behavioral context (Goel et al. 1997). In the light of our findings, one can speculate that such patients have difficulties in adapting their motor actions to external events. Apparently, the disturbances exhibit hemispheric differences: right frontal-cortex lesions induce spatial hemineglect and interfere with voluntary movements or at least distort movement sequences (Heilman et al. 1985), while left prefrontal and left premotor lesions have been shown to induce semantic and syntactic language impairments as well as limb apraxia (Freund and Hummelsheim 1985; Friederici et al. 1997).

The prominent engagement of the dorsolateral prefrontal cortical areas during conscious behavior (Table 1) and of the medial parietal cortex during fixation (Heide et al. 1999) should be regarded in the light of a recent report by Shulmann et al. (1997), in which it was shown that these areas are predominantly activated during control conditions, but less active during visual-activation tasks. Similarly, during a first PET-scanning condition, these areas and medial prefrontal and lateral parietal cortical areas had a higher regional cerebral metabolism than later scans when the subjects had become fully aware of the scanning conditions (Seitz and Roland 1992b; Stapleton et al. 1997). In motor-learning tasks, a prominent involvement of prefrontal areas was observed during the early stage of skill acquisition, as compared with a simple motor task in the control condition (Jenkins et al. 1994; Shadmer and Holcomb 1997; Sakai et al. 1998). It is likely that the performance of the simple task in the control condition led to a similar behav-

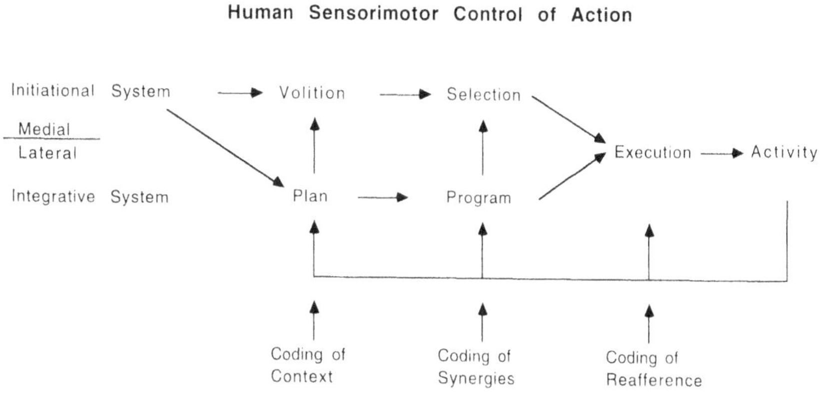

Fig. 5 Schematic view of control of action as mediated by the frontal cortex in humans

ioral state of the different subjects. In comparison, during the so-called resting state, prefrontal cortical areas are probably engaged to a very heterogeneous degree among the subjects, which may result from individual differences in monitoring the situation and in strategy of coping with the experimental situation. Consequently, a common engagement of prefrontal cortex was not possible during studies using rest as a control condition (Seitz and Roland 1992a; Shibasaki et al. 1993; Kawashima et al. 1994; Jahanshahi et al. 1995; Sadato et al. 1997). This explanation is substantiated by the observation that, during delayed-response conditions, the hemodynamic response curves in even-related fMRI are polyphasic and different among different cortical areas due to differences in timing and engagement of information processing (D'Esposito et al. 1997; Menon and Kim 1999).

Cingulate gyrus

In any discussion about the frontal lobe, the cingulate gyrus has to be mentioned, although it is considered to be part of the limbic cortex (Devinsky et al. 1995). The anterior cingulate cortex anterior to the frontal plane through the anterior commissure has been shown by a number of neuroimaging studies to be significantly activated during conscious selection of action in response to divergent cues (Pardo et al. 1990; George et al. 1994). More recently, evidence was presented suggesting that this activity is not related to the impeding behavior, but to error detection as such (Carter et al. 1998). We observed activation of the anterior cingulate during motor imagery (Seitz et al. 1997; Fig. 2) and during conscious tapping to an acoustic stimulus (Table 1 , Fig. 3). The relevance of the rostral cingulate cortex for behavior can also be appreciated from the neurological abnormalities following brain damage. Bilateral damage of the medial prefrontal cortex and the adjacent cingulate gyrus results in severe akinesia, while unilateral lesions of this sort induce the transient "alien hand syndrome" (Feinberg et al. 1992). In this condition, the contralesional hand feels alien and moves purposelessly around, being unresponsive to conscious selection of action as long as the hand is out of sight.

It should be noted that the activation of the midportion of the cingulate in healthy volunteers performing bilateral finger movements as well as motor imagery was in a more caudal position, ventrally adjacent to the supplementary motor area (Table 1) and probably including the cingulate motor area, which accommodates corticospinal projections (Dum and Strick 1991; Shima et al. 1991; Tanji 1994). Accordingly, bimanual phase coordination was disturbed in patients with lesions of the midportion of the cingulate (Stephan et al. 1999a). Figure 1 shows that the bihemispheric interactions necessary for bilateral limb coordination are multifold. However, a focal lesion of the cingulate motor area is sufficient to interrupt cross-talk of the right and left motor cortex, leading to decoupling of bilateral motor acts.

Conclusions

Figure 5 shows a hypothetical and simplistic scheme of information flow in the medial and lateral portions of prefrontal and premotor cortex related to control of motor behavior. The figure suggests that the cortical areas on the lateral aspects of the brain are engaged with the integration of external information. Sensory information is processed at different levels, allowing for influence on behavior with the highest level of abstraction in the prefrontal cortex. Accordingly, the lateral premotor cortical areas code how to act in response to perceptual cues, but also of what to do in relation to cue-movement associations (Halsband and Freund 1990; Jeannerod et al. 1995). The medial information stream subserves the initiation of movement from the internal world of the acting subject. The medial premotor subareas F6 and F7 are engaged during selection and internal generation of motor acts (Kurata and Wise 1988; Lang et al. 1990; Deiber et al. 1991; Rao et al. 1997b). Due to the massive input from the prefrontal cortex (Luppino et al. 1990), this initiative route stands under the continuous influence of information from the external world, which allows for strategic selection of action and goal-directed selection of movement. It must be emphasized that, at this stage, cortico-subcortical connections have not been included into this scheme of cortical information flow for reasons of simplicity. Nevertheless, the intense cortico-striatal loop is acknowledged for its supposed role for movement preparation, as evident from animal experiment and studies in patients with Parkinskon's disease (Alexander et al. 1986; Mink and Thach 1993). Similarly, subcortical feedback loops through the cerebellum allow for automatic adaptation of movement execution to imposed perturbations (Allen and Tsukahara 1974; Mai et al. 1988; Flament et al. 1996).

Acknowledgements The work presented in the article was supported by the Sonderforschungsbereich 194 of the Deutsche Forschungsgemeinschaft.

References

Alexander GE, DeLong MR, Strick PL (1986) Parallel organization of functionally segregated circuits linking basal ganglia and cortex. Annu Rev Neurosci 9:357–381

Allen GI, Tsukahara N (1974) Cerebrocerebellar communication systems. Physiol Rev 54:957–1006

Binkofski F, Seitz RJ, Arnold S, Claßen J, Benecke R, Freund H-J (1996) Thalamic metabolism and integrity of the pyramidal tract determine motor recovery in stroke. Ann Neurol 39:460–470

Binkofski F, Buccino G, Posse S, Seitz RJ, Rizzolatti G, Freund H-J (1999) A fronto-parietal circuit for object manipulation in man. Evidence from an fMRI-study. Eur J Neurosci 11:3276–3286

Bonda E, Petrides M, Frey S, Evans A (1995) Neural correlates of mental transformations of the body-in-space. Proc Natl Acad Sci USA 92:11180–11184

Bortoff GA, Strick PL (1993) Corticospinal terminations in two new-world primates: further evidence that corticomotoneuronal connections provide part of the neural substrate for manual dexterity. J Neurosci 13:5105–5118

Brinkman C (1984) Supplementary motor area of the monkey's cerebral cortex: short- and long-term deficits after unilateral ablation and the effects of subsequent callosal sections. J Neurosci 4:918–929

Carter CS, Braver TS, Barch DM, Botvinick MM, Noll D, Cohen JD (1998) Anterior cingulate cortex, error detection, and online monitoring of performance. Science 280:747–749

Deiber MP, Passingham RE, Colebatch JG, Friston KJ, Nixon PD, Frackowiak RSJ (1991) Cortical areas and the selection of movement: a study with positron emission tomography. Exp Brain Res 84:392–402

D'Esposito M, Aguirre GK, Zarahn E, Ballard D (1997) Functional MRI studies of spatial and non-spatial working memory. Cogn Brain Res 7:1–13

Devinsky O, Morrell M J, Vogt BA (1995) Contributions of anterior cingulate cortex to behaviour. Brain 118:279–306

Dum RP, Strick PL (1991) The origin of corticospinal projection from the premotor areas in the frontal lobe. J Neurosci 11:667–689

Duncan J, Owen A (2000) Dissociative methods in the study of frontal lobe function. In: Monsell S, Driver J (eds) Attention and performance XVIII. MIT Press, Cambridge (in press)

Feinberg TE, Schindler RJ, Flanagan NG, Haber LD (1992) The alien hand syndrome. Neurology 42:19–24

Fink GR, Marshall JC, Halligan PW, Frith CD, Driver J, Frackowiak RSJ, Dolan RJ (1999) The neural consequences of conflict between intention and the senses. Brain 122:497–512

Flament D, Ellermann JM, Kim S-G, Ugurbil K, Ebner TJ (1996) Functional magnetic resonance imaging of cerebellar activation during the learning of a visuomotor dissociation task. Hum Brain Map 4:210–226

Fogassi L, Gallese V, Pellegrino G di (1992) Space coding by premotor cortex. Exp Brain Res 89:686–690

Foerster O (1936) Motorische Felder und Bahnen. In: Bumke O, Foerster O (eds) Handbuch Neurology, Vol 6. Allgemeine Neurologie. Springer, Berlin. pp 1–357

Freund H-J, Hummelsheim H (1985) Lesions of premotor cortex in man. Brain 108:697–733

Friederici AD (1997) Autonomy of syntactic processing and the role of Broca's area. Behav Brain Sci 19:634–635

Funahashi S, Bruce CJ, Goldman-Rakic PS (1989) Mnemonic coding of visual space in the monkey's dorsolateral prefrontal cortex. J Neurophysiol 61:331–349

Fuster JM (1993) Frontal lobes. Curr Opin Neurobiol 3:160–165

Galea MP, Darian-Smith I (1994) Multiple corticospinal neuron populations in the macaque monkey are specified by their unique cortical origins, spinal terminations, and connections. Cereb Cortex 4:166–194

Gallese V, Fadiga L, Fogassi L, Rizzolatti G (1996) Action recognition in the premotor cortex. Brain 119:593–609

Gaymard B, Rivaud S, Pierrot-Deseilligny C (1993) Role of the left and right supplementary motor areas in memory-guided saccade sequences. Ann Neurol 34:404–406

George MS, Ketter TA, Parekh PI, Rosinsky N, Ring H, Casey BJ, Trimble MR, Horwitz B, Herscovitch P, Post RM (1994) Regional brain activity when selecting a response despite interference: an $H_2{}^{15}O$ PET study of the Stroop and an emotional Stroop. Hum Brain Map 1:194–209

Georgopoulos AP, Kalaska JF, Caminiti R, Massey JT (1982) On the relations between the direction of two-dimensional arm movements and cell discharge in primate motor cortex. J Neurosci 2:1527–1537

Georgopoulos AP, Ashe J, Smyrnis N, Taira M (1992) The motor cortex and the coding of force. Science 256:1692–1695

Georgopoulos AP, Taira M, Lukashin A (1993) Cognitive neurophysiology of the motor cortex. Science 260:47–52

Gentilucci M, Fogassi L, Luppino G (1988) Functional organization of inferior area 6 in the macaque monkey. I. Somatotopy and the control of proximal movements. Exp Brain Res 71:475–490

Godschalk M, Lemon RN, Kuypers HGJM, Ronday HK (1984) Cortical afferents and efferents of monkey postarcuate area: an anatomical and electrophysiological study. Exp Brain Res 56:410–424

Goebel R, Khorram-Sefat D, Muckli L, Hacker H, Singer W (1998) The constructive nature of vision: direct evidence from functional magnetic resonance imaging studies of apparent motion and motion imagery. Eur J Neurosci 10:1563–1573

Goel V, Grafman J, Tajik J, Gana S, Danto D (1997) A study of the performance of patients with frontal lobe lesions in a financial planning task. Brain 120:1805–1822

Grafton ST, Fagg AH, Woods RP, Arbib MA (1996) Functional anatomy of pointing and grasping in humans. Cereb Cortex 6:226–237

Halsband U, Freund H-J (1990) Premotor cortex and conditional motor learning in man. Brain 113:207–222

He S-Q, Dum RP, Strick PL (1993) Topographic organization of corticospinal projections from the frontal lobe: motor areas on the lateral surface of the hemisphere. J Neurosci 13:952–980

Heide W, Binkofski F, Posse S, Seitz RJ, Kömpf D, Freund H-J (1999) Cortical control of sequences of memory guided saccades. In: Becker W, Deubel H, Mergner T (eds) Current oculomotor research – physiological and psychological aspects. Plenum Press, New York, pp 223–233

Heilman KM, Bowers D, Coslett B, Whelan H, Watson RT (1985) Directional hypokinesia: prolonged reaction times for leftward movements in patients with right hemispheric lesions and neglect. Neurology 35:855–859

Herzog H, Seitz RJ, Tellmann L, Müller-Gärtner H-W (1996) Quantification of regional cerebral blood flow with ^{15}O-butanol and positron emission tomography in humans. J Cereb Blood Flow Metab 16:645–649

Hummelsheim H, Bianchetti M, Wiesendanger M, Wiesendanger R (1988) Sensory inputs to the agranular motor fields: a comparison between precentral, supplementary-motor and premotor areas in the monkey. Exp Brain Res 69:289–298

Jahanshahi M, Jenkins H, Brown RG, Marsden CD, Passingham RE, Brooks DJ (1995) Self-initiated versus externally triggered movements. I. An investigation using measurement of regional cerebral blood flow with PET and movement-related potentials in normal and Parkinson's disease subjects. Brain 118:913–933

Jeannerod M, Arbib MA, Rizzolatti G, Sakata H (1995) Grasping objects: the cortical mechanism of visuomotor transformation. Trends Neurosci 18:314–320

Jenkins IH, Brooks DJ, Nixon PD (1994) Motor sequence learning: a study with positron emission tomography. J Neurosci 14:3775–3790

Kawashima R, Roland PE, O'Sullivan BT (1994) Fields in human motor areas involved in preparation for reaching, actual reaching, and visuomotor learning: a positron emission tomography study. J Neurosci 14:3462–3474

Keizer K, Kuypers HGJM (1989) Distribution of corticospinal neurons with collaterals to the lower brain stem reticular formation in monkey (*Macaca fascicularis*). Exp Brain Res 74:311–318

Kleinschmidt A, Nitschke MF, Frahm J (1997) Somatotopy in the human motor cortex hand area. A high-resolution functional MRI study. Eur J Neurosci 9:2178–2186

Kozennikow O, Wicki U, Corboz M (1994) Temporal structure of a bimanual goal-directed movement sequence in monkeys. Eur J Neurosci 6:203–210

Kurata K, Wise SP (1988) Premotor and supplementary motor cortex in rhesus monkeys: neuronal activity during externally and internally instructed motor tasks. Exp Brain Res 72:237–248

Lang W, Obrig H, Lindinger G (1990) Supplementary motor area activation while tapping bimanually different rhythms in musicians. Exp Brain Res 79:504–514

Luppino G, Matelli M, Rizzolatti G (1990) Cortico-cortical connections of two electrophysiologically identified arm representations in the mesial agranular frontal cortex. Exp Brain Res 82:214–218

Luppino G, Matelli M, Camarda RM (1991) Multiple representations of body movements in mesial area 6 and the adjacent cingulate cortex: an intracortial microstimulation study in the macaque monkey. J Comp Neurol 311:463–482

Mai N, Bolsinger P, Averello M, Diener H-C, Dichgans J (1988) Control of isometric finger force in patients with cerebellar disease. Brain 111:973–998

Massion J, Viallet F, Massarino R, Khalil R (1989) La région de l'aire motrice supplémentaire est impliquée dans la coordination entre posture et mouvement chez l'Homme. CR Acad Sci [III] 308:417–423

Matelli M, Luppino G, Rizzolatti G (1991) Architecture of superior and mesial area 6 and the adjacent cingulate cortex in the macaque monkey. J Comp Neurol 311:445–462

McInthosh AR, Rajah MN, Lobaugh NJ (1999) Interactions of prefrontal cortex in relation to awareness in sensory learning. Science 284:1531–1533

Menon RS, Kim S-G (1999) Spatial and temporal limits in cognitive neuroimaging with fMRI. Trends Cogn Sci 3:207–216

Mink JW, Thach WT (1993) Basal ganglia intrinsic circuits and their role in behavior. Curr Opin Neurobiol 3:950–957

Oldfield RC (1971) The assessment and analysis of handedness: the Edinburgh inventory. Neuropsychologia 9:97–104

Pardo JV, Fox PT, Janer KW, Raichle ME (1990) The anterior cingulate cortex mediates processing selection in the Stroop attentional conflict paradigm. Proc Natl Acad Sci USA 87:256–259

Parsons LM, Fox PT, Downs JH, Glaas T, Hirsch TB, Martin CC, Jerabek PA, Lancaster JL (1995) Use of implicit motor imagery for visual shape discrimination as revealed by PET. Nature 375:54–58

Pellegrino G di, Wise SP (1993) Visuospatial versus visuomotor activity in the premotor and prefrontal cortex of a primate. J Neurosci 13:1227–1243

Pendlebury ST, Blamire AM, Lee MA, Style P, Matthews PM (1999) Axonal injury in the internal capsule correlates with motor impairment after stroke. Stroke 30:956–962

Penfield W, Boldrey E (1937) Somatic motor and sensory representation in the cerebral cortex of man as studied by electrical stimulation. Brain 60:389–443

Petit L, Orssaud C, Tzourio N, Salamon G, Mazoyer B, Berthoz A (1993) PET study of voluntary saccadic eye movements in humans: basal ganglia – thalamocortical system and cingulate cortex involvement. J Neurophysiol 69:1009–1017

Rao SR, Rainer G, Miller EK (1997a) Integration of what and where in the primate prefrontal cortex. Science 276:821–824

Rao SM, Harrington DL, Haaland KY, Bobholz JA, Cox RW, Binder JR (1997b) Distributed neural systems underlying the timing of movements. J Neurosci 15:5528–5535

Rauch SL, Savage CR, Brown HD, Curran T, Alpert NM, Kendrick A, Fischman AJ, Kosslyn SM (1995) A PET investigation of implicit and explicit sequence learning. Hum Brain Map 3:271–286

Rizzolatti G, Camarda R, Fogassi L (1988) Functional organization of inferior area 6 in the macaque monkey. II. Area F5 and the control of distal movements. Exp Brain Res 71:491–507

Rizzolatti G, Gentilucci M, Camarda R (1990) Neurons related to reaching-grasping arm movements in the rostral part of area 6 (area 6aß). Exp Brain Res 82:337–350

Rizzolatti G, Luppino G, Matelli M (1998) The organization of the cortical motor system: new concepts. Electroencephalogr Clin Neurophysiol 106:283–296

Sadato N, Yonekura Y, Waki A, Yamada H, Ishii Y (1997) Role of the supplementary motor area and the right premotor cortex in the coordination of bimanual finger movements. J Neurosci 15:9667–9674

Sakai K, Hikosaka O, Miyauchi S, Takino R, Sasaki Y, Pütz B (1998) Transition of brain activation from frontal to parietal areas in visuomotor sequence learning. J Neurosci 18:1827–1840

Sanes JN, Donoghue JP, Thangaraj V, Edelman RR, Warach S (1995) Shared neural substrates controlling hand movements in human motor cortex. Science 268:1775–1777

Schieber MH, Hibbard LS (1993) How somatotopic is the motor cortex hand area? Science 261:489–492

Schlag J, Schlag-Rey M (1987) Evidence for a supplementary eye field. J Neurophysiol 57:179–200

Seitz RJ, Roland PE (1992a) Learning of finger movement sequences: a combined kinematic and positron emission tomography study. Eur J Neurosci 4:154–165

Seitz RJ, Roland PE (1992b) Variability of the rCBF measured with [^{11}C]-fluoromethane and positron emission tomography (PET) in rest. Comp Med Imag Graph 5:311–322

Seitz RJ, Canavan AGM, Yagüez L, Herzog H, Tellmann L, Knorr U, Huang Y, Hömberg V (1997) Representation of graphomotor trajectories in human parietal cortex: evidence for controlled processing and skilled performance. Eur J Neurosci 9:378–389

Seitz RJ, Höflich P, Binkofski F, Tellmann L, Herzog H, Freund H-J (1998) Role of the premotor cortex for recovery from middle cerebral artery infarction. Arch Neurol 55:1081–1088

Seitz RJ, Knorr U, Azari NP, Herzog H, Freund H-J (1999) Visual network activation in recovery from sensorimotor stroke. Restor Neurol Neurosci 14:25–33

Shadmehr R, Holcomb HH (1997) Neural correlates of motor memory consolidation. Science 277:821–825

Shibasaki H, Sadato N, Lyshkow H, Yonekura Y, Honda M, Nagamine T, Suwazono S, Magata Y, Ikeda A, Miyazaki M, Fukuyama H, Sato R, Konishi J (1993) Both primary motor cortex and supplementary motor area play an important role in complex finger movement. Brain 116:1387–1398

Shima K, Aya K, Mushiake H (1991) Two movement-related foci in the primate cingulate cortex observed in signal-triggered and self-paced forelimb movements. J Neurophysiol 65:188–202

Shulman GL, Fiez JA, Corbetta M, Buckner RL, Miezin FM, Raichle ME, Petersen SE (1997) Common blood flow changes across visual tasks. II. Decreases in cerebral cortex. J Cogn Neurosci 9:648–663

Stapleton JM, Morgang MJ, Liu X, Yung BCK, Phillips RL, Wong DF, Shaya EK, Dannals RF, London ED (1997) Cerebral glucose utilization is reduced in second test session. J Cereb Blood Flow Metab 17:704–712

Stephan KM, Binkofski F, Halsband U, Dohle C, Wunderlich G, Schnitzler A, Tass P, Posse S, Herzog H, Sturm V, Zilles K, Seitz RJ, Zilles K (1999a) The role of ventral medial wall motor areas for bimanual coordination: a combined lesion and activation study. Brain 122:351–368

Stephan KM, Binkofski F, Posse S, Seitz RJ, Freund H-J (1999b) Cerebral midline structures in bimanual coordination. Exp Brain Res [Suppl] (in press)

Stephan KM, Binkofski F, Posse S, Seitz RJ, Freund H-J (1999c) Cerebral midline structures in bimanual coordination. Exp Brain Res 128:243–249

Stepniewska I, Preuss TM, Kaas J (1993) Architectonics, somatotopic organization, and ipsilateral cortical connections of the primary motor area (M1) of Owl monkey. J Comp Neurol 330:238–271

Talairach J, Tournoux P (1988) Co-planar stereotactic atlas of the human brain. Thieme Medical, Stuttgart New York

Tanji J (1994) The supplementary motor area in the cerebral cortex. Neurosci Res 19:251–268

Tootell RBH, Reppas JB, Dale AM, Look RB, Sereno MI, Malach R, Brady TJ, Rosen BR, Belliveau JWJ (1995) Functional analysis of human MT and related visual cortical areas using magnetic resonance imaging. J Neurosci 15:3215–3230

Watson JDG, Myers R, Frackowiak RSJ, Hajnal JV, Woods RP, Mazziotta JC, Shipp S, Zeki S (1993) Area V5 of the human brain: evidence from a combined study using positron emission tomography and magnetic resonance imaging. Cereb Cortex 3:79–94

Weinrich M, Wiese SP, Mauritz K-H (1984) A neurophysiological study of the premotor cortex in the rhesus monkey. Brain 107:385–414

Wise SP (1991) What are the specific functions of the different motor areas? In: Humphrey DR, Freund H-J (eds) Motor control: concepts and issues. John Wiley and Sons, New York, pp 463–485

Wunderlich G, Knorr U, Stephan KM, Azari NP, Tellmann L, Herzog H, Seitz RJ (1997) Dynamic scanning of ^{15}O-butanol with positron emission tomography can identify regional cerebral activations. Hum Brain Map 5:364–378

Glyn W. Humphreys · M. Jane Riddoch

One more cup of coffee for the road: object–action assemblies, response blocking and response capture after frontal lobe damage

Published online: 25 May 2000

Abstract We report data from a patient, FK, who manifested 'utilisation' behaviour after bilateral lesions of the medial frontal and anterior temporal lobes. In tasks requiring actions to be made with the hand compatible with the orientation of a cup, FK was able to ignore irrelevant distractors that fell in the path of action to the target. However, errors were made when the distractors were other cups. These errors reflected the hand selected on the basis of the properties of the target, suggesting that distractors competed to control the action after selection of the target. When similar in kind to the target, distractors sometimes captured the action. However, distractors that were associated with an action related to the target blocked the usual hand response. These results suggest a complex interlocking of attention and action when grasping responses are made to a target amongst distractors. There is initial selection of the target, but distractors on the path of a reach can then compete for control of the action. Distractors can be inhibited if they do not match the properties of the specified target, and there can also be inhibition of concurrently activated responses. We show that the magnitude of the inhibition is proportional to the strength of learned object–action associations.

Key words Frontal lobes · Affordance · Vision–action links · Distractor inhibition · Object–action association

On the selection of objects and actions

Imagine being seated at a table containing a kettle, a milk jug, a jar of instant coffee, a coffee pot and a cup. You are very used to making coffee directly in the cup, but you are told that today you must use the pot. How are you able to implement these instructions so that you perform the action as instructed and not in the over-learned way? One possibility is that the instructions set up some form of 'goal template' that acts to guide an initial visual selection process to the appropriate target (the coffee pot, not the cup). If there is little activation of actions associated with the stimuli present until they are selected visually, then competition from task-inappropriate objects having a strong response-association can be minimised. The coffee pot will be selected visually without the cup competing strongly for the action. On this view, selection of the object for a response largely precedes selection of the response to the object, as in traditional models of early selection (e.g. Broadbent 1958; see Riddoch et al. 2000). A somewhat different view is that all the objects present activate their associated responses in parallel. These object–action associations compete with one another, with the outcome of the competition determined by both the familiarity of the associations and the pertinence of the instructions. When an action must then be directed to an object, the object selected will be determined to some degree by the strength of object–action associations. This account is similar in spirit to pre-motor theories of attention (Rizzolatti et al. 1987, 1994), which hold that object selection is influenced by activation of a motor response to a particular stimulus.

Insights into the factors that determine our ability to select objects and actions in complex environments can be gained by studying patients who have difficulties in overriding over-learned actions to familiar objects. Such difficulties are encountered in patients who display so-called 'utilisation behaviour' after damage to the frontal lobes. Florid examples of utilisation behaviour were described by Lhermitte (1983), who documented instances in which patients made over-learned actions in relation to environmental objects in a manner unconstrained by task goals. For example, a patient may pick up a pair of spectacles from a table and place them on his nose, even if another pair of glasses is already positioned there and even if the task instructions required a completely different behaviour. This loosening of the effects of task goals on performance may enable us to study how object se-

G.W. Humphreys (✉) · M.J. Riddoch
Behavioural and Brain Sciences Centre, School of Psychology, University of Birmingham, Edgbaston, Birmingham B15 2TT, UK
e-mail: g.w.humphreys@bham.ac.uk
Fax: +44-1214144897

lection relates to action selection and whether properties of the object, the action, or both, play a dominant role in the control of behaviour.

An attempt to investigate the factors that influence behaviour of this type was recently carried out by Riddoch et al. (1998), using a patient, ES, with cortical basal degeneration. ES had great difficulty in effecting voluntary control over both of her hands, which could act in an unintentional manner (e.g. one hand reaching to open a door, the other to close it). Riddoch et al. used a simple task in which reaching or pointing responses had to be made to cups that were positioned to the right or left of ES's midline. The task instructions were to respond to the target cup using the hand that was on the same side of space relative to the body midline (right hand to right-side cups, left hand to left-side cups). The cups were positioned so that their handles fell either on the left or right side, but the instructions emphasised that the position of the handle on the cup was irrelevant. ES was able to repeat back the instructions throughout the study, and she was able to discriminate the left and right positions relative to her body. Despite this, she made frequent errors in which she reached with the hand that matched the position of the handle relative to the cup and not the hand aligned with the position of the cup relative to her body (e.g. reaching with the right hand to a cup on the left side but with its handle turned to the right). Riddoch et al. termed these errors 'manual interference responses'. They noted that manual interference responses were modulated by the nature of both the stimulus and the action. Interference responses, especially with ES's right hand, were most frequent when the targets were cups placed in their usual (upright) orientation. Interference responses decreased when cups were inverted. They also decreased when the target was a cup-like non-object (a small container attached like a handle to the side of a larger container), and when the task required pointing rather than reaching and grasping. Riddoch et al. (1998) suggested that these responses occurred when the action based on the task instructions was overridden by competing actions that were affected by (1) the familiarity of the object (with the cup rather than the cup-like non-object), (2) the familiarity of the object's orientation (with upright rather than inverted cups), (3) the spatial relation between the critical object part and the effector (the handle on the right, relative to the right hand), and (4) the strength of association between the object and the action required (for grasping rather than pointing).

The present paper is concerned with situations in which task goals are set against competing stimulus and response associations. Hence it is of interest that ES was sensitive to some forms of task instruction, such as using a pointing rather than a grasping response, and that, when this instruction set was active, manual interference responses were reduced in frequency. Presumably a pointing response was less strongly associated with the position of the handle on a cup than a grasping response. Consequently, for pointing, a right-hand response was less likely to be evoked to a left-side cup whose handle was on the right. Nevertheless, under conditions in which the stimulus did evoke a strong competing response from the set of actions established for the task, ES was profoundly impaired in her ability to select the action specified by the task instructions.

Riddoch et al. (2000a, 2000b) went on to explore whether, despite the problems in action selection, ES was able to use instructions to select the object for the action. For these studies ES was presented with two objects in a trial and instructed just to respond to one, the target, based on some pre-defined property (e.g. its colour). As in the previous experiments, ES had to respond using the hand on the same side of her body as the target. In some instances, the target object had a relatively weak association with the required action and the distractor had a stronger association. For example, the target might be an upside down cup and the distractor an upright one, and the task might require that the target be grasped. Here, using the evidence from manual interference responses to define when an object had a pre-potent action association, we expected the (upright) distractor to evoke a stronger response than the (inverted) target. If selection of the target is contingent on the most strongly activated response, as suggested by the pre-motor theory of attention, then errors should have occurred in which ES grasped the distractor rather than the target. However, Riddoch et al. (2000a, 2000b) found very few 'distractor errors' of this sort. ES continued to make errors, showing some failure to implement the task instructions, but the errors were overwhelmingly manual interference responses. ES responded to the correct object (the target) but did so frequently using the hand most strongly associated with the action and not the hand appropriate to the instruction (e.g. reaching with her right hand to a left-side target with its handle on the right). Thus ES was able to implement some but not all of the components making up the task set. She could select the object for the action, even though she was subsequently impaired in selecting the action appropriate to the object. This result is consistent with the notion that object selection can precede action selection rather than being contingent on it. Riddoch et al. (2000a, 2000b) interpreted the data in terms of Posner and Petersen's (1990) distinction between a posterior and an anterior attentional system concerned broadly with stimulus and response selection. The data are consistent with ES having a relatively intact posterior attentional system, which enabled her to select the object in accord with the task instructions; however, damage to the anterior attentional system would leave behaviour vulnerable to pre-potent responses associated with the selected object.

Blocking and distractor inhibition

Riddoch et al. (2000a, 2000b) also noted one surprising instance in which a distractor object actually facilitated performance, in that ES then used the hand appropriate to the task rather than the hand invoked more strongly by the stimulus. This behaviour occurred when the distractor was positioned close to the reach trajectory to the target and the two stimuli differed in kind (e.g. when the target was a light that ES had to point to and the distractor was a cup). To account for this finding, Riddoch et al. (2000a, 2000b) suggested that the following sequence of events took place. The first stage involved ES selecting the target object (the light). This was followed by competition between the actions evoked by the stimulus and those based on the task instructions; this competition for action was often won by the stimulus-associated but task-inappropriate hand. After this came a third selection process when distractors fell close to the reach path to the target. In this third selection process, distractors were attended to because they could constitute possible obstacles for the reaching action. The intact process of stimulus selection enabled ES to reject these distractors as the targets for the action, and these items were consequently inhibited in the ensuing competition with representations activated by the instruction set (e.g. 'respond to the inverted cup'). However, to explain why there was then blocking of the response to the target, it was argued that inhibition was applied not only to the representations of distractor stimuli but also to what we term object–action assemblies, which are set up between co-active stimulus and response representations. These object–action assemblies may contain links between currently attended objects (the distractor in the reach path) and actions recently activated (including actions activated by the target but not yet effected). Suppression of an assembly involving an attended distractor can lead to inhibition of the appropriate hand response (invoked by the target), allowing the hand biased by the instruction set sometimes to win the competition for action. On this account the inhibition of the distractor in turn blocked the action to the target.

This view, that actions to targets are selected by inhibiting competing actions associated with distractors, fits with evidence from normal subjects on both hand and eye movements (e.g. Tipper et al. 1997, 2000; Sheliga et al. 1995). For example, Tipper et al. (1997) have reported that several parameters of hand movements made to far targets, including the times to initiate and complete the movements, and the reach trajectories, are influenced by distractors placed near the hand of action. Interestingly, reach trajectories can be displaced away from distractors (see also Sheliga et al. 1994, for similar data on eye movement trajectories). This suggests that inhibition of competitor representations can bias a vector representation of the movement to a target so that it is activated more strongly in directions away from the distractor. There is some controversy, however, over whether these distractor effects arise as a natural part of the competition to select the target in the first place, or whether they arise only when distractors themselves are attended to. Castiello (1996) found effects on hand reaches to targets only when subjects had to attend to the distractors (the task was to count the number of times a light fell on the distractor prior to the occurrence of the cue to reach to the target). The data on response blocking, reported by Riddoch et al. (2000a, 2000b), are consistent with distractor inhibition arising only once distractors are allocated some attention.

The present study

In the present paper we examine in further detail the factors that determine when over-learned responses are made to stimuli, using again a patient who has difficulty in overriding such responses. The patient, FK, suffered lesions to the medial frontal and anterior temporal lobes bilaterally, which resulted in a number of neuropsychological disorders. Most relevant to the present study, FK shows disturbances in his performance of everyday actions, in which he uses objects in the wrong order and in a perseverative fashion (see Humphreys and Forde 1998). At least some of FK's errors in such tasks can be attributed to a failure to use goal-based activation (e.g. representing a task such as 'make a cup of coffee using the coffee pot') to override pre-potent responses to stimuli (placing coffee granules in a cup). In addition, in an experimental analysis of such behaviours, Humphreys and Forde (1998) and Humphreys et al. (2000) demonstrated that FK made errors specifically in which he used objects in an over-learned manner rather than following task instructions, even when he could subsequently report back the instructions. For example, FK might be given a visual array containing the objects cup, saucer, bread, sandwich bag, bow and wrapping paper, along with instructions which required the use of two of the objects in a novel rather than a familiar manner (e.g. 'put the cup onto the sandwich bag'). FK frequently made errors in which he made a familiar rather than the novel response (e.g. he might put the cup on the saucer rather than on the sandwich bag), whilst still being able to repeat back the instructions correctly after the action. Such errors are consistent with FK's behaviour being driven by vision–action associations unconstrained by task rules held in verbal working memory. Riddoch et al. (2000a) went on to confirm that FK also made errors in even simpler experimental situations in which grasp responses had to be made using the hand on the side where a cup was placed. Like patient ES (see above), FK could discriminate the spatial positions of objects and he could remember the task instructions ('reach with the hand that is on the side where the cup is presented'). Nevertheless, he would sometimes reach incorrectly, using the hand compatible with the position of the handle of the cup even though the instructions emphasised the position of the whole cup with respect to the body. These errors were particularly pronounced with FK's right (dominant) hand, indicating that they arose not simply because there was temporary loss of the instructions (which should affect both hands) but because a very familiar stimulus–response pairing could 'win' the competition for action.

In the present study, we assessed FK's ability to select a target for action under conditions in which two stimuli were presented. We ask, what are the circumstances in which a distractor influences FK's responses to a target, and do such influences reflect competition between targets and distractors for object selection, competition for response selection, or selection of a distractor after selection of the target? We also investigated the distractor 'blocking effect' reported by Riddoch et al. (2000a, 2000b). We ask, what properties of the distractor determine whether a distractor 'captures' or 'blocks' an action to a target? The data we report suggest that distractors influence FK's performance after target selection, and distractors either capture or block responses depending on their similarity to targets and the familiarity of their object–action associations. Blocking is most pronounced when distractors have a different identity to targets whilst being strong competitors for action. We discuss the results in terms of models of competition for object and action selection.

Case report

FK (date of birth 19.9.68), a right handed male, was 30 years old at the time of testing. He suffered carbon monoxide poisoning in 1989 when he was an engineering student at university. This resulted in bilateral lesions of the anterior and medial temporal lobe (superior and middle temporal gyri) regions, the lateral occipital gyri and medial frontal regions (superior and middle frontal gyri) (see Humphreys and Forde 1998, for an MRI scan). He presents with a number of neuropsychological disturbances. After the lesions, FK had a full IQ score of 58 on the Wechsler Adult Intelligence Scale (64 verbal, 56 performance), and a National Adult Reading Test-predicted IQ score of 94. His ability to learn new information was impaired, scoring <50 on the Wechsler Memory Scale. His digit span forwards, however, was 7 (2 backwards). He has a problem in visual object recognition linked to impaired stored knowledge about objects. He is able to copy objects and to perform perceptual categorization tasks [he scored 24 and 22/25 respectively on the minimal feature and foreshortened views test from the Birmingham Object Recognition Battery (BORB); Riddoch and Humphreys 1993]. However, his object decision responses were close to chance (38/64, combining easy and hard object decisions from BORB), he was poor at matching a head of an object to its body (the 'heads' test, 19/30 on a four-choice version; mean controls 27.5; see Humphreys and Rumiati 1998; Riddoch and Humphreys 1987), at matching associatively related objects (20/30; BORB test 12), and at pointing to a named picture amongst semantically and visually related distractors (29/40, test 13 from the Psycholinguistic Assessment of Language Processing in Aphasia; Kayet al. 1992). Object naming was impaired for both visual and tactile presentations (24 and 21/44 respectively, with real objects), as was his naming in response to auditory definition (though this was somewhat better for verbal definitions than for definitions stressing visual/perceptual properties of objects: 12 and 1/38 respectively, control means 35 and 33 respectively). In addition to these problems in object recognition and naming, he had deficits in 'executive' functions. On the Wisconsin Card Sorting task, FK was able to complete only one category. He had a raw score of 27 on the clinical version of the Stroop test (probability of deficit 0.99). He performed poorly on subtests from the Behavioural Assesment of the Dysexecutive Syndrome screen of dysexecutive symptoms (rule shift cards 0; action program 0; temporal judgement 0), and there was poor verbal fluency (within a 1-min period for each category he produced 9 animals, 5 sports, 6 countries, 4 vegetables, 1 vehicle). In the fluency tests, FK would stray beyond the boundaries of the category given; for instance, when asked to produce the names of vegetables he produced ten other food names (sandwich, orange juice, cereal, tea, etc.). FK's word reading was good. He named 40/40 concrete words correctly, with an average reaction time of about 850 ms.

In summary, FK has marked deficits in his knowledge about objects and in 'executive' processes, consistent with damage to the temporal and frontal lobes. In the experiments described below, we used objects from a constrained class of objects (kitchen utensils), and FK was able to name all of the objects involved (cup, teapot, jug). He also showed good memory for the task instructions throughout testing when asked to repeat back what the task was, and the data demonstrate that overt errors were not due to forgetting the task but rather to the goal-based response being overridden by a stronger object–action association.

The present studies

An initial set of studies of FK's ability to make novel location-dependent responses to familiar objects (cups) has been reported by Riddoch et al. (2000a). The present studies use a similar paradigm to explore distractor interference effects in action in more detail, so we begin by summarising the experiments already reported.

Experiment A: reaching to single cups

A first study employed the procedure introduced by Riddoch et al. (1998) in their investigation of manual interference in patient ES. This involved placing a cup 15 cm to the left or right side of the patient's midline, with the primary task being to pick up the cup by its handle, using the hand that was on the same side of the cup relative to the midline (right hand for right-side cup, left hand for left-side cup). It was emphasised that these responses should be made irrespective of the positions of the handles of the cups. In addition, in order to test that FK could localise the stimuli, we conducted a block of trials in which he made pointing rather than reach and grasp responses to the cups (this was interspersed between two blocks of reach and grasp trials). Riddoch et al. (1998) showed that manual interference responses, in which the patient grasped the cup with the contralateral hand aligned with the handle, were reduced for a pointing response (which should not be so strongly associated with the position of the handle on the cup). In each block there were 30 trials for each combination of cup side (left, right) and handle (left, right) in the reach and grasp trials, and 20 trials in the pointing task. FK was asked to respond as quickly as possible once the experimenter lifted a wooden partition that prevented FK from viewing the stimuli before the beginning of the trial.

On reach and grasp trials FK made no errors with his right hand; he always reached and grasped a right-side cup using his right hand, irrespective of whether the handle of the cup was on the right or left (30/30 for both conditions). However he made errors with left-side cups. There were 27/30 correct left-hand responses when the handle was on the left but only 9/30 when the handle was on the right. In the last case, all of the errors involved FK reaching to pick up the cup with his right hand. On pointing trials FK made no errors.

The data demonstrate that, like patient ES (Riddoch et al. 1998), FK was prone to making responses that contravened a task rule, based on the strength of association between the object and the response. He made many incorrect grasp responses with his right hand, reaching to a left-side cup with its handle on the right. These errors occurred despite the fact that FK was able to repeat back the task rule, and even though he was able to implement the same rule for a pointing task. This last result rules out the possibility that errors were due to mislocalisation of left-side targets or due to FK forgetting the task rule. Rather the task-rule was overridden in circumstances where the target had a strong association with the response for the task. FK has impaired selection of actions according to novel task rules.

Experiment B: initial distractor effects

Riddoch et al. (2000a) also examined the effect of a distractor on FK's reaching and grasping of target cups. Distractors were either a wooden block (approximately the same size as the target cup) or a distractor cup of a different colour to the target (target red, distractor green; the cups were otherwise identical), and, on each trial, the distractor could be placed either in the reach trajectory to the target (if FK used the correct hand, as signalled by the target) or on the opposite side of the midline (in the reach trajectory for the other hand). The target cup was always placed in the centre of a table, aligned with the mid-position of FK's body. The task was changed from that in Experiment A so that, here, FK had to respond with the hand associated with the position of the handle (if the handle was on the right, use the right hand; if the handle was on the left, use the left hand). When the distractor fell in the reach path, this meant that FK had to make a slight shift in his reach trajectory, to avoid the distractor. Work with both normal subjects (Tipper et al. 1997) and neuropsychological patients (Riddoch et al. 2000a, 2000b) indicates that distractors may have most effect when they fall close to the reach trajectory to a target. Experiment B assessed whether this held for FK.

Experiment B also tested whether FK's reaches were affected by the properties of the target or the distractor. Consider the case in which the central target cup has its handle on the left and the distractor is a cup with a right-facing handle that falls in the near-right location (aligned with the reach path of FK's right hand to the target). There may be competition for selection based on both the properties of the stimuli (e.g. which colour is consistent with the instruction set for the target) and their associated responses (e.g. which response is most strongly activated). If the stimulus properties alone are dominant, then FK should select the target, and any subsequent effects should be contingent on factors such as the position of the handle of the target (associated with a left-hand response). However, if response properties also take part in the competition for selection (as suggested by the premotor theory of attention; Rizzolatti et al. 1987), then the distractor may be selected in these circumstances. This is because the distractor is both nearer than the target and, judging by the asymmetry in the interference responses found in Experiment A, the right-facing handle has a stronger pre-potent response.

The target was positioned 40 cm from FK, aligned with the centre of his body. The distractor was placed 20 cm away, with its nearest edge 6 cm to the right or left of FK's midline. Prior to each block of experimental trials, FK was given 40 practice trials in which the target was presented alone and he had to reach and grasp it with the hand aligned with the position of the handle. FK made no errors in these practice trials. There followed a block of experimental trials in which the target cup was presented along with either a distractor cup or a distractor block. There were five trials per block according to whether the target had its handle on the left or right, the position of the distractor was on the left or right of the midline, and the position of the handle of the distractor was left or right (when the distractor was a cup; when it was a wooden block then there were simply ten trials when it was on the left and ten when it was on the right, per block of trials). The conditions with the distractor cup and wooden block were presented in an ABBA fashion.

The results were clear. FK made only one error when the distractor was a wooden block: when the target had its handle on the left and the distractor was positioned on the right, FK reached with his right hand to pick up the target; on all other trials he reached with the correct hand as cued by the target (79/80 correct). Thus FK could bypass the distractor when it fell in the reach trajectory to the target. In contrast, when the distractor was a cup, he sometimes made errors by picking up the distractor. Interestingly, these errors were affected by the position of the handle *on the target*, not the position of the handle *on the distractor*, and they occurred when the distractor was in the reach trajectory for the hand cued by the target. When the distractor fell on the side opposite to the hand cued by the target (e.g. target handle left, distractor in near-right location), FK made 34/40 correct responses. The errors in these trials were all due to FK picking up the target by the rim rather than the handle, using the correct hand. However, when the distractor fell on the side cued by the target (e.g. target handle left, distractor in near-left location), he made only 2/40 correct responses. All of the errors on these trials consisted of FK picking up the distractor.

The data demonstrate that distractors affected FK's reaching and grasping responses, but predominantly after selection of the target. This conclusion follows because performance was influenced by the position of the target's handle, not the handle of the distractor cup. If the response properties of the distractor were important for object selection, then errors should have arisen when the target had a weak hand-response association and the distractor a strong one (e.g. target facing left and the distractor facing right in the near-right location). No such errors arose. Indeed, distractor errors were equally likely irrespective of whether the distractor's handle was in a position that was incompatible with the response actually made – there were 18 trials with an incompatible reach to a distractor and 20 with a compatible reach (an example of incompatible reach is where the target faced left and the distractor faced right and was in the near-left position, when FK used his left hand to pick up the distractor). These incompatible reaches suggest that FK first selected and activated a response associated with the target, and that errors were caused by distractors in the reach trajectory becoming linked to this response. Distractors in the reach trajectory may normally be selected in order that they are avoided during the reach – as shown by FK's behaviour with the wooden blocks. However, when distractors have properties that are part of the instruction set ('reach to the cup'), they may 'capture' the response so that FK picks up distractors rather than targets.

In addition to the distractor errors, FK made some errors (six in total) by grasping the target in the wrong manner. These errors occurred on trials where distractor cups fell on the opposite side of FK's midline relative to the arm compatible with the target. We attribute these errors to general effects of the task load, which is increased when distractors and targets share properties (both cups). Under load conditions, FK sometimes failed to implement the response-end of the instruction set (grasping the incorrect part of the object), though again the target was selected rather than the distractor. This last point, when coupled with the fact that distractor errors were contingent on the position of the handle on the target, also emphasises that FK was relatively good at selecting the target despite his having an impaired ability to select novel actions for tasks (as shown in Experiment A). Object selection can be relatively spared even when action selection is disrupted (see also Riddoch et al. 2000a, 2000b).

Experiments 1–4: overview

Here we conducted four further experiments to assess the factors that influence distractor effects on FK's reaching and grasping. Experiment 1 is similar in design to Experiment B (Riddoch et al.2000a), except that we varied the start position of FK's hands (they were crossed so that the left hand started from the right side of his body and the right hand from the left side). This allows us to assess whether the position of the distractor relative to the hand cued by the target is important or whether it is the position relative to the side of the body cued. If the distractor is selected because it falls in the reach trajectory to the target, then the distractor should affect performance when it falls between the cup and the hand used for the action. Consider the case when the handle of the target cup faces left and FK's left hand starts on the right of his midline. Here a distractor cup on the right should interfere with left-hand reaches evoked by the target, since the right-side distractor lies between the hand activated by the target and the target itself.

Experiments 2–4 evaluated the relations between the target and distractor. Rather than using a distractor with the same function as the target (a cup), we had distractors that were both semantically related to and used in conjunction with targets (a coffee pot in Experiment 2, and a jug in Experiment 3). Would the distractor 'capture' errors shown by FK (see Experiment B above) generalise from functionally identical objects to objects that are semantically related and/or used in conjunction with targets? Interestingly, with related distractors we found response-blocking by distractors rather than capture, suggesting that related distractors were subject to strong inhibition. Experiment 4 attempted to tease apart effects due to semantic relatedness and effects due to object–action associations by having FK reach to a jug when the distractor was a cup. These items are both semantically related, but the action association from one object to the other is greater from a jug to a cup (since liquid is usually poured from a jug into a cup) than from the cup to the jug. Do action associations, from one object onto another, influence competition for action selection?

Experiment 1: distractor capture and hand position

In Experiment 1 we used a procedure similar to that in Experiment B (Riddoch et al.2000a), except that we had FK make responses from a start position in which his hands were crossed. The task was again to pick up a central cup using the hand cued by the position of its handle. However on this occasion FK's left hand began from a position on his right side, and his right hand began from a position on his left side. From Experiment B we expected to observe distractor capture errors in which FK sometimes picked up the distractor with the hand cued by the target. By having FK cross his hands at the outset, we test whether the target cues the hand for the response or the side of the body. Tipper et al. (1992) examined interference effects from distractor lights on a pointing response to a central target. Distractor lights appeared just beyond the target or in front of it, with respect to the subject's body. The hand used for the pointing response could either start from in front of the nearest distractor or from behind the farthest distractor. Tipper et al. found that interference effects were a function of the start position of the hand. Distractor lights affected performance more when they fell between the response hand and the target than when they fell on the opposite side. Thus distractors that were further from the subject affected performance more than close distractors, if the hand started from the 'far' location. Tipper et al. (1992) proposed that distractors were coded in terms of an 'action-based' frame of reference, in which their positions were localised with respect to the hand of action rather than the subject's body. We examine whether the same holds in the present situation.

Method

There were 10 trials for each combination of target handle position (left, right), distractor handle position (left, right) and distractor location (left or right of FK's midline), making 80 trials in total. These were conducted in a single block, preceded by 40 practice trials in which FK was given just the target and told to make reaches with the hand that matched the position of the handle (right hand to pick up a right handle). At the start of each trial his hands were placed on opposite sides of his body, 6 cm from midline, and a wooden partition placed between his hands and the target and distractor stimuli. As soon as the partition was lifted, FK was told to reach to the target. The target was a red cup and the distractor a green cup that was otherwise identical in shape and structure. Each cup was 8 mm in diameter and 9 mm in height. The target was centred 40 cm in front of FK's midline and the distractor with its nearest edge 6 cm from his midline at a distance of 20 cm. He was given no feedback during the experiment.[1]

Results and discussion

The numbers of correct responses are presented in Table 1. As in the study reported by Riddoch et al. (2000a, see Experiment B above), FK made errors by picking up the distractor rather than the target. These errors again occurred when the distractor was on the side closest to the hand cued by the target, even though this was now when the distractor fell on the opposite side of FK's body relative to Experiment B. For example, FK made errors here when the target's handle was on the left and the distractor was in the near-right location, close to FK's left hand but on the right side of his body (he made only 6/40 correct responses when the distractor fell close to the reach trajectory for the hand cued by the target, with all the errors being due to 'distractor capture'). These distractor errors were unaffected by the position of the handle on the distractor (only 4/20 correct responses on trials where the hand used was incompatible with the handle on the distractors vs 2/20 when it was compatible). In addition to the errors due to distractor capture, FK made five other errors in the trials where the distractor fell on the side opposite to the hand cued by the target, and in each case he reached to the rim rather than the handle of the target.

These results essentially replicate those in Experiment B. Again FK appeared to select the target (and hence showed strong effects of the position of the handle on the target), but then transferred the response activated by the target to the distractor, when the distractor fell in the reach path to the target. Once more performance was unaffected by the position of the handle on the distractor. Interestingly, errors were affected by the position of the distractor relative to the hand cued by the target and not by its position relative to FK's body. Previously FK made no right- (or left-) hand grasp errors to left (or right) side distractors. Here, when his hands were crossed, all of the capture errors were of this type.

[1] For ease of presentation we report the data from Experiment 1 before those from the subsequent experiments. However Experiment 1 was actually conducted after the other experiments, as a partial replication of earlier experiments on distraction capture errors in FK (Riddoch et al. 2000a)

Table 1 Number of correct responses made by FK, starting with hands crossed so that the left hand was in the right spatial position (and vice versa for the right hand) (Experiment 1)

Target handle:	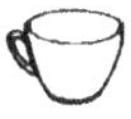		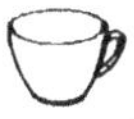	
Distractor position	Left	Right	Left	Right
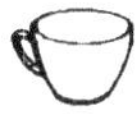	9/10	2/10	2/10	8/10
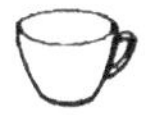	9/10	1/10	1/10	9/10
Totals	18/20	3/20	3/20	17/20

Experiment 2: target cup and distractor coffee pot

In Experiment 2, we returned to the situation in which FK's hands were uncrossed at the start of the trial but, on this occasion, we used a coffee pot rather than a cup distractor. The coffee pot is semantically related to the cup, both being found within the context of a meal. Coffee pots and cups are also used together; for example, a coffee pot is used to pour liquid into a cup. We ask whether either of these factors is sufficient to cause transfer of the response from the target to the distractor, to generate the 'capture' errors observed in Experiment 1 and Experiment B (Riddoch et al. 2000a).

Method

FK took part in a single block of trials in which the task was to pick a red target cup placed 40 cm in front of his body, using the hand compatible with the position of the handle. He was given 40 practice trials at the outset, during which he made no errors. The target was then presented along with a brown distractor coffee pot, which had its nearest edge 6 cm from FK's midline and which was 20 cm from FK. The teapot was 10 cm in diameter and 12 cm high, and was closer in colour to the target than the green distractor cup used in Experiment 1. There were 20 trials for each combination of target handle position (left, right) x distractor location (left vs right of FK's midline) x distractor handle position (left, right), making 160 trials in total.

Results and discussion

Table 2 gives the number of correct responses in each condition. As in the previous studies, FK performed well when the distractor fell on the side opposite to the hand cued by the target (e.g. target handle left, distractor near right): 80/80 correct trials. As before, the only errors arose when the distractor lay close to the reach trajectory of the hand cued by the target. However, unlike Experiment 1 (and also unlike Experiment B, Riddoch et al. 2000a), the errors here were of the 'distractor blocking' rather than 'capture' type. Fourteen out of fifteen of the

Table 2 Number of correct responses made by FK as a function of the position of the target's handle, the position of the distractor (coffee pot), and the position of the distractor's handle (Experiment 2)

Target handle:	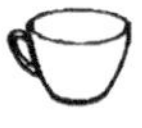		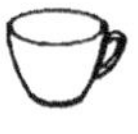	
Distractor position	Left	Right	Left	Right
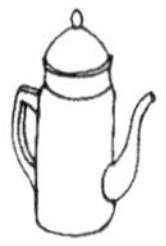	17/20	20/20	20/20	16/20
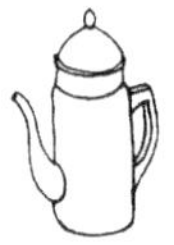	17/20	20/20	20/20	15/20
Totals	34/40	40/40	40/40	31/40

errors arose because FK responded with the hand that was incompatible with the handle of the target (e.g. due to him picking up with his right hand a target with its handle facing left, when the distractor lay in the reach path of the left hand). These errors were unrelated to the position of the handle on the distractor (eight were when the distractor's handle was compatible with the target handle, six when they were incompatible). The one remaining error occurred because he picked up the target cup by its rim, using the hand cued by the handle.

These results are both striking and surprising. Previously FK had never made errors in which he reached to the target using the wrong hand when the distractor lay in the path of action to the correct hand. In this study, though, this was the dominant mistake. The errors did not arise because the task here generated a greater load on selection than previously, generally increasing the error rate. Errors were generally decreased and wrong-hand errors were even eliminated in the conditions in which the distractor was on the side opposite to that cued by the target. It is also not the case that the present data reflect a temporary phenomenon that arose in this session because FK became aware of his sometimes making distractor capture errors (e.g. as in Riddoch et al. 2000a). In the subsequent experiments reported here we show that blocking errors arose consistently when distractors were associated and used in actions to targets; the effect was not confined to a particular test session. In addition, we conducted Experiment 1 here after the other experiments, and showed that distractor capture errors could be reinstated under the appropriate conditions. The change across the experiments does not reflect the order of administration.

Rather the results suggest that the related distractor blocked rather than captured the response activated by the target when it fell in the reach trajectory. To account for this, we suggest the following. First, there is selection of the target object based on its visual properties (the green cup), along with activation of an action cued by the position of the target's handle. Subsequently, distractors close to the reach trajectory are selected, but rejected as targets for action if they have inappropriate properties (e.g. being coffee pots rather than cups). Tipper et al. (2000) propose that competition for action selection involves both excitation of target representations and inhibition of distractor representations. The amount of inhibition involved will be proportional to the activation level of the distractor representations, and so may be increased when distractors are related to targets and/or to the task set (given that distractor activation is boosted when it is related to or used in conjunction with targets). Now if this inhibition is applied to action responses that are co-active at the same time as the competition taking place, there may be blocking of the target response. This blocking of the target response enables activation for the opposite hand response to be dominant, with the result that incompatible hand responses are made. This account is similar to the argument made by Riddoch et al. (2000b) concerning the blocking effects with patient ES, except that here we extend the proposal to suggest that inhibition of distractor representations is greater when they are related to and/or used in conjunction with targets.

A somewhat different account is that blocking arose because the coffee pot distractors here were larger than the distractors used hitherto. Large amounts of inhibition might be applied to prevent any response where there is a danger of the subject's hand colliding with the distractor, and this might underlie the blocking of the target response (see Tresilian 1998). To assess this suggestion, we repeated Experiment 2 but used a small jug as the distractor rather than a coffee pot. The target cup was about the same size as the distractor jug, so that, on this score, inhibition should be no greater in Experiment 3 than in Experiments 1 and B (with a cup distractor). Nevertheless cups and jugs are semantically related and frequently used together. If these last factors are crucial, and lead to strong inhibition of the distractor, then a blocking effect should emerge in Experiment 3, as in Experiment 2.

Experiment 3: Target cup and distractor jug

Method

The task was to pick up a green target cup and to ignore a brown jug. The cup was approximately the same size as the cup and it was placed with its nearest edge 6 cm to the left or right of FK's midline, 20 cm from his body. The target cup was placed 40 cm away in line with the centre of his body. There were 40 practice trials (target alone) followed by a single block of 160 experimental trials. There were 20 trials for each combination of target handle (left, right) x distractor location (left, right of midline) x distractor handle (left, right).

Results and discussion

The results were similar to those found in Experiment 2, with the distractor teapot. FK made no errors when the

Table 3 Number of correct responses made by FK as a function of the position of the target's handle, the position of the distractor (jug), and the position of the distractor's handle (Experiment 3)

Target handle:	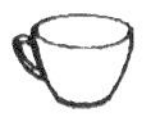		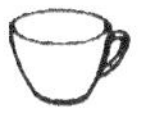	
Distractor position	Left	Right	Left	Right
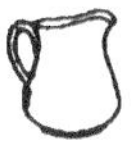	18/20	20/20	20/20	17/20
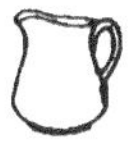	18/20	20/20	20/20	16/20
Totals	36/40	40/40	40/40	33/40

distractor was on the opposite side of midline relative to the hand cued by the target (80/80 correct). He made 11 errors altogether when the distractor fell in the reach path to the hand cued by the target, and these all involved him reaching with the opposite hand (incompatible with the position of the target handle) to pick up the target. The numbers of correct responses are given in Table 3.

The jug distractor in Experiment 3 was about the same size as the cup distractor in Experiment 1. In Experiment 1 FK often made errors by picking up the distractor lying in the reach trajectory using the hand cued by the target. In Experiment 3 he never made these errors and instead made errors where he responded to the target using the opposite hand, when the distractor fell in the cued reach trajectory. The data from Experiment 3 match those from Experiment 2, where we again employed a distractor that was both related to and used in conjunction with the target, but one that was somewhat larger than either the cup or the jug (a coffee pot). Since the present results resemble those using the different rather than the same-size distractor, the data are difficult to understand simply in terms of object size and seem more related to whether the distractor fulfils part of the instruction set (in particular, having the identity of a cup). A distractor that does not fulfil part of the instruction set can be rejected in selecting the action on a trial, so that it does not capture the response activated by the target. We suggest that distractor rejection is based on inhibition that is applied not only to the representation of the distractor stimulus but also to co-active responses. As a result, there is blocking of the response activated by the target, and rebound selection of the opposite hand to make the response to the target.

In the final experiment, we evaluated the response-blocking effect in order to assess whether it reflected the semantic relations between targets and distractors or the strength of the associated action between stimuli. We have found response-blocking effects on target cups from distractor coffee pots and jugs. These stimuli are all semantically related, tending to be found together in the same contexts and they are used to carry out a common function (making coffee). In addition to this, though, the actions made with the objects are directional, in that coffee pots and jugs tend to be used to pour liquid into cups, and (usually) cups are not used to pour liquid into coffee pots or jugs. It may be that there is strong suppression of coffee pot and jug distractors (and any co-active response) in order to overcome an over-learned action in which these stimuli are used in conjunction with the target. This produces a stronger blocking effect than is found, for example, with neutral distractors of a similar size (e.g. the wooden blocks in Experiment B). To test this in Experiment 4 we simply reversed the roles of the cup and jug: the jug was the target and the cup the distractor. We assume that cups are used less often in actions connected with jugs than jugs are in actions connected with cups. Consequently, reaching to a cup distractor paired with a jug target should be a weaker competitor for action selection than reaching to a jug distractor paired with a cup target. If inhibition for action selection to the target is proportional to the activation of the distractor (Tipper et al. 2000), then inhibition effects (and response blocking) should be reduced here.

Experiment 4: target jug and distractor cup

Method

The method was exactly the same as for Experiment 3, except that the target and distractor stimuli were reversed. The instruction was to pick up the jug using the hand compatible with the handle, and to ignore the distractor cup. The number of trials matched those in Experiment 3.

Results and discussion

FK made only two errors in the study (overall 158/160 correct). There was one error when the distractor was in the reach trajectory cued by the target, when he made an incompatible hand response to the target (target right, distractor handle right in near-right location; response: left-hand reach). There was one error when the distractor was opposite to the cued side and FK used the correct hand but reached to the top of the jug. When the distractor fell in the path of the action cued by the target, performance was better in Experiment 4 than in Experiment 3 (P=0.003, Fisher exact probability).

FK performed better when the task required reaching to a target jug paired with a distractor cup than when he had to reach to a target cup and the distractor was a jug. This result occurred even though FK had participated in a number of previous sessions in which he had had to make reaching responses to target cups, which ought to have increased the potency of the cup as a distractor. The data were not due to FK altering the temporal dynamics of his performance in the task, nor to a general improvement in his condition. In all the present experiments FK responded promptly on a trial and showed few signs of hesitation or alteration of the action once it was set underway. To test for general improvements, we subsequently repeated the procedure with the cup as target and the jug as distractor. FK again made response blocking errors when the distractor fell in the reach trajectory cued by the target, when he used the hand incompatible with the handle on the target (these arose in 13/80 trials; $P<0.001$, Fisher exact probability, for the comparison relative to performance in the comparable conditions in Experiment 4). There were no other errors (80/80 correct when the distractor fell on the opposite side to the hand cued by the target).

The semantic relatedness between the cup and jug should be equivalent irrespective of which is deemed the target and which the distractor. However, since effects of target-distractor assignment affected performance, we conclude that general semantic relatedness is less important than the strength of the action association between one object (the jug) and the other (the cup). When there is a strong association, there is increased inhibition of the distractor and any co-active action, and blocking of the response cued initially by the handle of the target.

General discussion

We have examined target and action selection in a patient FK with impaired control of action selection after damage to the medial and anterior temporal lobes and to medial frontal regions. Two patterns of error have been demonstrated in simple tasks requiring reaching to and grasping the handle of a target cup or jug in the context of an irrelevant distractor.

First, when the distractor had a similar functional identity to the target (both being cups, though differing in colour), FK made errors by sometimes grasping the distractor rather than the target: distractor capture errors. However, these errors were not due to the distractor winning any initial competition for selection. Errors were contingent on the orientation of the handle of the target, not that of the distractor. As a consequence, distractor capture errors were equally likely irrespective of whether the distractor's handle was compatible or incompatible with the actual response (Experiment B, Riddoch et al. 2000a; Experiment 1 here). In contrast, when the task was to respond to the same target according to novel task instructions, FK had difficulty making incompatible responses and often made compatible responses in error (Experiment A, where he had to use the hand on the side where a cup was placed; see Riddoch et al. 2000a). The difficulty FK had in effecting incompatible responses under a novel instruction set emphasises that, here, capture errors were not incompatible responses evoked by distractors; rather they were compatible responses evoked by the target that happened to be taken up by distractors. In Experiment 1 here, we further showed that errors were determined by the position of the target's handle with respect to FK's right and left hands, not the position relative to the left and right sides of his body. Below we outline a more detailed account of how distractor capture comes about.

Second, when the distractor differed in kind from the target, but was used in relation to it (e.g. jug->cup), response blocking errors occurred. These errors were present in trials where the distractor fell in the reach path cued by the target (e.g. target handle right, distractors near-right position), when FK sometimes reached to the target using the hand incompatible with its handle (e.g. using his left hand). We suggest that these errors occurred in trials where the distractor was subjected to strong inhibition in order for the target to be selected. However, why should inhibition of the distractor lead to blocking of the compatible response activated by the target? To account for this we propose that inhibition is applied to perceptual-motor assemblies established on the basis of concurrent excitation in stimulus and response representations. If response activation from the target is concurrent with excitation of stimulus representations for distractors, inhibition from the target and the instruction set is carried over to the compatible target response. Blocking errors were reduced when we reversed targets and distractors so that the distractors tended not to be used in relation to targets (cups to jugs, rather than jugs to cups; Experiment 4). This last result indicates that semantic relatedness per se is less important than the strength of the learned action between objects. There is strong inhibition if the distractor is habitually used in conjunction with the target.

A framework for object and action selection

Object and action selection

The present findings point to behaviour even in simple reaching tasks being dependent on a complex sequence of events, involving competition between target and distractor representations for the control of action. FK shows poor task-based selection of actions, so that response instructions cannot easily be used to overrule learned actions to stimuli (see Experiment A). Nevertheless, he remains able to use the instruction set to select the target object for an action. This suggests that object selection can precede action selection, and be relatively spared in a patient such as FK even when action selection is impaired (see also Riddoch et al. 2000a, 2000b). A framework illustrating this suggestion is presented in Fig. 1. In this framework, we propose that there is an 'early' process of object selection and a 'late' process of action selection. These processes of object and action selection determine the momentary dominance of, respectively, one stimulus and one response, during action. Both forms of selection may be realised within 'winner take all' networks, which have been used to simulate aspects of human selective attention (e.g. Humphreys and Heinke 1998; Koch and Ullman 1985; Mozer 1991). Within such networks, selection is determined by increasing the activation of target representations and inhibiting those of distractors. In some realisations, excitation and inhibition are controlled by separate mecha-

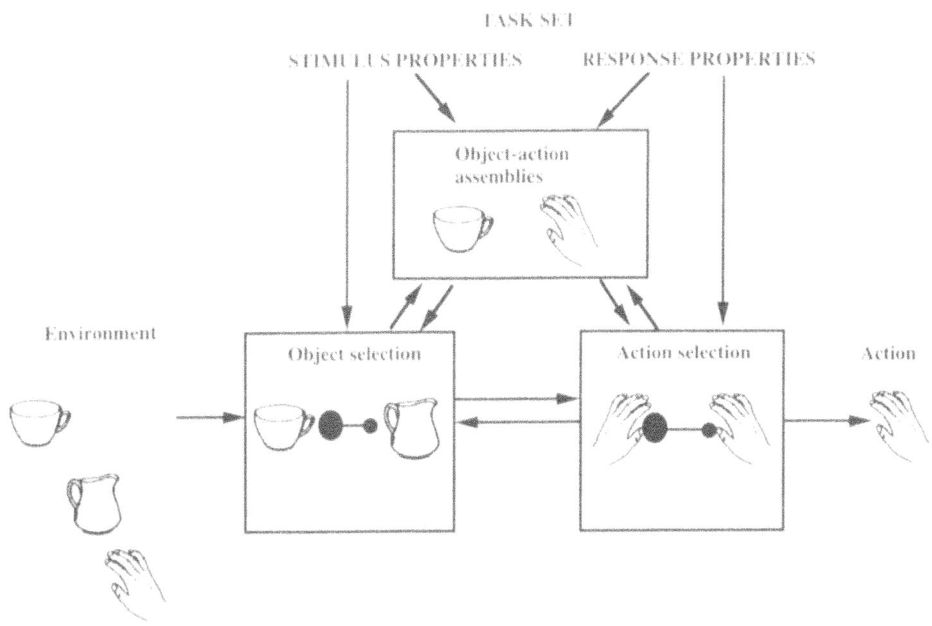

Fig. 1 A framework illustrating the relations between object selection, action selection, and object–action assemblies. In this figure we illustrate the task of reaching to a cup using the hand associated with its handle, where a related distractor (the jug) lies in the reach trajectory. We suggest that the cup and the associated response are selected and linked in an object–action assembly. Subsequently, the distractor is selected (shown here by increased inhibition of the target) so that it can direct influence action parameterization. Nevertheless, maintenance of the object–action assembly for the target enables the action to be made to the target but influenced by (and by-passing) the distractor

nisms (e.g. Houghton and Tipper 1994; Houghton et al. 1996). Within models of this type, a distractor may be activated on the basis of learned contextual relations with a target whilst concurrently being inhibited as a competitor by the target representation. The degree of inhibition required to select the target would then be a function of the activation of the distractor. The stronger the distractor is as a candidate, the greater the inhibition required to bias selection in favour of the target.

Object selection will be affected by task criteria specifying the perceptual attributes of targets, and by factors such as the perceptual similarity between targets and distractors. Action selection will be determined by the strength of the learned response to the stimulus, and it will be affected by the relative activations of responses evoked by the stimulus and the task set (e.g. between a left or a right hand action, between a power or a precision grip etc.). We suggest that object selection precedes action selection. Thus a patient with impaired selection of unfamiliar responses in a task can nevertheless show reasonable object selection based on novel criteria (Riddoch et al. 2000a, 2000b). This is not to state, however, that the two processes would necessarily proceed as discrete stages. For instance, planning of a motor response to a location may bias object selection to the same location (Deubelet al. 1998), due to feed-forward from the action system to the object-selection system. The present studies used targets that were relatively easy to discriminate, at relatively separate spatial locations, and under these conditions we propose that there was little influence on object selection of the relative strength of response activation by targets and distractors. Targets were selected according to their perceptual properties (e.g. their colour), and a response associated to the target was activated. Nevertheless distractors did influence performance subsequently, when they fell in the reach trajectory to targets. To account for this, we need to account for how selection and action evolve over time; this account relies on the idea of object–action assemblies.

Object–action assemblies

In addition to the transitory processes of object and action selection, we propose that there are longer-lasting representations of selected objects and actions that serve to guide behaviour when it involves multiple steps. We term these object–action assemblies. For example, take a situation in which one wants to walk across a crowded room to reach a target. Here one might initially select the target and aspects of the action (walk across the room, in a given direction). In addition, en route other objects will need to be selected so that they can be avoided, and these other objects need to influence the motor programs being computed. The object- and action-selection processes will constantly be updated over time. Now it would not do to have behaviour determined solely by each object as it is selected without also (1) maintaining a representation of the eventual target and (2) allowing aspects of this representation (e.g. the location of the target) to influence the selection of ongoing actions (e.g. so that actions are updated in respect to the directional parameter provided by the target). Without this form of longer-lasting representation, an actor would wander in a goal-less state, with behaviour determined only by each new object that is selected. Within the framework shown in Fig. 1, longer-lasting representations of targets and linked actions are held in object–action assemblies, which continue to influence immediate object and action selection processes as behaviour evolves over time. The object–action assemblies provide a form of hierarchical control over motor behaviour, maintaining the correct goal structure whilst lower-order parameters are altered according to which objects are subsequently selected. In our terms, action selection involves competition for these lower-level parameters, a process affected partly by the object momentarily being selected and by the object represented in the object–action assembly. This separation, of transient object- and action-selection processes, and a more sustained representation of an object–action assembly, enables distractors to be selected and to influence the evolving action to the target rather than becoming targets for actions in their own right. Of course distractors, once selected, may also compete to be represented at the highest level in the object–action assembly, but they will usually be overruled by activation from the representation of the target.

This framework can be applied to simpler situations, such as reaching to grasp a cup when a distractor jug falls along the path of action. Here we suggest that the cup is initially selected, and this is followed by activation of the associated action. However after this the distractor object is selected perhaps because attention is applied to the spatial area between the effector and the target object, to avoid possible collisions. During this second object-selection process an object–action assembly is maintained for the target, so that this remains the goal of the action and so that movement parameters are selected with respect to target, not distractor, properties (e.g. the hand selected should be appropriate to the target rather than the distractor). This object–action assembly is then used to guide the subsequent selection and parameterization of the action over time, as a hand movement is made to the target but avoiding the distractor.

To account for the patterns of performance with FK we suggest the following. First, consider capture errors. It appears that FK is able to implement the task set to enable the target object to be selected. There is then activation of the response associated with the target, based on relatively direct links between the representation of the object and its over-learned response (e.g. grasp the handle of the cup with the hand compatible with the position of the handle; see Riddoch et al. 1998). At a later moment in time, the distractor is selected. We propose that FK is impaired in his ability to maintain the longer-duration object–action assemblies that would allow the reach to the target to be made normally. Instead we suggest that only parts of the object representation are used in any object–action assembly (e.g. that it is a cup but not a red cup). This makes the object representation vulnerable to replacement by a distractor that shares the same part-representation (e.g. when the distractor is a green cup). Capture errors result in which the action is directed to the similar distractor though aspects of the object–action assembly set up by the target may be carried over (e.g. using the hand selected on the basis of the target).

Second, consider the response-blocking effect. Here we suppose again that the target is initially selected (along with selection of the hand for the action), and this is followed by selection of the distractor. Now at this stage a distractor that is used habitually to act upon the target will be activated particularly strongly, and may even become linked to parts of the dominant object–action assembly in a patient who is impaired in ability to maintain a stable representation of the target at this level. We presume this is the case for FK. Nevertheless, distractors with a different identity to the target will contravene the instruction set (not having the appropriate target properties), and so be subject to inhibition from this source so that the distractor representation never determines the action. On the other hand, inhibition of the distractor representation will also lead to inhibition of the associated action assembly, when both have become linked. Due to inhibition of this assembly, there is suppression of the action parameterized at the time – even though this was initially activated by the target. A blocking error then occurs.

Our framework, separating object selection, action selection and the maintenance of object–action assemblies, has several attributes. In particular it allows us to explain both capture and blocking errors in a single model. It can also account for both (1) why FK's performance is determined by the initial selection of the target, and (2) why distractors nevertheless affect the evolving target response. Furthermore, the account can also be related to physiological data on the role and properties of cells in the prefrontal cortex. For example, Fuster (1995) and Goldman-Rakic (1990) have both argued that the lateral prefrontal cortex acts as a form of working memory, maintaining information over temporal intervals whilst other stimuli are being presented. This may contrast with earlier cortical areas where activation is dictated by the stimulus currently present or being attended to. Miller (1999) further points out that cells in lateral prefrontal cortex can help to establish links between object identity, spatial location and properties of the action (e.g. saccade left or right), similar to our proposal for object–action assemblies being formed that may direct the selection of parameterised actions in motor cortex. FK has damage to his medial frontal lobes, rather than to more lateral frontal areas. Nevertheless, this damage may disrupt the influence of object–action assemblies on action. These assemblies may normally direct action selection via medial areas of frontal cortex, including the supplementary motor cortex, which are involved in task-based control of action (see Passingham 1993). As a consequence, FK's performance is highly vulnerable to effects of distractors even in simple reaching tasks of the type we have explored.

Acknowledgements The work was supported by grants from the Medical Research Council and the Wellcome Trust (UK). We thank FK for his kind participation in the study.

References

Broadbent DE (1958) Perception and communication. Pergamon Press, London

Castiello U (1996) Grasping a fruit: Selection for action. J Exp Psychol Hum Percept Perform 22:582–603

Deubel H, Schneider WX, Paprotta I (1998) Selective diorsal and ventral processing: Evidence for a common attentional mechanism in reaching and perception. Vis Cogn 5:81–108

Fuster, J.M. (1995) Memory in the cerebral cortex. MIT Press, Cambridge, Mass.

Goldman-Rakic PS (1990) Cellular and circuit basis of working memory in prefrontal cortex of nonhuman primates. Prog Brain Res 85:325–335

Houghton G, Tipper SP (1994) A model of inhibitory mechanisms in selective attention. In: Dagenbach D, Carr T (eds) Inhibitory mechanisms in attention, memory and language. Academic Press, Orlando, Fl.:

Houghton G, Tipper SP, Weaver B, Shore, D.I. (1996) Inhibition and interference in selective attention: Some tests of a neural network model. Vis Cogn 3:119–164

Humphreys GW, Forde E (1998) Disordered action schema and action disorganization syndrome. Cogn Neuropsychol 15:771–811

Humphreys, GW, Heinke D (1998) Spatial representation and selection in the brain: Neuropsychological and computational constraints. Vis Cogn 5:9–47

Humphreys GW, Rumiati RI (1998) Agnosia without prosopagnosia or alexia: Evidence for stored visual memories specific to objects. Cogn Neuropsychol 15:243–278

Humphreys GW, Forde, EME, Francis D (2000) The organisation of sequential action. In: Monsell S, Driver J (eds) Attention and performance XVIII. MIT Press, Cambridge, Mass., in press

Kay J, Lesser R, Coltheart M (1992) PALPA. Lawrence Erlbaum, London

Koch C, Ullman S (1985) Shifts in selective visual attention: Towards the underlying neural circuitry. Hum Neurobiol 4:219–227

Lhermitte F (1983) 'Utilisation' behaviour and its relation to lesions of the frontal lobes. Brain 106:237–255

Miller, E.K. (1999) Prefrontal cortex and the neural basis of executive functions. In: Humphreys GW, Duncan J, Treisman A (eds) Attention, space and action: Studies in cognitive neuroscience. Oxford University Press, Oxford

Mozer MC (1991) The perception of multiple objects: A connectionist approach. MIT Press, Cambridge, Mass.

Passingham R (1993) The frontal lobes and voluntary action. Oxford University Press, Oxford

Posner MI, Petersen SE (1990) The attention system of the human brain. Ann Rev Neurosci 13:25–42

Riddoch MJ, Humphreys GW (1987) Visual object processing in optic aphasia: A case of semantic access agnosia. Cogn Neuropsychol 4:131–185

Riddoch MJ, Humphreys GW (1993) BORB: The Birmingham Object Recognition Battery. Psychology Press, London

Riddoch MJ, Edwards MG, Humphreys GW, West R,. Heafield T (1998) An experimental study of anarchic hand syndrome: Evidence that visual affordances direct action. Cogn Neuropsychol 15:645–683

Riddoch MJ, Humphreys GW, Edwards MG (2000a) Visual affordances and object selection. In: Monsell S, Driver J (eds) Attention and performance XVIII. MIT Press, Cambridge, Mass., in press

Riddoch MJ, Humphreys GW, Edwards MG (2000b) Neuropsychological evidence distinguishing object selection from action (effector) selection. Cogn Neuropsychol, in press

Rizzolatti G, Riggio L, Dascola I, Umilta C (1987) Reorienting of attention across horizontal and vertical meridians. Neuropsychologia 25:31–40

Rizzolatti G, Riggio L, Sheliga BM (1994) Space and selective attention. In: Umilta C, Moscovitch M (eds) Attention and performance XV. MIT Press, Cambridge, Mass.

Sheliga BM, Riggio L, Rizzolatti G (1994) Orienting of attention and eye movements. Exp Brain Res 98:507–522

Tipper SP, Lortie C, Baylis GC (1992) Selective reaching: Evidence for action-centred attention. J Exp Psychol Hum Percept Perform 18:891–905

Tipper SP, Howard LA. Jackson SR (1997) Selective reaching to grasp: Evidence for distractor interference effects. Vis Cogn 4:1–38

Tipper SP, Howard LA. Houghton G. (2000) Behavioural consequences of selection from neural population codes. In: Monsell S, Driver J (eds), Attention and performance XVIII. MIT Press, Cambridge, Mass.

Tresilian JR (1998) Attention in action or obstruction of movement? A kinematic analysis of avoidance behavior in prehension. Exp Brain Res 120:352–368

H.J. Markowitsch · J. Kessler

Massive impairment in executive functions with partial preservation of other cognitive functions: the case of a young patient with severe degeneration of the prefrontal cortex

Published online: 19 May 2000

Abstract Historical bases for the special role of the prefrontal cortex are outlined and the case of a 27-year-old woman with massive bilateral prefrontal damage of unknown etiology is then described. Frontal lobe degeneration was repeatedly examined with magnetic resonance imaging and fluoro-deoxy-D-glucose -positron emission tomography and was found to include both orbital and dorsolateral aspects of the frontal lobes. While the degeneration initially measured was limited to portions of the orbital, medial and dorsolateral parts of both frontal lobes, with right-sided predominance, a second brain scan 15 months later revealed massive shrinkage of both frontal lobes, together with additional involvement of the posterior association cortices. The patient had completed her high-school education and had superior verbal long-term memory, normal short-term memory, and normal priming, but manifested grossly deficient scores in various frontal lobe-sensitive tests. Though a number of neurological examinations were performed, no plausible cause for the damage was established.

Key words PET · History of frontal lobe · Pick's disease · Frontotemporal dementia

Introduction

Since the beginning of modern brain research, the frontal lobes in particular have attracted scientists. Niessl von Mayendorf (1908, p 1175) termed the prefrontal cortex the most mythical part of the brain. The interest in the frontal lobes (or, more particularly, the prefrontal cortex; Owen 1868) originated from a number of diverse but influential sources. Among them were the observations of Fritsch and Hitzig (1870) that the frontal lobes were electrically non-excitable or 'silent'; that is, electrical stimulation of the area did not result in movements of the eyes or other body parts, and extirpation produced neither any form of paralysis nor loss of perceptual abilities, but rather defects of intelligence. Fritsch and Hitzig (1870) therefore termed the frontal lobes the 'organ for abstract reasoning'. Another important origin for their special role arose from Brodmann's (1912) description of a considerable expansion of the prefrontal cortex across mammals, culminating in the human prefrontal cortex (Table 1). Planning, foresight and decision-making were among the attributes assigned to this region, which Brodmann (1909, 1912) termed the 'regio frontalis' (Anton and Zingerle 1902; Bianchi 1895; Ferrier 1874; Ferrier and Yeo 1884). Even before Brodmann, Flechsig (1896a) had emphasized the roles of the prefrontal cortex in attentive processes and their consequences for personality ('active attention, contemplation, goal-directed ego'; p 63); furthermore Flechsig (1896b) considered the frontal association center as responsible for the control of drives, saying that animals and human infants with their still underdeveloped association areas are merely 'Affectwesen' (affective creatures) (p 103).

Personality dimensions were also placed in the foreground by the report of Welt (1888). She described several patients with prefrontal damage. One of them, a craftsman, had been described as a cheerful, relaxed man of good humor who due to a prefrontal tumor became very critical and annoying to his co-patients. When the professor of the clinic urged him to behave himself and told him that he received good meals and the best wine in the hospital, the patient answered that the other patients and the hospital staff were at fault and, concerning the wines, that he was used to drinking Chateau Lafitte and other French wines but not the sour stuff provided in the clinic.

Even before Welt's time, the astonishing story of Phineas Gage, the crowbar case, had appeared (Harlow 1848, 1869; Bigelow 1850; Damasio et al. 1994). Phineas Gage's maxillary bone was pierced by an iron

H.J. Markowitsch (✉)
Physiological Psychology, University of Bielefeld,
D-33501 Bielefeld, Germany
e-mail: hjmarkowitsch@uni-bielefeld.de

J. Kessler
Max-Planck-Institute for Neurological Research, Cologne,
Germany

Table 1 Surface area of the regio frontalis (in mm) and its relation to the total surface of the cerebral cortex (in %) for some mammals (based on Brodmann 1912). [In the heading of his table, Brodmann (1912) originally stated that values for the surface area of both the regio frontalis and the regio praecentralis would be provided; however, his table actually includes only values for the regio frontalis, as becomes clear from his discussion of these values in several species (e.g. p 196)]

Order	Species	Total cortical surface of one hemisphere (in mm^2)	Regio frontalis	Proportion of the regio frontalis to the total cortical surface (in %)
Primates	Man, *Homo sapiens*	135,470	39,287	29.0
	Chimpanzee, *Pan troglodytes*	39,572	6,719	16.9
	Great gibbon, *Symphalangus syndactylus*	16,302	1,839	11.3
	Mandrill, *Papio sphinx*	21,321	2,168	10.1
	Baboon, *Papio hamadryas*	20,594	1,967	9.5
	Baboon, *Papio cynocephalus*	20,376	2,111	10.3
	Moor macaque, *Macaca maurus*	15,308	1,733	11.3
	Guenon, *Cercopithecus sp.?*	14,641	1,625	11.1
	Capuchin monkey, *Cebus capucinus*	13,682	1,260	9.2
	Black pencilled marmoset, *Callithrix penicillata*	1,649	148	8.9
Prosimii	Red-bellied lemur, *Lemur rubriventer*	4,054	337	8.3
	Greater dwarf lemur, *Cheirogaleus major*	921	70	7.2
Chiroptera	Flying fox, *Pteropus edwarsi geoffroy*	1,097	26	2.3
Carnivora	Dog, *Canis familiaris*	9,527	657	6.9
	Cat, *Felis domestica*	4,474	152	3.4
Lagomorphes	Common rabbit, *Oryctolagus cuniculus*	1,627	36	2.2
Insectivora	Hedgehog, *Erinaceus europaeus*	575	–	–
Edentata	Hairy armadillo, *Chaetophractus villosus*	2,010	–	–
Marsupialia	White-eared opossum, *Didelphis albiventris azarae*	804	–	–

rod of more than one meter in length and roughly 6 kg in weight. Due to a dynamite explosion this rod passed first through his left eye, then through the frontal lobes and exited at the beginning of the right upper cranium. Harlow (1848) described the man as 'Phineas P Gage, a foreman, engaged in building the road, 25 years of age, of middle stature, vigorous physical organization, temperate habits, and ... of considerable energy of character' (p 20). Phineas Gage was semi-comatose for more than two weeks, but then improved during the next month. His personality, however, had changed radically so that his friends said that he was 'no longer Gage' (Harlow 1869, p 14). In the years following the accident he worked in a livery stable and then in Chile 'to establish a line of coaches at Valparaiso' (p 14), where he remained for nearly eight years before returning to the United States. He died after several epileptic fits 'twelve years, six months and eight days after the date of his injury' (p 15f).

Harlow's (1869, p 13f) description of the behavioral changes in Phineas Gage is particularly impressive: 'The equilibrium or balance, so to speak, between his intellectual faculties and animal propensities, seems to have been destroyed. He is fitful, irreverent, indulging at times in the grossest profanity (which was not previously his custom), manifesting but little deference for his fellows, impatient of restraint or advice when it conflicts with his desires, at times pertinaciously obstinate, yet capricious and vacillating, devising many plans of future operation, which are no sooner arranged than they are abandoned in turn for others appearing more feasible. A child in his intellectual capacity and manifestations, he has the animal passions of a strong man'.

A number of other cases from the 19th century demonstrated bizarre social behavior, including religious delusions after massive prefrontal degeneration (Knörlein 1865; Voegelin 1897), and the second decade of the 20th century brought with the First World War numerous patients with prefrontal damage due to shrapnel or bullet injuries. The most extensive work in this respect was the monograph by Feuchtwanger (1923) who compared a wealth of data from 200 soldiers with definite frontal lobe damage with data from 200 other brain-damaged soldiers who most likely had no frontal lobe damage. He further subdivided the 200 frontal lobe patients into 153 with pure prefrontal damage and 47 in whom other brain regions (e.g. Broca's area, precentral cortex) were affected in addition. 'Moria' or 'Witzeln', meaning a grossly non-serious behavior with respect to one's own conditions of life, was observed nine times as often in frontal as in non-frontal damaged patients and was the symptom which most clearly differentiated the two groups. Table 2, which is translated from Feuchtwanger's Table 1, gives a summary of the frequency of occurrence of this and other symptoms.

Bianchi (1895) wrote that frontal lobe damage 'disaggregate[s] the personality, and incapacitate[s] for seriali-

Table 2 Overview of the symptoms observed in 200 frontal lobe and 200 non-frontal lobe damaged patients (based on Table 1 of Feuchtwanger 1923)

	Frontal lobe cases		Non-frontal cases	
	Total no.	%	Total no.	%
All cases	200	100	200	100
Cerebral disturbances of movement and sensation	38	19	92	46
Disturbances in balance	88	44	72	36
Cerebral language disturbances	22	11	62	31
Cerebral perceptual disturbances	2	1	45	23
Gnostic disturbances	–	–	27	14
Disturbances in remembering	60	30	71	36
Disturbances in learning	72	36	102	51
Disturbances in thinking	21	11	32	16
Disturbances in attention	117	59	93	47
Excitement and euphoria	119	60	72	36
Hastiness	8	4	3	2
Fatigue	35	18	52	26
Witzeln (moria)	9	5	1	1
Depression	54	27	30	15
Slowness and apathy	76	38	30	15
Epileptic attacks	43	22	55	28
Psychogenic disturbances	42	21	56	28

sing and synthetizing groups of representations' (p 522). Donath (1923) considered the frontal lobes to be 'the seat of the highest mental activity' (p 301). Early studies in animals discussed 'the frontal lobes as centres of inhibition' (Schäfer 1900) and as centers for intellectual states (Franz 1907). More recently, Stuss and Benson (1986) discouraged the use of animals for unraveling prefrontal functions; they considered only human case descriptions as valid, as in their eyes the human prefrontal cortex differs considerably in anatomy and functions from that of non-human species. All this work, however, demonstrates the need for ongoing investigations of the contributions of the frontal lobes to the processing of intellectual functions.

Feuchtwanger's (1923) ideas still represent major aspects of the modern state of the art. His summary of the psychological sector, given on pages 174 and 175, reads in translation: 'The various forms of damage in frontal lobe patients have in common the fact that their psychic disturbances are within the fields of emotion and performance, and not in the field of concrete actions, as with damage in more posteriorly situated parts of the cerebral cortex. Disturbances of concrete functions (perception, memory, thinking, movement, etc.), which can be found in pure prefrontal damage, are in the cases investigated not primarily but secondarily caused by the emotional or topical deficits.'

Additional aspects of the frontal lobes which have been discussed more recently, based on their marked evolutionary development and their late neuronal maturation (Fuster 1997; Jerison 1997), are self-awareness, metamemory, and conscious reflection (Shimamura 1995; Stuss 1991; Wheeler et al. 1997).

A major issue in the description of patients with prefrontal damage is the discrepancy between some who appeared little concerned, joyful, and alert, while others appeared depressed (Feuchtwanger 1923; Lahmeyer 1982; Ross and Stewart 1987). Such descriptions resulted in a differentiation between orbitofrontal portions of the frontal lobes, damage to which was associated with disinhibited behavior, changed personality traits and emotional flatness, and dorsolateral ones, damage to which produced an inhibited, depressed, or even compulsive personality (Eisen et al. 1997; Harrington et al. 1997; Röhrenbach and Markowitsch 1997). The right frontal hemisphere seems especially related to emotional but also to attentive processing (Heilman and Van den Abell 1980; Rueckert and Grafman 1996; Schuster 1902; Starkstein et al. 1989).

Biochemical alterations in the prefrontal cortex and changes in its connectivity may alter physiological and cognitive reactions to stress (Frith and Done 1988; Markowitsch 1999). There are also single case reports on severe cognitive impairments after bilateral frontal lobe damage (Eslinger and Damasio 1985).

In conclusion, the prefrontal cortex has a major role in the control of cognitive and affective behavior. Consequently, a patient with major and bilateral prefrontal degeneration can be expected to have severe impairments in these behavioral dimensions. In the next part of this paper, neuroanatomical and neuropsychological data will be reported on a young adult patient who came to our attention because of certain bizarre behaviors in her everyday life.

Case report

The mother of a 27-year-old woman reported that her daughter sometimes behaved in an odd manner – failing to detect obvious items, storing garbage in the car, or 'seeing' people who in fact did not exist. The patient had finished high-school education and had engaged in a number of different professional activities, from starting to study foreign languages to secretarial assistant jobs. She had no long-term friend, though she and her mother said that she had had a few partners for short periods. Some weeks prior to her first neurological examination, her failure to organize her private life became so obvious that she had to give up living in a

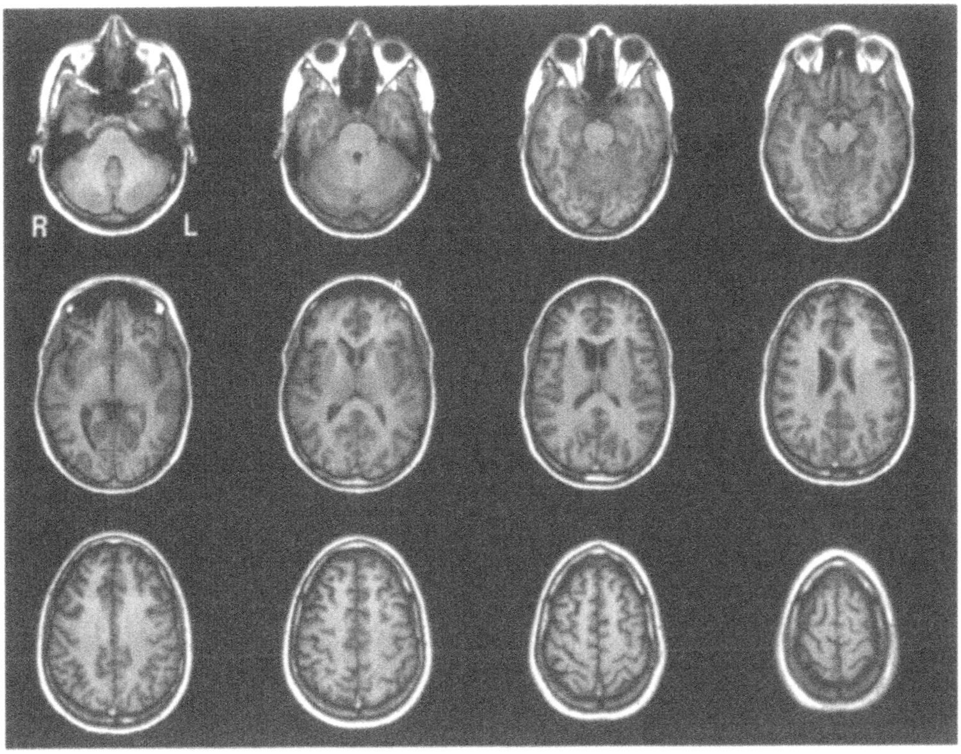

Fig. 1 Horizontal T1-weighted MRI-sections at the first neuropsychological and neuroradiological examination of the patient described in this paper. The cortical atrophy is principally restricted to the prefrontal regions and to the right hemisphere

shared household in a major city and return to her mother's home in a city about three hours away from her former residence.

The patient was studied neuropsychologically and neuroradiologically at two time points separated by 15 months. At her first examination, she already appeared unconcerned about her condition and denied any changes or abnormalities in her behavior. Standard and special laboratory tests yielded no pathological results. There were no pathological signs in EEG. Brain scanning was done with a magnetic resonance scanner (MRI; 1T Siemens Magnetom Impact; T1 and T2 images of 2 or 2.5 mm thickness). A three-dimensional fast low-angle shot mode (repetition time 32 ms, echo time 6 ms, flip angle 40°) provided 64 contiguous slices with a slice thickness of 2.5 mm. MRI disclosed bilateral atrophy of the prefrontal cortex with predominance in the right frontal lobe. Structural involvement of other cortical areas or subcortical gray matter was absent (Fig. 1).

Positron emission tomography (PET) was performed on a high resolution scanner (Siemens ECAT EXACT HR) (Wienhard et al. 1994) with septa retracted in 3D acquisition mode. The PET scan was then co-registered to the MRI. All images were displayed and inspected on transaxial, coronal and sagittal planes. Fluoro-deoxy-D-glucose-PET confirmed the degeneration, which included orbitofrontal and dorsolateral portions of the prefrontal cortex while the rest of the brain appeared normal.

For the right frontal lobe, brain damage was seen all along the basal prefrontal cortex, sparing however its lateral aspect. The degeneration followed the frontal pole upwards to include all of the medial frontal gyrus up to the level of the precentral gyrus (which appeared normal). Furthermore, anterior portions of the superior frontal gyrus were affected as well. In the left frontal lobe, degeneration was less pronounced but included medial orbitofrontal, frontopolar, and medial frontal gyral portions as well. The posterior end of the degeneration was limited by the border between the medial and inferior frontal gyri.

Neuropsychologically, the patient was characterized by – at first glance – largely normal intellectual performance: her short-term memory was average, her verbal long-term memory (Verbal Selective Reminding Test of Buschke 1973; Logical Memory subtest of the Wechsler Memory Scale – revised; Wechsler 1987) even above average; in the Benton test and in a language test she performed normally as well (Table 1). Her visual priming was also normal. However, all visuo-constructive tests, including all relevant portions of intelligence tests (Progressive Matrices of Raven; mosaic test of the Shortened Wechsler Intelligence Test; Dahl 1986), and all tests measuring cognitive flexibility, reasoning, or fluency, were far below average and sometimes in an extremely subnormal range (Table 3).

Measuring her personality traits (Freiburger Personality Inventory; Fahrenberg et al. 1989) revealed a person without much ambition or competition, who otherwise appeared largely in the normal range. The patient was, however, completely anosognosic with respect to her deficits. When confronted with her poor test results she simply said that she either did not like the respective tests or that they were irrelevant to her life.

Fifteen months after the first detailed examination the patient was studied again, using principally the same methods, both neuropsychologically and neuroradiologically. As is evident from Table 3, she initially had preserved verbal memory functions (Selective Reminding Test, Logical Memory of the Wechsler Memory Scale-revised), while at her second examination verbal memory had considerably deteriorated as well. The only test results within normal range were some language abilities (writing to dictation, oral repetition), digit span forward, and picture priming.

When asked about her situation she responded that she was well and comfortable, though her mother said she could no longer read and was even unable to select TV programs. She still managed to go for short periods to a fitness center and also went out with her dog. Interestingly, from a short conversation her deficits would not immediately become apparent.

On the anatomical side, her degeneration had markedly increased, with the prefrontal cortex being considerably shrunken. MRI, done with the identical technique as initially, disclosed a progressive cortical atrophy that predominantly affected frontotemporal cortical areas, but also affected the parietal cortex bilaterally. The progressive atrophy is obvious from the enlargement of the cerebral sulci (Fig. 2). In contrast to the previous MRI-scan, the cortical atrophy had extended to the temporal and parietal lobes, and the initial asymmetry in frontal atrophy had disap-

Table 3 Neuropsychological test performance of the patient at first and second examination. *min* minutes; *C* centile score, *PC* percentile, *T* T score, *LPS* Leistungs-Prüf-System, *FAS* production of substantives starting with the letters F, A, or S, *WCST* Wisconsin Card Sorting Test. If not stated otherwise, all scores for the control subjects refer to means ± one standard deviation

Test	Performance		Remarks (control scores)
	1st examination	2nd examination (15 months later)	
Mini Mental State examination	Not assessed	19	Demented
Selective Reminding Test			
Immediate recall	6.6±1.2	4.4±0.5	7.87±0.9
After delay (15 min)	8	3	7.11±1.3
Rey-Osterrieth Figure			
Copy	9	4	35.1±1.5
After delay	8.5	3	22.7±7
Logical memory			
Immediate recall	32 (PC=70)	16 (PC=0)	(28.5) (PC=50)
Delayed recall	25 (PC=60)	18 (PC=17)	(24) (PC=50)
Digit span			
Forwards	5	4	5
Backwards	3	3	4–5
Block span	Not assessed	Impossible	5
Benton test (multiple choice)	2 errors	11 errors	2 errors
Raven progressive matrices	19 (PC<5)	Impossible	44 (PC=50)
Mosaic test	1 (PC=0)	Impossible	31.6±7.6 (PC=50)
Fragmented picture test			
A	26	24	22.1±4.2
B	15	16	11.8±2.2
Reasoning (LPS-IV)	1 (C=5)	Impossible	(C=5)
Fluency test			
FAS	25	7	45.3
Animals	13	7	18.6
Stroop test, interference condition	222 s (T=23)	Impossible	78 s (T=50)
Modified trail making test	255 s (PC=0)	Impossible	75 s (PC=50)
Tower of Hanoi, 3 discs	Impossible	Impossible	
WCST, error ratio	325	Impossible	<50
Items of Ghent's overlapping figures	Not assessed	13/40	>35
Aachener aphasia test			
Token test	0 errors	Impossible	1.3 (1.6)
Naming	117	90	111.1 (5.4)
Reading	Not assessed	Impossible	29.7 (0.6)
Writing to dictation	Not assessed	29	Unimpaired 29.3 (0.7)
Oral repetition	Not assessed	148	Unimpaired 147.1 (3.3)
Written numeral transcoding			
Arabic numerals to number words	Not assessed	0	9.9 (0.1)
Number words to arabic numerals	Not assessed	0	9.7 (0.3)
Elaborated calculation C 301 R [n]			
Mental calculation	Not assessed	2	15.9 (0.5)
Written calculation	Not assessed	0	14.4 (0.9)

peared. Furthermore, there was a moderate symmetrical atrophy of the head of the caudate nucleus and a moderate enlargement of the lateral ventricles, indicating progressive inner atrophy. Neither finding had been obvious in the first MRI scan (Fig. 1).

Figures 1 and 2 provide images of the patient's brain at the time of the first and second examinations.

Discussion

The patient shows the typical cognitive and affective consequences of combined dorsal and orbital prefrontal damage: in general, preserved cognitive functions for those abilities which do not require flexible adjustments and adaptations to environmental changes, reduced abili-

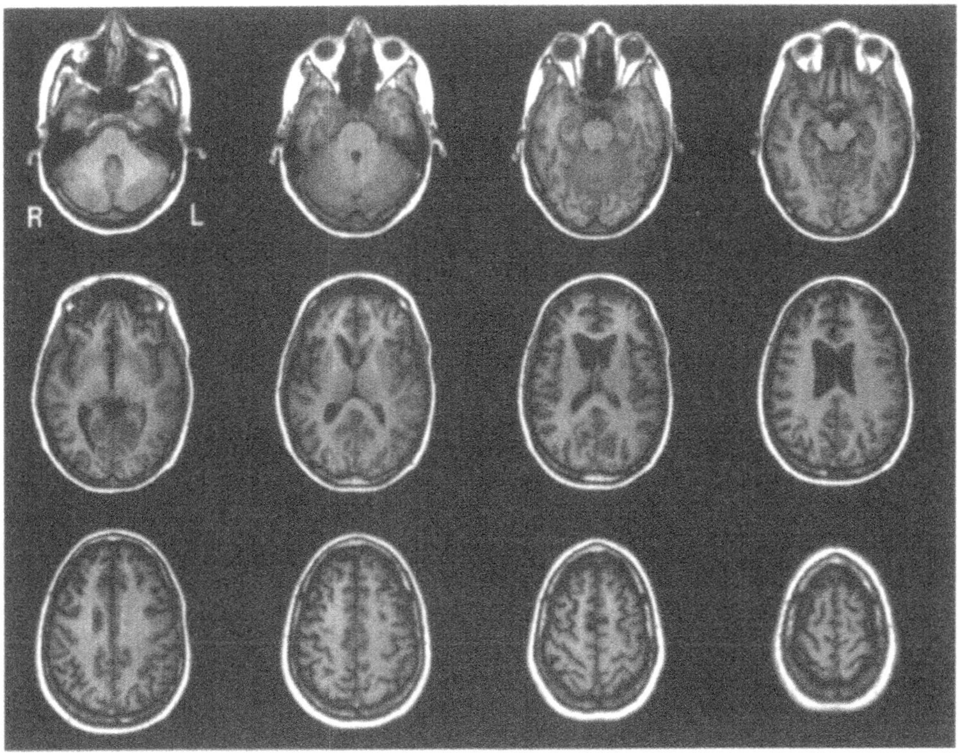

Fig. 2 Horizontal T1-weighted MRI-sections at the second neuropsychological and neuroradiological examination, about 15 months after the initial examination. Note the rapid progression of the cortical atrophy as well as the extension of the disease process into subcortical white matter structures. The atrophy now extends to the temporal and parietal lobes. The progressive atrophy is also evident from the enlargement of the cerebral sulci. The follow-up MRI also discloses atrophy of the caudate nuclei and an enlargement of the lateral ventricles

ties in executive functions and self-generated tasks, and grossly impaired performance in newly presented situations which require the development and preservation of strategies and sustained concentration (Burgess and Shallice 1996; Gershberg and Shimamura 1995; Godefroy and Rousseaux 1996, 1997; Goel et al. 1997; Miotto and Morris 1998; Röhrenbach and Markowitsch 1997; de Zubicaray et al. 1998). On the affective side, an emotional attenuation which manifested itself especially as unconcern and anosognosia was prominent.

This case resembles a number of earlier-described patients with prefrontal damage who manifested emotional flattening or hypomania (Schuster 1902; Ackerly 1935; Stuss and Benson 1983; Cicerone and Tanenbaum 1997; Hornak et al. 1996). There is also evidence for anatomical alterations in the prefrontal cortex of patients with mood disorders (Öngür et al. 1998; Sax et al. 1999) and for a changed prefrontal glucose metabolism in deviant personalities (Raine et al. 1998).

The patient is of especial interest as she was well educated, had lived on her own for several years, and had managed to lead a more or less ordinary life, though she never succeeded in long-term relationships with respect to either her professional or her social life. In this way she paralleled Phineas Gage.

Executive functions

The discrepancy in this patient between some normal or even supra-average cognitive capacities and her sometimes complete inability to deal with tasks requiring some strategic thinking or manipulating is astonishing. She had been totally unable to work with even the three-disc version of the Tower-of-Hanoi, a test which in this basic version is even managed by patients with Alzheimer's disease or Down's syndrome (Kessler et al. 1988). Similarly, in the mosaic test she was unable to construct even the most simple pattern and her copy of the Rey-Osterrieth Figure differed grossly from the original.

In these and other respects her behavior strongly resembled that of an equally young patient with severe cortical and cerebellar atrophy of unknown etiology who was unable to perform the Tower of London test, the Rey-Osterrieth Figure, or even simpler drawing tasks such as copying the required figure in the Mini Mental Status Examination (Markowitsch et al. 2000). Nevertheless, that patient had a much more generalized cortical degeneration and consequently had grossly deteriorated within two years along most cognitive dimensions.

Anosognosia

Bisiach and Geminiani (1991) noted that the earliest description of anosognosia is found in a letter of Seneca, where he described a friend of his wife who could no longer see but who let herself be guided everywhere and complained about the darkness in the house. A similar case was reported two thousand years later by Monakow (1885): His patient had extensive bilateral posterior cortical damage and could no longer see but failed to recognize his deficiency and instead attributed his behavior to the darkness of the environment. A few years later, Anton (1899) had a patient with similar characteristics.

Anton (1906) and Flechsig (1908) ascribed to the prefrontal cortex a special role in conscious reflection, and later it was indeed confirmed that patients with prefrontal damage lack introspection and self-reflection (Ackerly and Benton 1947; Brickner 1936). Recent findings confirm and extend this role of portions of the prefrontal cortex (Levine et al. 1999; Stuss 1991) and indicate furthermore that prefrontal damage may lead to anosodiaphoria – a lack of insight into one's own illness (Säring et al. 1988).

Our patient demonstrated exactly this kind of indifference, which again had been known for a long time (de Nobele 1835; Welt 1888; Feuchtwanger 1923; Sachs 1927). Her unconcern and lack of insight parallels that found in patients with orbitofrontal damage (Burgess and Shallice 1996; Nestor et al. 1992). The same is true for her reduced attentional functions (Nestor et al. 1992) and her inflexibility (Burgess and Shallice 1996; Morice and Delahunty 1996). Her reduced verbal fluency and her visuo-spatial problems are also observed in patients with lateral prefrontal damage (Park et al. 1995; Pascual-Leone et al. 1995) and, of course, in patients with dementia (Barr and Brandt 1996; Chan et al. 1997; Daum et al. 1996b; Passini et al. 1995).

Etiology

The etiology of the major prefrontal degeneration in this patient remains a riddle. Usually, frontal lobe degeneration is found especially in aged persons or in patients with age-related degenerative diseases such as Alzheimer's disease or Pick's disease or frontotemporal dementia (Gregory and Hodges 1996; Ball 1997; Frisoni et al. 1996; Giannakopoulos et al. 1997; Hachinski 1997; Levy et al. 1996; Liu et al. 1996; Raz et al. 1997; Markowitsch et al. 2000). In all these disease processes, however, the pattern of degenerated tissue deviates considerably from that observed in the present case. Though there has been a report on juvenile frontotemporal dementia, both the anatomical and behavioral aspects differed considerably from those seen in our patient (Nagaoka et al. 1995).

Recent reports also point to prefrontal changes in old people (Camiciolo et al. 1997; Chao and Knight 1997; Daum et al. 1996a; Nielsen-Bohlman and Knight 1995; Parkin et al. 1995). Exactly the same functions – complex attention, temporo-spatial information processing and controlled inhibition of action – were also strongly impaired in our patient and might suggest a phenomenon of strongly accelerated aging at the cognitive and brain levels.

Conclusions

The myth of the frontal lobes still exists in that it is regarded as the portion of the cerebral cortex which is involved in numerous non-sensory and non-motor functions, from attention concerning planning and execution to various social and personality dimensions. Patients such as the one described here illustrate quite clearly how and to what degree an individual may change, concomitant with degeneration along the prefrontal surface.

References

Ackerly S (1935) Instinctive, emotional and mental changes following prefrontal lobe extirpation. Am J Psychiatry 92:717–729

Ackerly SS, Benton AL (1947) Report of case of bilateral frontal lobe defect. Res Publ Assoc Res Nerv Ment Dis 27:479–504

Anton G (1899) Ueber die Selbstwahrnehmung der Herderkrankungen des Gehirns durch den Kranken bei Rindenblindheit und Rindentaubheit. Arch Psychiatr Nervenkrankh 32:86–127

Anton G (1906) Symptome der Stirnhirnerkrankung. Münch Med Wochenschr 53:1289–1291

Anton G, Zingerle H (1902) Bau, Leistung und Erkrankung des menschlichen Stirnhirnes. Leuschner and Lubensky, Graz

Ball MJ (1997) Frequency of stages of Alzheimer-related lesions in different age categories: concurrences and cautions. Neurobiol Aging 18:375–376

Barr A, Brandt J (1996) Word-list generation deficits in dementia. J Clin Exp Neuropsychol 18:810–822

Bianchi L (1895) The functions of the frontal lobes. Brain 18: 497–530

Bigelow HJ (1850) Dr. Harlow's case of recovery from the passage of an iron bar through the head. Am J Med Sci 39:13–22

Bisiach E, Geminiani G (1991) Anosognosia related to hemiplegia and hemianopia. In: Prigatano GD, Schacter DL (eds) Awareness of deficit after brain injury. Oxford University Press, New York, pp 63–83

Brickner RM (1936) Intellectual functions of the frontal lobes: A study based upon observation of a man after partial bilateral frontal lobectomy. Macmillan, New York

Brodmann K (1909) Vergleichende Lokalisationslehre der Grosshirnrinde in ihren Prinzipien dargestellt auf Grund des Zellenbaues. Barth, Leipzig

Brodmann K (1912) Ergebnisse über die vergleichende histologische Lokalisation der Grosshirnrinde mit besonderer Berücksichtigung des Stirnhirns. Anat Anz 41 (Suppl.):157–216

Burgess PW, Shallice T (1996) Response suppression, initiation and strategy use following frontal lobe lesions. Neuropsychologia 34:263–273

Buschke H (1973) Selective reminding for analysis of memory and learning. J Verb Learn Verb Behav 12:543–546

Camiciolo R, Howieson D, Lehman S, Kaye J (1997) Talking while walking: The effect of a dual task in aging and Alzheimer's disease. Neurology 48:955–958

Chan AS, Butters N, Salmon DP (1997) The deterioration of semantic networks in patients with Alzheimer's disease: A cross-sectional study. Neuropsychologia 35:241–248

Chao LL, Knight RT (1997) Prefrontal deficits in attention and inhibitory control with aging. Cereb Cortex 7:63–69

Cicerone KD, Tanenbaum LN (1997) Disturbance of social cognition after traumatic orbitofrontal brain injury. Arch Clin Neuropsychol 12:173–188

Dahl G (1986) WIP – Reduzierter Wechsler-Intelligenztest. Hain, Meisenheim

Damasio H, Grabowski T, Frank R, Galaburda AM, Damasio AR (1994) The return of Phineas Gage: Clues about the brain from the skull of a famous patient. Science 264:1102–1105

Daum I, Gräber S, Schugens MM, Mayes AR (1996) Memory dysfunction of the frontal type in normal ageing. NeuroReport 7:2625–2628

Daum I, Riesch G, Sartori G, Birbaumer N (1996) Semantic memory impairment in Alzheimer's disease. J Clin Exp Neuropsychol 18:648–665

de Nobele [no first name given] (1835) Observation de suicide. Annal Méd Belge Etrang Fev;113–117 de Zubicaray GI, Williams SCR, Wilson SJ, Rose SE, Brammer MJ, Bullmore ET, Simmons A, Chalk JB, Semple J, Brown AP, Smith GA, Ashton R, Doddrell DM (1998) Prefrontal cortex involvement in selective letter generation: A functional magnetic resonance imaging study. Cortex 34:389–401

Donath J (1923) Die Bedeutung des Stirnhirns für die höheren seelischen Leistungen. Dtsch Z Nervenheilkd 23:282–306

Eisen JL, Beer DA, Pato MT, Venditto TA, Rasmussen SA (1997) Obsessive-compulsive disorder in patients with schizophrenia or schizoaffective disorder. Am J Psychiatry 154:271–273

Eslinger PJ, Damasio AR (1985) Severe disturbance of higher cognition after bilateral frontal lobe ablation: Patient EVR. Neurology 35:1731–1741

Fahrenberg J, Hampel P, Selg H (1989) Die revidierte Form des Freiburger-Persönlichkeits-Inventar (FPI-R). Diagnostica 31: 1–21

Ferrier D (1874) The localisation of function in the brain. Proc R Soc Lond B 22:229–232

Ferrier D, Yeo GF (1884) A record of experiments on the effects of lesion of different regions of the cerebral hemispheres. Phil Trans R Soc 175:479–565

Feuchtwanger E (1923) Die Funktionen des Stirnhirns. Ihre Pathologie und Psychologie. Springer, Berlin

Flechsig P (1896a) Die Lokalisation der geistigen Vorgänge, insbesondere der Sinnesempfindungen des Menschen. Veit Leipzig

Flechsig P (1896b) Gehirn und Seele. Veit, Leipzig

Flechsig PE (1908) Bermerkungen über die Hörsphäre des menschlichen Gehirns. Neurol Zentralblatt 27:2–7, 50–57

Franz SI (1907) On the functions of the cerebrum. The frontal lobes. Arch Psychol 2:1–64

Frisoni GB, Beltramello A, Geroldi C, Weiss C, Bianchetti A, Trabucchi M (1996) Brain atrophy in frontotemporal dementia. J Neurol Neurosurg Psychiatry 61:157–165

Frith CD, Done DJ (1988) Towards a neuropsychology of schizophrenia. Br J Psychiatry 153:437–443

Fritsch G, Hitzig E (1870) Ueber die elektrische Erregbarkeit des Grosshirns. Arch Anatom Physiol Wiss Med 37:300–332

Fuster JM (1997) The prefrontal cortex, 3rd ed. Lippincott-Raven, Philadelphia, Pa.

Gershberg FB, Shimamura AP (1995) Impaired use of organizational strategies in free recall following frontal lobe damage. Neuropsychologia 13:1305–1333

Giannakopoulos P, Hof PR, Michel J-P, Guimon J, Brouras C (1997) Cerebral cortex pathology in aging and Alzheimer's disease: A quantitative survey of large hospital-based geriatric and psychiatric cohorts. Brain Res Rev 25:217–245

Godefroy O, Rousseaux M (1996) Divided and focused attention in patients with lesion of the prefrontal cortex. Brain Cogn 30:155–174

Godefroy O, Rousseaux M (1997) Novel decision making in patients with prefrontal or posterior brain damage. Neurology 49:695–701

Goel V, Grafman J, Tajik J, Gana S, Danto D (1997) A study of the performance of patients with frontal lobe lesions in a financial planning task. Brain 120:1805–1822

Gregory CA, Hodges JR (1996) Frontotemporal dementia: Use of consensus criteria and prevalence of psychiatric features. Neuropsychiatry Neuropsychol Behav Neurol 9:145–153

Hachinski V (1997) Frontotemporal degeneration, Pick disease, and corticobasal degeneration. Three entities or 1? Arch Neurol 54:1429

Harlow JM (1848) Passage of an iron rod through the head. Boston Med Surg J 39:389–393

Harlow JM (1869) Recovery from the passage of an iron bar through the head. Clapp, Boston

Harrington C, Salloway S, Malloy P (1997) Dramatic neurobehavioral disorder in two cases following bilateral anteromedial frontal lobe injury: Delayed psychosis and marked change in personality. Neurocase 3:137–149

Heilman KM, Van den Abell T (1980) Right hemisphere dominance for attention: The mechanisms underlying hemispheric asymmetries in attention (neglect). Neurology 30:327–330

Hornak J, Rolls ET, Wade D (1996) Face and voice expression identification in patients with emotional and behavioural changes following ventral frontal lobe damage. Neuropsychologia 34:247–261

Jerison HJ (1997) Evolution of prefrontal cortex. In: Krasnegor NA, Lyon GR, Goldman-Rakic PS (eds) Development of the prefrontal cortex: Evolution, neurobiology, and behavior. Brookes, Baltimore, pp 9–26

Kessler J, Markowitsch HJ, Denzler P, Klonner-Klopp M (1988) Cognitive functioning of juveniles with Down syndrome and other forms of mental retardation. Int J Neurosci 38,1–9

Knörlein [no first name given] (1865) Krankengeschichte und Sectionsbefund eines basalen Hirntumors. Allg Wien Med Z 15:250–252

Lahmeyer HW (1982) Frontal lobe meningioma and depression. J Clin Psychiatry 43:254–255

Levine B, Freedman M, Dawson D, Black S, Stuss DT (1999) Ventral frontal contribution to self-regulation: Convergence of episodic memory and inhibition. Neurocase 5:263–275

Levy ML, Miller BL, Cummings JL, Fairbanks LA, Craig A (1996) Alzheimer disease and frontotemporal dementias. Arch Neurol 53:687–690

Liu X, Erikson C, Brun A (1996) Cortical synaptic changes and gliosis in normal aging, Alzheimer's disease and frontal lobe degeneration. Dementia 7:128–134

Markowitsch HJ (1999) Neuroimaging and mechanisms of brain function in psychiatric disorders. Curr Opin Psychiatry 12: 331–337

Markowitsch HJ, Kessler J, Frölich L, Schramm U (2000) Severe degenerative cortical and cerebellar atrophy and progressive dementia in a young adult. Neurocase: in press

Miotto EC, Morris RG (1998) Virtual planning in patients with frontal lobe lesions. Cortex 34:639–657

Monakow A von (1885) Experimentelle und pathologisch-anatomische Untersuchungen über die Beziehung der sogenannten Sehsphäre zu den infracortikalen Opticuscentren und zum N. opticus. Arch Psychiatr 16:151–199

Morice R, Delahunty A (1996) Frontal/executive impairments in schizophrenia. Schizophrenia 22:125–137

Nagaoka S, Arai H, Iwamoto N, Ohwada J, Ichimiya Y, Nakamura M, Inoue R (1995) A juvenile case of frontotemporal dementia: neurochemical and neuropathological investigations. Progr Neuro-Psychopharmacol Biol Psychiatry 19:1251–1262

Nestor PG, Faux SF, McCarley RW, Penhune V, Shenton ME, Pollak S, Sands SF (1992) Attentional cues in chronic schizophrenia: Abnormal disengagement of attention. J Abnorm Psychol 101:682–689

Nielsen-Bohlman L, Knight RT (1995) Prefrontal alterations during memory processing in aging. Cereb Cortex 5:541–549

Niessl von Mayendorf E (1908) Casuistische Mittheilungen zur Pathologie des Stirnhirns. Arch Psychiat Nervenkrankh 43:1175–1192

Öngür D, Drevets WC, Price JL (1998) Glial reduction in the subgenual prefrontal cortex in mood disorders. Proc Natl Acad Sci USA 95:13290–13295

Owen R (1868) On the anatomy of vertebrates. Vol. III. Mammals. Longmans, Green, London

Park S, Holzman PS, Goldman-Rakic PS (1995) Spatial working memory deficits in the relatives of schizophrenic patients. Arch Gen Psychiatry 52:821–828

Parkin AJ, Walter BM, Hunkin NM (1995) Relationships between normal aging, frontal lobe function, and memory for temporal and spatial information. Neuropsychology 9:304–312

Pascual-Leone A, Grafman J, Hallett M (1995) Procedural learning and prefrontal cortex. Ann New York Acad Sci 769:61–70

Passini R, Rainville C, Marchand N, Joanette Y (1995) Wayfinding in dementia of the Alzheimer type: planning abilities. J Clin Exp Neuropsychol 17:820–832

Raine A, Stoddard J, Bihrle S, Buchsbaum M (1998) Prefrontal glucose in murderers lacking psychosocial deprivation. Neuropsychiatry Neuropsychol Behav Neurol 11:1–7

Raz N, Gunning FM, Head D, Dupuis JH, McQuain J, Briggs SD, Loken WJ, Thornton AE, Acker JD (1997) Selective aging of the human cerebral cortex observed in vivo: Differential vulnerability of the prefrontal gray matter. Cereb Cortex 7:268–282

Röhrenbach C, Markowitsch HJ (1997) Störungen im Bereich exekutiver und überwachender Funktionen – der Präfrontalbereich. In: Markowitsch HJ (ed) Klinische Neuropsychologie, Enzyklopädie der Psychologie, Bd C/I/2. Hogrefe, Göttingen, pp 329–493

Ross ED, Stewart RS (1987) Pathological display of affect in patients with depression and right frontal brain damage. J Nerv Ment Dis 175:165–172

Rueckert L, Grafman J (1996) Sustained attention deficits in patients with right frontal lesions. Neuropsychologia 34:953–963

Sachs E (1927) Symptomatology of a group of frontal lobe lesions. Brain 50:474–479

Säring W, Prosiegel M, Cramon, D. von (1988) Zum Problem der Anosognosie und Anosodiaphorie bei hirngeschädigten Patienten. Nervenarzt 59:129–137

Sax KW, Strakowski SM, Zimmerman ME, DelBello MP, Keck Jr PE, Hawkins JM (1999) Frontosubcortical neuroanatomy and the continuous performance test in mania. Am J Psychiatry 156:139–141

Schäfer EA (1900) Textbook of physiology, Vol. II. Pentland, Edinburgh

Schuster P (1902) Psychische Störungen bei Hirntumoren. Enke, Stuttgart

Shimamura AP (1995) Memory and the prefrontal cortex. Ann New York Acad Sci 769:151–159

Starkstein SE, Robinson RG, Honig MA, Parikh RM, Joselyn J, Price TR (1989) Mood changes after right hemisphere lesions. Br J Psychiatry 155:79–85

Stuss DT (1991) Self, awareness and the frontal lobes: A neuropsychological perspective. In: Strauss J, Goethals GR (eds) The self: An interdisciplinary approach. Springer, New York Berlin Heidelberg, pp 255–278

Stuss DT, Benson DF (1983) Emotional concomitants of psychosurgery. In: Heilman KM, Satz P (eds) Neuropsychology of human emotion. Guilford Press, New York, pp 111–140

Stuss DT, Benson DF (1986) The frontal lobes. Raven Press, New York

Voegelin H (1897) Beitrag zur Kenntnis der Stirnhirn-Erkrankungen. Allg Z Psychiat Grenzgeb 54:588–599

Wechsler D (1987) Wechsler Memory Scale – Revised. Psychological Corporation, New York

Welt L (1888) Ueber Charakterveränderungen des Menschen infolge von Läsionen des Stirnhirns. Dtsch Arch Klin Med 42:339–390

Wheeler MA, Stuss DT, Tulving E (1997) Towards a theory of episodic memory. The frontal lobes and autonoetic consciousness. Psychol Bull 121:331–354

Wienhard K, Dahlborn M, Eriksson L, Michel C, Bruckbauer T, Pietrzyk U, Heiss WD (1994) The ECAT EXACT HR: performance of a new high resolution positron scanner. J Comput Assist Tomogr 18:110–118

R.E. Passingham · I. Toni · M.F.S. Rushworth

Specialisation within the prefrontal cortex: the ventral prefrontal cortex and associative learning

Published online: 10 May 2000

Abstract This paper provides evidence that the ventral prefrontal cortex plays a role in the learning of tasks in which subjects must learn to associate visual cues and responses. Imaging with both positron-emission tomography (PET) and functional magnetic-resonance imaging (fMRI) reveals learning-related increases in activity when normal subjects learn visual associative tasks. Evidence is also presented from an event-related fMRI study that activity in this area is time-locked both to the presentation of the visual stimuli and also to the time of the motor response. Finally, it is shown in a study of monkeys that removal of the ventral prefrontal area 12 (including 45 A) impairs the ability of monkeys to relearn a visual associative task (visual matching), even though there were no demands on working memory. It is, therefore, proposed that the ventral prefrontal cortex constitutes part of the circuitry via which associations are formed between visual cues and the actions or choices that they specify. On the basis of the existing anatomical and electrophysiological data, it is argued that the prefrontal cortex is the only area that can represent cues, responses and outcomes.

Key words PET · fMRI · Ventral frontal cortex · Motor learning · Associative learning

Introduction

It has often been proposed that the prefrontal cortex is involved in decision making and in the selection of actions (Damasio 1991; Frith et al. 1991; Frith 2000; Passingham 1993, 1997). However, strictly speaking, it is the animal that selects, and not one area of the brain. It is, therefore, necessary to specify more precisely the operations that are performed by the prefrontal cortex. Hypotheses concerning these operations have been mainly based on data concerning the dorsal prefrontal cortex and, in particular, Brodmann area 46. Goldman-Rakic (1987, 1998) and Fuster (1997) stress the importance of "working memory" or "active memory" in response selection. By contrast, Shallice (1982; Shallice and Burgess 1998) argues that the prefrontal cortex can be regarded as a "supervisory attentional system", and Baddeley and Della Sala (1998) identify this with the "central executive" of working memory.

The present account redresses the balance by considering the ventral prefrontal cortex. In the macaque brain, this lies ventral to sulcus principalis and, in the human brain, it lies ventral to the inferior frontal sulcus. It comprises the inferior prefrontal convexity (areas 45 A, 12/47) and the orbital surface (11, 13, 14) (Petrides and Pandya 1995). This paper studies the functions of the ventral prefrontal cortex using functional brain imaging in humans and the lesion method in macaques.

R.E. Passingham (✉) · M.F.S. Rushworth
Department of Experimental Psychology, University of Oxford, South Parks Road, Oxford OX1 3UD, UK
e-mail: dick.passingham@psy.ox.ac.uk
Fax: 441 1865 310447

I. Toni
Wellcome Department of Cognitive Neurology, Institute of Neurology, University College London, 12 Queen Square, WC1N 3BG, UK

The learning of visuo-motor associations

Positron emission tomography

We required subjects to select between actions, moving one finger given stimulus A, another finger given stimulus B, and so on for the four fingers of the right hand (Passingham et al. 1998; Toni and Passingham 1999). This is a visuo-motor associative task. Since the appropriate movement is conditional on the stimulus presented, a task of this sort is often also referred to as a "visuo-motor conditional task" (Passingham 1993). The association between the stimulus and the appropriate movement is entirely arbitrary, and it must therefore be learned or acquired.

Using positron emission tomography(PET), we scanned human subjects while they learned such a visuo-motor con-

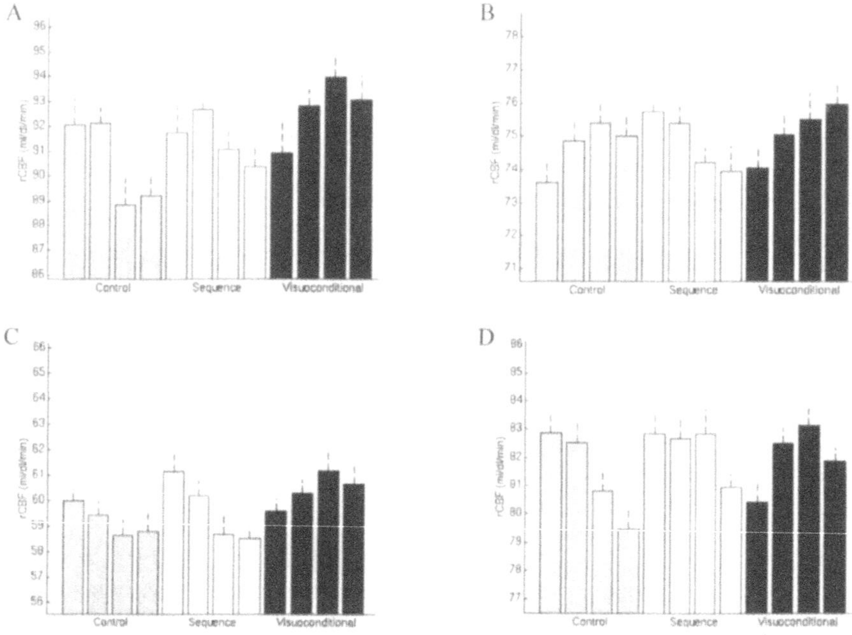

Fig. 1A–D Learning-related changes: baseline control (*grey*), motor sequence task (*white*), visuo-motor conditional task (*black*). The data are shown for four scans for each task. *rCBF* Relative cerebral blood flow. Data from Toni and Passingham (1999). **A** Lingual gyrus (MNI coordinate = 16, –60, –10). **B** Inferior frontal gyrus (36, 16, 20). **C** Caudate (–12, 8, 18); **D** Subiculum/parahippocampal gyrus (–24, –26, –8)

ditional task by trial and error (Toni and Passingham 1999). There were four sessions in which they learned, by trial and error, which finger to press given each of four nonsense figures (VMC). In another condition, the subjects learned a motor-sequence task, eight-moves long (SEQ); here, the nonsense figures served to pace performance, but not to specify *which* finger should be moved. Finally, in a baseline condition (BASE), the subjects were presented with a different set of nonsense figures, but no response was required. Comparison of the visuo-motor with the motor sequence condition allowed us to look for learning-related changes that were specific to the learning of visuo-motor transformations. Learning-related changes were assessed by investigating where there were differential changes in activation across the four sessions as the subjects learned.

As previously reported (Passingham et al. 1998), when we looked for interactions between the changes over time for the visuo-motor conditional task and the baseline condition (VMC vs. BASE), we found a learning-related change in the ventral temporal cortex (lingual gyrus) (Fig. 1A). We take this change to reflect the process of learning the identity of the visual stimuli. When we compared visuo-motor conditional learning with the learning of a sequence (VMC vs. SEQ), we found learning-related increases in the inferior prefrontal gyrus; as is shown in Fig. 1B, there was an increase in activation over time for the visuo-motor task, but a decrease for the motor-sequence task. We also found activation in the inferior prefrontal gyrus in a related study in which we scanned subjects while they performed a visuo-motor conditional task that they had already learned (Passingham et al. 1998).

Removal of the ventral prefrontal cortex in monkeys very severely impairs the learning of visuo-motor conditional tasks (Murray and Wise 1997; Murray et al. 2000), and it is known that this area derives its visual input from the infero-temporal cortex (Webster et al. 1994; Pandya and Yeterian 1998). Both the infero-temporal cortex (van Hoesen et al. 1981) and the ventral prefrontal cortex (Selemon and Goldman-Rakic 1985) also send subcortical projections to the caudate nucleus. We also found a learning-related increase in the caudate nucleus for the visuo-motor task (Fig. 1C) (Toni and Passingham 1999). Lesions in the nuclei of the ventral thalamus, to which the basal ganglia project, have been shown to severely impair the retention of a visuo-motor conditional task (Canavan et al. 1989).

There was also a learning-related increase in the parahippocampal gyrus (VMC vs BASE) (Fig. 1D). The peak lay on the borders between the subiculum and the parahippocampal gyrus. Lesions of hippocampus and parahippocampal gyrus have also been shown to severely impair the learning of visuo-motor conditional tasks (Murray and Wise 1996).

Functional magnetic resonance imaging

In the PET study described above (Toni and Passingham 1999), there were only four data points during learning. Using functional magnetic resonance imaging (fMRI), it is possible to scan for much longer during learning and, thus, to produce continuous curves for activity during learning (e.g. Toni et al. 1998). In a recent study, we scanned subjects while they learned a visuo-motor conditional task by trial and error (Toni et al. 1999a). In another condition, the subjects performed a pre-learned visuo-motor task. Here, the nonsense figures contained arrowheads: if the arrowhead pointed to the left, the subject moved the first finger; if the arrowhead pointed up and to the left, the subject moved the second finger;

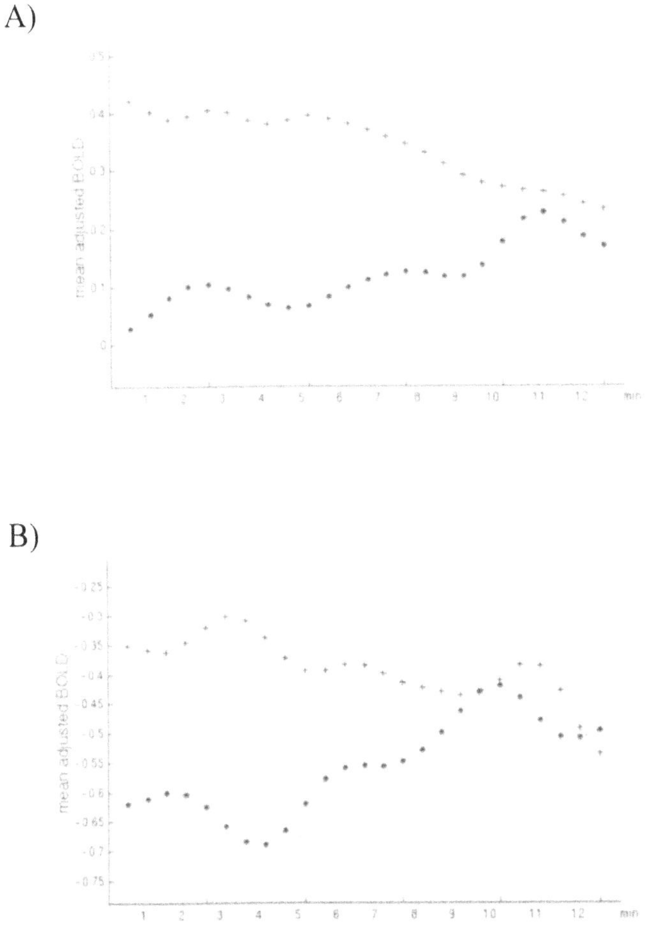

Fig. 2A, B Curves showing change in blood oxygen-level detection (*BOLD*) signal (mean adjusted) during learning of a visuo-motor conditional task (*stars*) and performance of a pre-learned visuo-motor task (*crosses*). Minutes during learning are plotted on the abscissa. Data from a study by Toni et al. (1999a). **A** Scans for infero-temporal cortex (MNI coordinate = –58, –54, –6); **B** Scans for ventral prefrontal cortex (–52, 40, –4)

and so on. Thus, in this control condition, the subjects also attended to visual stimuli and made movements on the basis of visual cues. This design allowed us to compare the *learning* of visuo-motor associations with the performance of a visuo-motor task in which the association had been pre-learned. Figure 2 shows that there were learning-related increases in the infero-temporal cortex (Fig. 2A) and in the inferior frontal gyrus (Fig. 2B), as well as in the orbitofrontal cortex. For the pre-learned motor task, there was a decrease in activation with time.

Representation of cue, response and outcome

To learn a visuo-motor conditional task, the subject has to associate the success of a particular response with the specific cue that is presented (Fig. 3). Response 1 is only successful (correct) in the presence of cue A. Here, we review evidence that prefrontal cortex can represent cues, responses and outcomes.

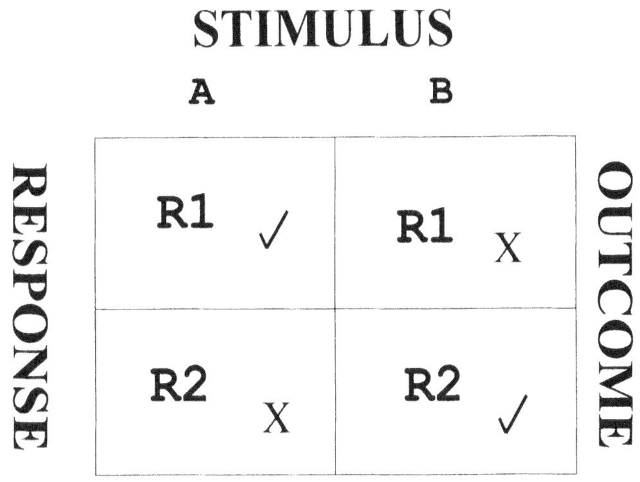

Fig. 3 The association of cues (*A* and *B*), responses (*R1* and *R2*) and outcomes (correct, incorrect) in the learning of a visuo-motor conditional task

There are two indications that cues can be represented in the ventral prefrontal cortex. First, it can be seen from Fig. 1A that, during learning, there was an increase of activation in the inferior frontal gyrus not only in the visuo-motor learning condition, but also over the four sessions of the baseline condition. In the latter condition, four new nonsense figures were repeatedly presented, one at a time, and thus the subjects had the opportunity to learn to identify which figure was presented on any trial. The learning-related increase in this area for the visuo-motor condition may, therefore, also be related to the learned identification of the figures. It is not suggested that this area is involved in the process via which stimuli are recognised as *familiar*, but rather in the process via which stimuli are *categorised* as the A, B, C or D figure. There are also cells in the inferior prefrontal convexity that respond to visual stimuli even when no explicit response is required (Wilson et al. 1993; Scalaidhe et al. 1997).

There is another way of showing that there is activity in the ventral prefrontal cortex that is related to the presentation of the cue. In a related study using event-related fMRI, we plotted the evoked hemodynamic responses when subjects selected a finger on the basis of visual cues (visuo-motor conditional task) (Toni et al. 1999b). Random delays were introduced between the presentation of the instruction cue and an auditory cue that triggered the response. This allowed us to align the evoked hemodyamic response either to the presentation of the instruction cue or to the presentation of the trigger cue. The response in the infero-temporal cortex could be shown to be statistically associated with the presentation of the instruction cue, but not with the response (Fig. 4A). Figure 4B shows the data for trials with a long delay (12.8 s); if the data are plotted for short delays, there is overlap between the evoked hemodynamic responses to the instruction cue and trigger stimulus. It will be seen that, in the inferior frontal gyrus, there was also a cue-related response.

There is also evidence that responses can be represented in the prefrontal cortex. First, it can be seen from Fig. 4B that, in the inferior frontal gyrus, there is also an evoked hemodynamic response that is time locked to the response. Movement-related activity has also been reported in the inferior prefrontal convexity in monkeys (Di Pellegrino and Wise 1991). We also found a second prefrontal peak in the frontal polar cortex (Fig. 4C), and here the movement-related activity started early before the tone, building up towards the time at which the movement was performed. It is not clear whether the peak should be classified as lying in dorsal or ventral prefrontal cortex. Pre-movement activity has also been reported for single cells in the dorsal prefrontal cortex (Fuster 1973; Kubota and Funahashi 1982; Funahashi et al. 1991). Other imaging studies have shown that the dorsal prefrontal cortex is activated when subjects select between finger movements (Frith et al. 1991; Jueptner et al. 1997) or prepare to make finger movements (Krams et al. 1998).

Finally, it can be shown using brain imaging that outcomes are represented in the prefrontal cortex. Elliott et al. (1997) report activation of the ventromedial frontal cortex when subjects are given either positive or negative feedback; the subjects were required to guess, and the feedback was unrelated to the actual guesses they made. The orbito-frontal cortex is also activated when subjects are scanned while they await negative outcomes: Chua et al. (1998) scanned subjects while they expected electric shocks and found activation in the orbito-frontal cortex that varied as a function of the degree of anxiety the different subjects felt. Cells have also been recorded in the inferior prefrontal convexity and orbital frontal cortex that respond to cues predicting a specific reward (reward A rather than reward B) (Watanabe 1996; Rolls 1998; Tremblay and Schultz 1999).

The level of representation

If two-dimensional shapes are to be associated with specific actions, both the stimuli and the actions must be represented at a high level, since there is no direct spatial correspondence between them. Wise et al. (1996) cites such associations as examples of "cross-domain mapping". A high-level representation of the response may differ little from the high-level representation of the cue. Thus, prefrontal cortex may specify the response by its target, irrespective of how that target can be achieved. It is, however, not clear how the prefrontal cortex can influence movement. Desimone and Duncan (1995) have suggested that the ventral prefrontal cortex may act to set

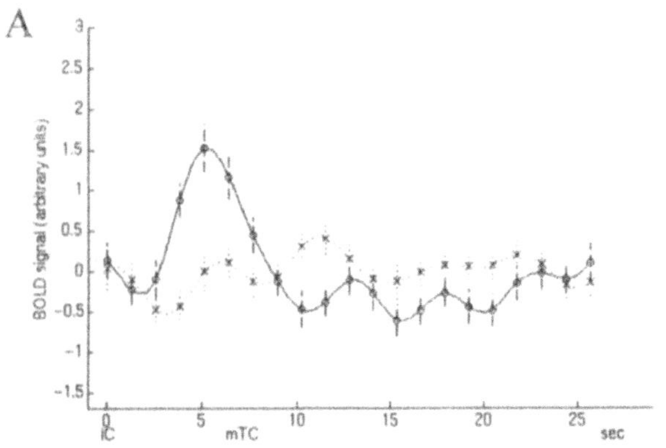

Fig. 4A–C Evoked hemodynamic responses. The ordinate shows the relative blood oxygen-level detection (*BOLD*) signal. The abscissa shows time during a trial in seconds. *IC* Presentation of instruction cue, *mTc* mean time of presentation of trigger cue, *TC* presentation of trigger cue. Data from Toni et al. (1999b). **A** Data for infero-temporal cortex (MNI coordinate = 52, –56, –20). The *solid line* shows the evoked hemodynamic response when the data are aligned to the time of presentation of the instruction cue. The *dotted line* shows the lack of an evoked hemodynamic response when the data are aligned to the time of presentation of the trigger cue. **B** Data for the inferior prefrontal cortex (*solid line*) (–30, 28, 12) and motor cortex (*dotted line*) (–36, –22, 60). The data are shown only for trials with a delay of 12.8 s. There is an evoked hemodynamic response for ventral prefrontal cortex at the time of the instruction cue and at the time of the movement. For motor cortex, there is only a response at the time of the movement. **C** Data for the frontal polar cortex (*solid line*) (34, 58, 20) and motor cortex (*dotted line*) (–36, –22, 60). The data are shown only for trials with a delay of 12.8 s. The hemodynamic response for the frontal cortex rises before the time of presentation of the trigger

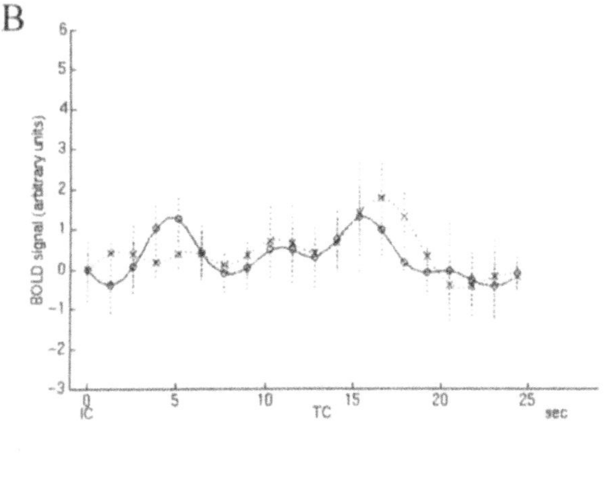

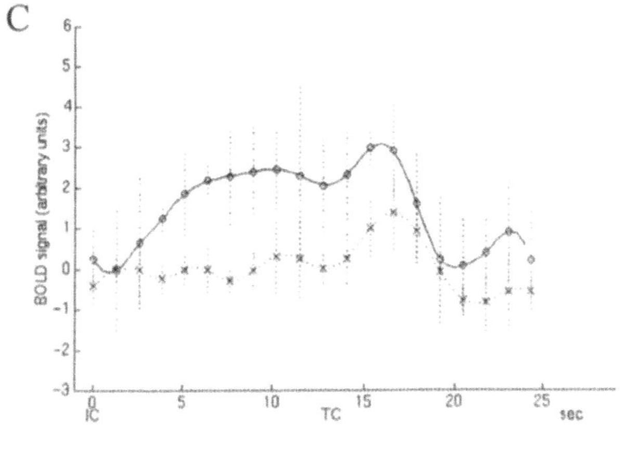

up an "attentional template" for objects and their unique features in the infero-temporal cortex. This acts to "highlight" the cues that are behaviourally significant and to bias competition in favour of the representation of one stimulus. It is possible that the prefrontal cortex selects movements in the same way, by biasing competition between the representations of movement in the premotor areas (Frith 2000).

The role of the ventral prefrontal cortex is not restricted to the learning of visuo-motor associations. Monkeys with lesions of the inferior prefrontal convexity are severely impaired in relearning a visual matching task, in which they must choose A rather than B if the sample is A (Rushworth et al. 1997). Disconnection of the inferotemporal and prefrontal cortex also severely impairs the learning of associations between one visual stimulus and another (Eacott and Gaffan 1992), between an auditory stimulus and a visual stimulus (Gaffan and Harrison 1991) and between presentation of a reward and choice of a visual stimulus (Parker and Gaffan 1998). Hasegawa et al. (1998) taught monkeys to associate two visual stimuli and reported that, if the cue was presented to one hemisphere, the anterior callosum must be intact if the other hemisphere is to select the correct response. The ventral prefrontal cortex is also activated when human subjects either encode (Dolan and Fletcher 1997) or retrieve (Rugg et al. 1996) verbal paired-associates and when they categorise items such as tools (Vandenberghe et al. 1996).

Associations

The fact that cues, responses and outcomes can be represented in the prefrontal cortex does not show that the *associations* between these are also explicitly represented in the prefrontal cortex. Figure 4B shows that there is a cue-related and a movement-related response in the inferior frontal gyrus; but the hemodynamic responses represent the activity of a whole population of cells, and there may be separate subpopulations representing *only* the cue *or* the response. However, Asaad et al. (1998) have shown that single cells in the dorsal and ventrolateral prefrontal cortex can code a specific cue-response association. These authors trained monkeys to look to the left or right, depending on the identity of an instruction cue. They report that many of the task-related cells coded a specific cue-response relation. For example, a cell might fire when the monkey looked to the left given cue A, but not when it looked to the right given A; at the same time, the same cell might fire less or not at all if the monkey was taught to look to the left given cue B.

This leaves open the questions of where these associations are first formed and where they are stored. There are interconnections between and within the ventrolateral, orbital and dorsal sectors of the prefrontal cortex (Barbas 1988; Pandya and Yeterian 1998). It could thus be argued that associations can be formed by interconnections *within* the prefrontal cortex. To learn a visual conditional task, it is necessary to associate the success of a specific response with the presentation of a specific cue (Fig. 2). It has been argued that representations of the cue, response and reward are available to the prefrontal cortex.

These associations may be learned in interaction with the basal ganglia and the hippocampal system. There were learning-related increases in the caudate nucleus (Fig. 1B) and parahippocampal gyrus (Fig. 1C) that were specific for the establishment of visuo-motor associations. Several authors have proposed that the basal ganglia are involved in procedural motor learning and, more specifically, in the process via which the contexts of the movements are learned (Hikosaka 1993; Passingham 1993; Dominey et al. 1995; Houk and Wise 1995). The nigral dopamine cells sends projections to the same medium spiny neurones in the striatum on which the cortical afferents terminate (Groves et al. 1995), and it has been shown that these synapses are modifiable (Calabresi et al. 1996). Furthermore, changes have been shown in the firing of the nigral dopamine cells (Hollerman and Schultz 1998) and of the striatal cells (Kawagoe et al. 1998; Tremblay et al. 1998) when monkeys are reinforced for making specific responses. The association between cue and response may be reinforced by the dopamine system at the level of the striatum. It is important to note that no assumption need be made that there is an interaction between the prefrontal and premotor loops (Alexander et al. 1991). If both the cue and the response can be represented in the prefrontal cortex, the association can be established by projections onto striatal cells within a prefrontal-striatal loop.

There is evidence that the hippocampal system is also involved in the acquisition of the association. Lesions that include both the hippocampus and parahippocampal gyrus severely impair the learning of visual conditional tasks, while leaving unimpaired the retention of such tasks if learned before surgery (Murray and Wise 1996). Similarly, transection of the fornix impairs the ability of monkeys to learn a visuo-spatial conditional task (Rupniak and Gaffan 1987). Furthermore, the parahippocampal gyrus is activated when human subjects encode verbal paired associates in episodic memory (Dolan and Fletcher 1997). There are suggestions that the hippocampal system may be involved in the process by which the context of episodic memories is established (Dore et al. 1998; Parker and Gaffan 1998). Further work is needed to directly compare the contribution of the basal ganglia and hippocampal system with the learning of visual conditional tasks. Furthermore, studies need to be conducted to identify the pathways that are involved in overlearned performance.

Working memory

It could be argued that the ventral prefrontal cortex is involved not in the association of the cue and the response, but in the working-memory. Though the cue is available

Fig. 5A, B Performance on visual matching task for monkeys with ventral prefrontal lesions. The histograms give the means for pre-operative and post-operative trials; *dots* data for individual animals. Data from Rushworth et al. (1997).
A Errors in a relearn task to criterion before (*Pre-Op1*) and after (*Post-Op*) surgery.
B Errors at 0 s (*0 s*) and for four delays (*2, 4, 6, 8 s*). The histograms give the means for pre-operative (*dark hatched*) and post-operative (*light hatched*) performance; the data for the individual animals are given by *dots*

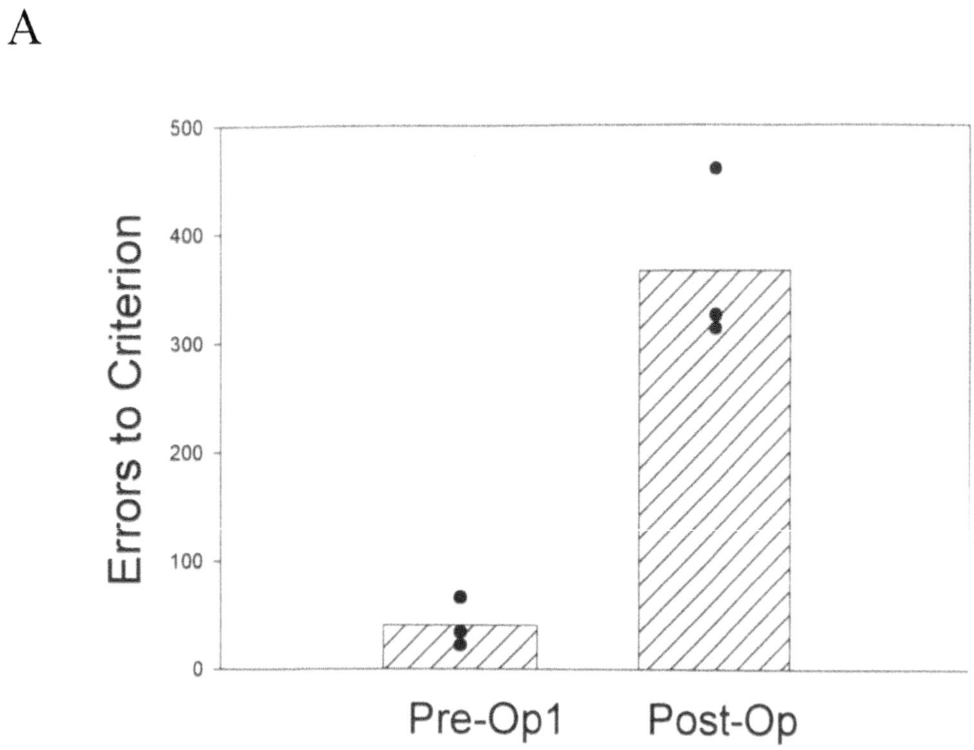

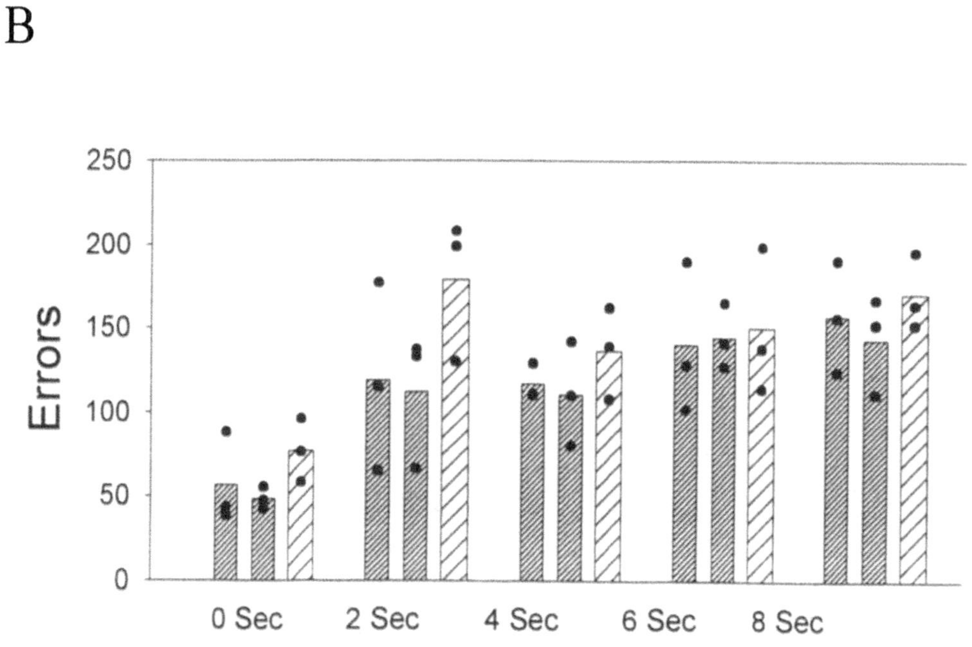

at the time of response, it might be supposed that, nonetheless, subjects first remember the cue, before deciding on the appropriate response.

It has long been known that monkeys with bilateral lesions in dorsal prefrontal area 46 are impaired on delayed-response tasks, but not impaired if the same responses are required without a delay (Goldman and Rosvold 1970; Funahashi et al. 1993). Rushworth et al. (1997) therefore assessed the ability of monkeys with lesions of the inferior prefrontal convexity to remember across delays. The monkeys were trained on a visual matching task. After surgery, they were severely impaired, even when the sample was present at the same time that the choice was made (Fig. 5A). The animals were, however, able to relearn the task with extended training. They were then tested with delays interposed between the presentation of the cue and the time of response, and they were able to perform as well as they had done pre-operatively (Fig. 5B). It cannot, therefore, be argued that the impairment of the animals on the simultaneous condition was due to a working-memory impairment. This experiment (Rushworth et al. 1997) makes two points. First, the ventral prefrontal cortex is not essential for working memory. Second, there is a difference in specialisation between the ventral and dorsal prefrontal cortex, since lesions of the dorsal prefrontal cortex do not impair visual matching (Passingham 1975; Mishkin and Manning 1978).

The connected brain

There are two findings from single-unit studies that might be thought to challenge the first of these conclusions. First, on a delayed-response task, it is possible to record continuous cell activity during the delay period not only in area 46, but also in the inferior prefrontal convexity (area 12) (Rosenkilde 1981; Rao et al. 1997). However, White and Wise (1999) have recorded cell activity on a visuo-motor conditional task with no working memory requirement, and they were able to record task-specific activity in the prefrontal cortex. It is true that there are cells in the ventral prefrontal cortex which respond differentially when a stimulus is presented for the second time after a delay filled with other stimuli (Chelazzi et al. 1993). But the results of the study by Rushworth et al. (1997) suggest that the change in activity could reflect the comparison that is made, and that it may not be crucial that the comparison be made between the stimuli that are presented at different times.

There are also single-unit studies which appear to challenge the conclusion that there is specialisation between the ventral and dorsal prefrontal cortex. For example, in a visuo-motor conditional task, White and Wise (1999) recorded task-related cells in the dorsolateral as well as the ventrolateral prefrontal cortex (caudal third). In the studies by Rao et al. (1997) and Asaad et al. (1998), cell activity was recorded on conditional tasks both in area 46 and in the ventrolateral prefrontal cortex below. One possible explanation for the difference between the results of lesions and recording studies relies on the fact that there are strong interconnections between the dorsal and ventral prefrontal cortex (Barbas 1988; Pandya and Yeterian 1998). Both cell recording and functional brain-imaging studies are conducted in a "connected brain", that is one with intact interconnections. Thus, it is not possible to distinguish whether the activity of a cell in the dorsal prefrontal cortex depends on the activity of a cell in the ventral prefrontal cortex, and vice versa. In a lesion study, one of the areas is removed, and behavioural tests demonstrate whether that area is essential for the task. In other words, in the interconnected frontal lobe, the activity of a cell in one sector may be *derived* from the other. In a lesion study, one of the areas is removed, and behavioural tests demonstrate whether that area is essential for the task. After a lesion of, say, the ventral prefrontal cortex, the activity of the cells in the dorsal prefrontal cortex can no longer be derived from the activity in the ventral prefrontal cortex. If this explanation is correct, it should be possible to demonstrate a change in the pattern of activity in one area when the other is removed or temporarily inactivated.

Specialisation of ventral and dorsal prefrontal cortex

There have been two views as to the specialisation of the dorsal and ventral prefrontal cortex. The first is that they perform the same operations, but for different inputs (Goldman-Rakic 1998). The second is that the ventral and dorsal prefrontal cortex perform different operations (Owen et al. 1996; Owen 1997; Petrides 1998). The data presented in this paper are consistent with the second of these views.

That there may be differences in specialisation is suggested by the pattern of anatomical connections. The dorsal area 46 and the ventral areas 12/47 and 45 A differ in their inputs and outputs. The inferior prefrontal convexity and orbital prefrontal cortex receives inputs from all sensory modalities. The ventral prefrontal cortex derives visual information from the infero-temporal cortex (Webster et al. 1994; Pandya and Yeterian 1998), auditory information from superior temporal cortex (Pandya and Yeterian 1998) and somatic information from SII and 7b (Cavada and Goldman-Rakic 1989; Preuss and Goldman-Rakic 1989; Carmichael and Price 1995); and the orbital prefrontal cortex derives information about taste from the insula and smell from the pyriform cortex (Rolls 1998). There are also interconnections between the ventral and orbital prefrontal cortex (Barbas and Pandya 1989), and both are connected with the amygdala (Aggleton et al. 1980; Porrino et al. 1981; Amaral and Price 1984; Barbas and De Olmos 1990). In both ventrolateral and orbital prefrontal cortex, there are cells that respond to cues predicting a specific reward (reward A rather than reward B) (Watanabe 1996; Rolls 1998; Schultz and Tremblay 1998).

The dorsal prefrontal cortex, on the other hand, derives its visual input from inferior parietal cortex in the dorsal visual system and is also connected with somatic area parietal 7b. There are motor outputs from area 46 to the dorsal and ventral premotor cortex (Dum and Strick 1997; Matelli et al. 1986) and to the pre-SMA and cingulate motor area CMAr (Lu et al. 1994). There are also outputs from area 46 to the superior colliculi (Goldman and Nauta 1976; Fries 1984) and to the cerebellum via the pons (Schmahmann and Pandya 1997). There are no projections to the pons from the ventral prefrontal area 12 (Schmahmann and Pandya 1997), and it is disputed whether the origin of the projections to the ventral premotor cortex is restricted to the ventral bank of sulcus principalis (area 46) (Matelli et al. 1986; Luppino et al. 1998) or includes the ventral convexity cortex (area 12) (Pandya and Yeterian 1998).

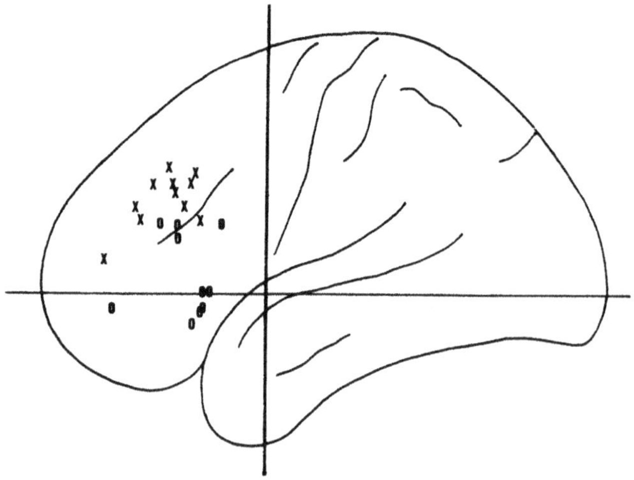

Fig. 6 A comparison of the peaks for visual conditional tasks (*0*) and free-selection and motor-preparation tasks (*X*), plotted on the Talairach and Tournoux (1988) brain. Some of the studies normalised the brains using the Talairach and Tournoux (1988) template and others using the MNI template (Montreal Neurological Institute); this introduces minor errors when the peaks for MNI data are plotted on the Talairach and Tournoux (1988) brain. Data from Paus et al. (1993), Deiber et al. (1997), Jueptner et al. (1997), Krams et al. (1998), Spence et al. (1998), Toni et al. (1999b) and Rushworth et al. (in preparation)

These anatomical differences underlie the functional specialisation of the ventral and dorsal prefrontal cortex. The ventral prefrontal cortex receives information concerning the identity of a visual stimulus, since it is the infero-temporal cortex that analyses the shape or colour that identifies an object (Ungerleider and Mishkin 1982; Milner and Goodale 1997). It is the inferior prefrontal cortex that is activated when subjects categorise items by making semantic judgements about them (Vandenberghe et al. 1996). By contrast, the dorsal prefrontal cortex receives an input from the inferior parietal cortex in the dorsal visual system. Milner and Goodale (1997) have reviewed evidence that suggests that parietal cortex operates on sensory information for the purposes of action. This includes the generation of both hand and eye movements (Snyder et al. 1998) as well as the direction of covert attention, where subjects prepare to make eye movements, but do not actually make them (Nobre et al. 1997, 1998).

This functional difference between the ventral and dorsal prefrontal cortex is highlighted by contrasting the activations on two types of task. In the first, visual cues are presented that specify the appropriate response (visual conditional task). In the second, the subject must either arbitrarily select between responses ("free selection") (Deiber et al. 1991; Frith et al. 1991; Jueptner et al. 1997) or are required to attend while they prepare to move a finger (Krams et al. 1998). Figure 6 shows that there is a difference between the peaks of activation. They tend to lie more ventrally for performance of visual conditional tasks and more dorsally for the tasks on which subjects must represent actions to themselves.

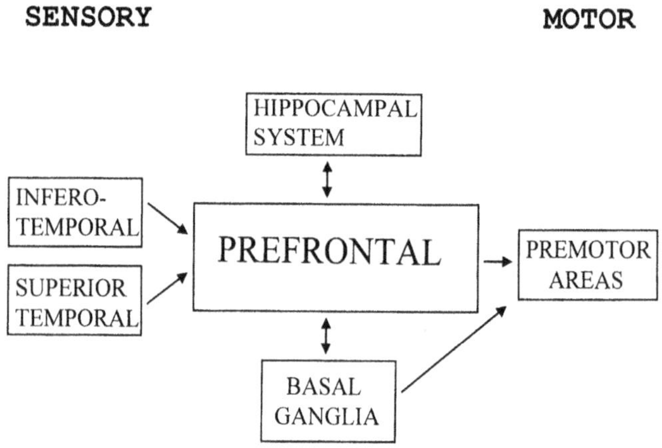

Fig. 7 Anatomical connections of the prefrontal cortex showing that it lies at the top of the sensory hierarchy and at the top of the motor hierarchy

Conclusions

It has been argued that the prefrontal cortex has an associative role that can be missed by the concentration in the literature on the functions of the dorsal prefrontal cortex. Both Passingham (1993) and Petrides (1987) have previously argued for a role of the prefrontal cortex in conditional learning, and Murray et al. (2000) also argue that the prefrontal cortex is involved in the process by which rules are learned that govern the production of responses on the basis of visual cues. White and Wise (1999) have demonstrated that there are cells in the ventrolateral and dorsolateral prefrontal cortex that show a different pattern of activity, depending on whether the rule concerns the association between a visual pattern and an eye movement or the association between a spatial location and an eye movement.

The prefrontal cortex is a position that associates high-level representations of cues and actions. As also noted by Fuster (1997), the prefrontal cortex lies at the top of the sensory hierarchy and at the top of the motor hierarchy (Fig. 7). The question arises why these associations are not learned by a direct interaction between the infero-temporal cortex and the premotor areas. As far as we know, there are no direct projections from the infero-temporal cortex to premotor area 6 (Boussaoud et al. 1996, and pers. comm.). The behavioural relevance of a visual stimulus can only be determined by detecting the association of a successful response with the presence of that stimulus. This means that there must be associations between the visual stimuli, the responses and the outcomes. While infero-temporal cortex has information about visual stimuli and premotor cortex can represent actions, *only* the prefrontal cortex can represent stimuli, actions and outcomes.

Acknowledgements Dr I. Toni was supported by a European BIOMED grant. The work was supported by a grant from the Wellcome Trust.

References

Aggleton JP, Burton MJ, Passingham RE (1980) Cortical and subcortical afferents to the amygdala of the rhesus monkey (*Macaca mulatta*). Brain Res 190:347–368

Alexander GE, Crutcher MD, DeLong MR (1991) Basal ganglia-thalamocortical circuits: parallel substrates for motor, oculomotor, "prefrontal" and "limbic" functions. Prog Brain Res 85:119–146

Amaral DG, Price JL (1984) Amygdalo-cortical projections in the monkey (*Macaca fascicularis*). J Comp Neurol 230:465–496

Asaad WF, Rainer G, Miller EK (1998) Neural activity in the primate prefrontal cortex during associative learning. Neuron 21:1399–1407

Baddeley A, Della Sala S (1998) The domain of supervisory processes and the temporal organization of behaviour. In: Roberts AC, Robbins TW, Weiskrantz L (eds) The prefrontal cortex. Oxford University Press, Oxford, pp 9–21

Barbas H (1988) Anatomical organization of basoventral and mediodorsal visual recipient prefrontal region in the rhesus monkey. J Comp Neurol 276:313–342

Barbas H, De Olmos J (1990) Projections from the amygdala to basoventral and mediodorsal prefrontal regions in the rhesus monkey. J Comp Neurol 300:549–571

Barbas H, Pandya DN (1989) Architecture and intrinsic connections of the prefrontal cortex in the rhesus monkey. J Comp Neurol 286:353–375

Boussaoud D, Di Pellegrino G, Wise SP (1996) Frontal lobe mechanisms subserving vision-for-action versus vision-for-perception. Behav Brain Res 72:1–15

Calabresi P, Pisani A, Mercuri NB, Bernardi G (1996) The cortico-striatal projection: from synaptic plasticity to dysfunctions of the basal ganglia. Trends Neurosci 19:19–24

Canavan AGM, Nixon P, Passingham RE (1989) Lesions in motor thalamus and motor learning in monkeys (*Macaca fascicularis*). Exp Brain Res 77:113–126

Carmichael ST, Price JL (1995) Sensory and premotor connections of the orbital and medial prefrontal cortex of macaque monkeys. J Comp Neurol 363:642–664

Cavada C, Goldman-Rakic PS (1989) Posterior parietal cortex in rhesus monkeys. II. Evidence for segregated corticocortical networks linking sensory and limbic areas with the frontal lobe. J Comp Neurol 28:422–445

Chellazi L, Miller EK, Lueschow A, Desimone R (1993) Dual mechanisms of short-term memory: ventral prefrontal cortex. Soc Neurosci Abstr 19:975

Chua P, Krams M, Toni I, Passingham RE, Dolan R (1999) A functional neuroanatomy of anticipatory anxiety. Neuroimage 9:563–572

Damasio AR (1991) Concluding comments. In: Levin HS, Eisenberg HM, Benton AL (eds) Frontal lobe function and dysfunction. Oxford University Press, Oxford, pp 401–407

Deiber MP, Passingham RE, Colebatch JG, Friston KJ, Nixon PD, Frackowiak RSJ (1991) Cortical areas and the selection of movement: a study with PET. Exp Brain Res 84:393–402

Deiber M-P, Wise SP, Honda M, Catalan MJ, Grafman J, Hallett M (1997) Frontal and parietal networks for conditional motor learning: a positron emission tomography study. J Neurophysiol 78:977–991

Desimone R, Duncan J (1995) Neural mechanisms of selective visual attention. Annu Rev Neurosci 18:193–222

Di Pellegrino G, Wise SP (1991) A neurophysiological comparison of three distinct regions of the primate frontal lobe. Brain 114:951–978

Dolan RJ, Fletcher PC (1997) Dissociating prefrontal and hippocampal function in episodic memory encoding. Nature 388: 582–585

Dominey P, Arbib M, Joseph JP (1995) A model of corticostriatal plasticity for learning oculomotor associations and sequences. J Cogn Neurosci 7:311–336

Dore FY, Thornton JA, White NM, Murray EA (1998) Selective hippocampal lesions yield nonspatial memory impairments in rhesus monkeys. Hippocampus 8:323–329

Dum RP, Strick PL (1997) Cortical inputs to the digit representations in the primary motor cortex and the dorsal premotor area of the cebus monkey. Soc Neurosci Abstr 23:502.12

Eacott MJ, Gaffan D (1992) Inferotemporal-frontal disconnections: the uncinate fascicle and visual associative learning in monkeys. Eur J Neurosci 4:1320–1332

Elliott R, Frith CD, Dolan RJ (1998) Differential neural response to positive and negative feedback in planning and guessing tasks. Neuropsychology 15:1395–1404

Fries W (1984) Cortical projections to the superior colliculus in the macaque monkey: a retrograde study using horseradish peroxidase. J Comp Neurol 230:55–76

Frith CD (2000) The role of the dorsolateral prefrontal cortex in the selection of action. In: Monsell S, Driver (eds) Control of cognitive processes. Attention and Performance XVIII. MIT Press, Cambridge (in press)

Frith CD, Friston K, Liddle PF, Frackowiak RSJ (1991) Willed action and the prefrontal cortex in man: a study with PET. Proc Roy Soc Lond B Biol Sci 244:241–246

Funahashi S, Bruce CJ, Goldman-Rakic PS (1991) Neuronal activity related to saccadic eye movements in the monkey's dorsolateral prefrontal cortex. J Neurophysiol 65:1464–1482

Funahashi S, Bruce, CJ, Goldman-Rakic PS (1993) Dorsolateral prefrontal lesions and oculomotor delayed-response performance: evidence for mnemonic "scotomas". J Neurosci 13: 1479–1497

Fuster JM (1973) Unit activity in prefrontal cortex during delayed-response performance: neuronal correlates of transient memory. J Neurophysiol 36:61–78

Fuster JM (1997) The prefrontal cortex. Lippincott-Raven, Philadelphia

Gaffan D, Harrison S (1991) Auditory-visual associations, hemispheric specialization and temporal-frontal interaction in the rhesus monkey. Brain 114:2133–2144

Goldman PS, Nauta WJH (1976) Autoradiographic demonstration of a projection from prefrontal association cortex to the superior colliculus in the rhesus monkey. Brain Res 116:145–149

Goldman PS, Rosvold HE (1970) Localization of function within the dorsolateral prefrontal cortex of the rhesus monkey. Exp Neurol 27:291–304

Goldman-Rakic P (1987) Circuitry of primate prefrontal cortex and regulation of behaviour by representational memory. In: Plum F, Mountcastle V (eds) Handbook of physiology: the nervous system, Vol 5. American Physiological Society, Bethesda, pp 373–417

Goldman-Rakic PS (1998) The prefrontal landscape: implications of functional architecture for understanding human mentation and the central executive. In: Roberts AC, Robbins TW, Weiskrantz L (eds) The prefrontal cortex. Oxford University Press, Oxford, pp 117–130

Groves PM, Garcia-Munoz M, Linder JC, Manley MS, Martone ME, Young SJ (1995) Elements of intrinsic organization and information processing in the neostriatum. In: Jouk JC, Davis JL, Beiser DG (eds) Models of information processing in the basal ganglia. MIT Press, Cambridge, pp 51–96

Hasegawa I, Fukushima T, Ihara T, Miyashita Y (1998) Callosal window between prefrontal cortices: cognitive interaction to retrieve long-term memory. Science 281:814–818

Hikosaka O (1993) Role of the basal ganglia in motor learning: a hypothesis. In: Ono T, Squire LR, Raichle ME, Perrett DI, Fukuda M (eds) Brain mechanisms of perception and memory: from neuron to behavior. Oxford University Press, Oxford, pp 497–513

Hollerman JR, Schultz W (1998) Dopamine neurons report an error in the temporal prediction of reward during learning. Nature Neurosci 1:304–308

Hoesen G van, Yeterian EH, Lavizzo-Mourey R (1981) Widespread corticostriate projection from temporal cortex of the rhesus monkey. J Comp Neurol 199:205–219

Houk JC, Wise SP (1995) Distributed modular architectures linking basal ganglia, cerebellum, and cerebral cortex: their role in planning and controlling action. Cereb Cortex 5:95–110
Jueptner M, Frith CD, Brooks DJ, Frackowiak RSJ, Passingham RE (1997) Anatomy of motor learning. II. Subcortical structures and learning by trial and error. J Neurophysiol 77:1325–1337
Kawagoe R, Takikawa Y, Hikosaka O (1998) Expectation of reward modulates cognitive signals in the basal ganglia. Nature Neurosci 1:411–416
Krams M, Rushworth M, Deiber M-P, Frackowiak RSJ, Passingham RE (1998) The preparation, execution and suppression of copied movements in the human brain. Exp Brain Res 120:386–398
Kubota K, Funahashi IS (1982) Direction specific activation of dorsolateral prefrontal and motor cortex pyramidal tract neurons during visual tracking. J Neurophysiol 47:362–376
Lu M-T, Preston JB, Strick PL (1994) Interconnections between the prefrontal cortex and the premotor areas in the frontal lobe. J Comp Neurol 341:375–392
Luppino G, Govoni P, Matelli M (1998) Prefrontal and cingulate afferents to the rostral premotor areas in the macaque monkey. Soc Neurosci Abstr 24:257.11
Matelli M, Camarda M, Glickstein M, Rizzolatti G (1986) Afferent and efferent projections of the inferior area 6 in the macaque monkey. J Comp Neurol 251:281–298
Milner AD, Goodale MA (1997) The visual brain in action. Oxford University Press, Oxford
Mishkin M, Manning FJ (1978) Nonspatial memory after selective prefrontal lesions in monkeys. Brain Res 143:313–323
Murray EA, Wise SP (1996) Role of the hippocampus plus subjacent cortex but not amygdala in visuomotor conditional learning in rhesus monkeys. Behav Neurosci 110:1261–1270
Murray EA, Wise SP (1997) Role of orbitoventral prefrontal cortex in conditional motor learning. Soc Neurosci Abstr 23:12.1
Murray EA, Bussey T, Wise SP (2000) Role of prefrontal cortex in a network for arbitrary visuomotor mapping. Exp Brain Res DOI 10.1007/s002210000406
Nobre AC, Sebestyen GN, Gitelman DR, Mesulam MM, Frackowiak RSJ, Frith CD (1997) Functional localization of the system for visuospatial attention using positron emission tomography. Brain 120:515–533
Nobre AC, Dias EC, Gitelman DR, Mesulam MM (1998) The overlap of brain regions that control saccades and covert spatial attention revealed by fMRI. Neuroimage 7:S9
Owen AM (1997) The functional organization of working memory processes within human lateral frontal cortex: the contribution of functional neuroimaging. Eur J Neurosci 9:1329–1339
Owen AM, Evans AC, Petrides M (1996) Evidence for a two-stage model of spatial working memory processing within the lateral frontal cortex: a positron emission tomography study. Cereb Cortex 6:31–38
Pandya DN, Yeterian EH (1998) Comparison of prefrontal architecture and connections. In: Roberts AC, Robbins TW, Weiskrantz L (eds) The prefrontal cortex. Oxford University Press, Oxford, pp 51–66
Parker A, Gaffan D (1998) Memory after frontal/temporal disconnection in monkeys: conditional and non-conditional tasks, unilateral and bilateral frontal lesions. Neuropsychol 36:259–271
Passingham RE (1975) Delayed matching after selective prefrontal lesions in monkeys. Brain Res 92:89–102
Passingham RE (1993) The frontal lobes and voluntary action. Oxford University Press, Oxford
Passingham RE (1997) The organization of the motor system. In: Frackowiak RSJ (ed) Human brain functions. Academic Press, New York, pp 243–274
Passingham RE, Toni I, Schluter N, Rushworth MFS (1998) How do visual instructions influence the motor system? In: Goode J, Glickstein M (eds) Sensory guidance of movement, Wiley, Chichester, pp 129–141
Paus T, Petrides M, Evans AC, Meyer E (1993) Role of the human anterior cingulate cortex in the control of oculomotor, manual, and speech responses: a positron emission tomography study. J Neurophysiol 70:453–469
Petrides M (1987) Conditional learning and primate frontal lobes. In: Perecman E (ed), The frontal lobes revisited. IBRN press, New York, pp 91–108
Petrides M (1998) Specialized systems for the processing of mnemonic information within the primate frontal cortex. In: Roberts AC, Robbins TW, Weiskrantz L (eds) The prefrontal cortex. Oxford University Press, Oxford, pp 103–116
Petrides M, Pandya DN (1995) Comparative architectonic analysis of the human and macaque frontal cortex. In: Grafman J, Boller F (eds) Handbook of neuropsychology, Vol 9. Elseverier, Amsterdam, pp 17–58
Porrino LJ, Crane AM, Goldman-Rakic PS (1981) Direct and indirect pathways from the amygdala to the frontal lobe in rhesus monkeys. J Comp Neurol 198:121–136
Preuss TM, Goldman-Rakic PS (1989) Connections of the ventral granular frontal cortex of macaques with perisylvian premotor and somatosensory areas: anatomical evidence for somatic representation in primate frontal association cortex. J Comp Neurol 282:293–316
Rao SC, Rainer G, Miller EK (1997) Integration of what and where in the primate prefrontal cortex. Science 276:821–824
Rolls ET (1998) The orbitofrontal cortex. In: Roberts AC, Robbins TW, Weiskrantz L (eds) The prefrontal cortex. Oxford University Press, Oxford, pp 67–86
Rosenkilde CE, Bauer RH, Fuster JM (1981) Single unit activity in ventral prefrontal cortex of behaving monkeys. Brain Res 209:375–394
Rugg MD, Fletcher PC, Frith CD, Frackowiak RSJ, Dolan RJ (1996) Differential activation of the prefrontal cortex in successful and unsuccessful memory retrieval. Brain 119:2073–2083
Rupniak NMJ, Gaffan D (1987) Monkeys hippocampus and learning about spatially directed movements. J Neurosci 7:2331–2337
Rushworth M, Nixon PD, Eacott MJ, Passingham RE (1997) Ventral prefrontal cortex is not essential for working memory. J Neurosci 17:4829–4838
Scalaidhe PE, Wilson FAW, Goldman-Rakic PS (1997) Area segregation of face-processing neurons in prefrontal cortex. Science 278:1135–1138
Schmahmann JD, Pandya DN (1997) The cerebrocerellar system. In: Schmahmann JD (ed) The cerebellum and cognition. Academic Press, San Diego, pp 31–60
Schultz W, Tremblay L (1998) Reward processing in primate orbitofrontal cortex. Eur J Neurosci 10[Suppl 10]:127.04
Selemon LD, Goldman-Rakic PS (1985) Longitudinal topography and interdigitation of corticostriatal projections in the rhesus monkey. J Neurosci 5:776–794
Shallice T (1982) Specific impairments of planning. Philos Trans Roy Soc Lond B 298:199–209
Shallice T, Burgess P (1998) The domain of supervisory processes and the temporal organization of behaviour. In: Roberts AC, Robbins TW, Weiskrantz L (eds) The prefrontal cortex. Oxford University Press, Oxford, pp 22–35
Snyder LH, Batista AP, Andersen RA (1997) Coding of information in the posterior parietal cortex. Nature 386:167–170
Spence SA, Hirsch SR, Brooks DJ, Grasby PM (1998) Prefrontal cortex activity in people with schizophrenia and control subjects. J Psychiatr 172:1–8
Talairach J, Tournoux P (1988) Co-planar stereotaxic atlas of the human brain. Thieme, Stuttgart
Toni I, Passingham RE (1999) Prefrontal-basal ganglia pathways are involved in the learning of arbitrary visuomotor associations: a PET study. Exp Brain Res 127:19–32
Toni I, Krams M, Turner R, Passingham RE (1998) The time-course of changes during motor sequence learning: a whole-brain fMRI study. Neuroimage 8:50–61
Toni I, Shah J, Grosse-Ruyken M-L, Passingham RE, Zilles K (1999a) Dissociation of signal-, set-, and movement-related activity: a replication. Neuroimage 9:S417

Toni I, Schluter ND, Josephs O, Friston K, Passingham RE (1999b) Signal-, set- and movement-related activity in the human brain: an event-related fMRI study. Cereb Cortex 9:35–49

Tremblay L, Schultz W (1999) Relative reward preference in primate orbitofrontal cortex. Nature 398:704–708

Tremblay L, Hollerman JR, Schultz W (1998) Modifications of reward expectation-related neuronal activity during learning in primate striatum. J Neurophysiol 80:964–977

Ungerleider LG, Mishkin M (1982) Two cortical visual systems. In: Ingle DJ, Goodale MA, Mansfield RJW (eds). Analysis of visual behavior. MIT Press, Cambridge, pp 549–586

Vandenberghe R, Price C, Wise R, Josephs O, Frackowiak RSJ (1996) Functional anatomy of a common semantic system for words and pictures. Nature 383:254–256

Watanabe M (1996) Reward expectancy in primate prefrontal neurones. Nature 382:629–632

Webster MJ, Bachevalier J, Ungerleider LG (1994) Connections of inferior temporal areas TEO and TE with parietal and frontal cortex in macaque monkeys. Cereb Cortex 4:471–483

White IM, Wise SP (1999) Rule-dependent neuronal activity in the prefrontal cortex. Exp Brain Res 126:315–335

Wilson FAW, Schalaidhe SP, Goldman-Rakic PS (1993) Dissociation of object and spatial processing domains in primate prefrontal cortex. Science 260:1955–1958

Wise SP, Di Pellegrino G, Boussaoud G (1996) The premotor cortex and nonstandard sensorimotor mapping. Can J Physiol Pharmacol 74:469–482

Elisabeth A. Murray · Timothy J. Bussey
Steven P. Wise

Role of prefrontal cortex in a network for arbitrary visuomotor mapping

Published online: 16 May 2000

Abstract In arbitrary visuomotor mapping, an object instructs a particular action or target of action, but does so in a particular way. In other forms of visuomotor control, the object is either the target of action (termed *standard* mapping) or its location provides the information needed for targeting (termed *transformational* mapping). By contrast, in *arbitrary* mapping, the object's location bears no systematic spatial relationship with the action. Neuropsychological and neurophysiological investigation has, in large part, identified the neural network that underlies the rapid acquisition and performance of arbitrary visuomotor mappings. This network consists of parts of the premotor (PM) and prefrontal (PF) cortex, the hippocampal system (HS), and the basal ganglia (BG). Here, we propose specialized contributions of the network's different components to its overall function. To do so, we invoke the concept of distributed information-processing architectures, or modules, which may involve a variety of neural structures. According to this view, recurrent neural networks involving cortex, basal ganglia, and thalamus operate largely in parallel. Each of these interacting networks can be termed a cortical-BG module. A large number of these modules include PM neurons, and they can be termed PM cortical-BG modules. A comparable number include PF neurons, termed PF cortical-BG modules. We propose that PM and PF cortical-BG modules compute specific object-to-action mappings, in which the network learns the action associated with a given input. These mappings serve as specific solutions to arbitrary visuomotor mapping problems. However, they are also exemplars of more abstract rules, such as the knowledge that nonspatial visual information (e.g., color) can guide the choice of action. We propose that PF cortical-BG modules subserve abstract rules of this kind, along with other problem-solving strategies. This view should not be taken to imply that the PF network lacks the capacity to compute specific mappings, but rather that it has higher-order mapping functions in addition to its lower-order ones. Furthermore, it seems likely that PF provides PM with pertinent sensory information. The hippocampal system appears to play a role parallel to that of both neocortical-BG networks discussed here. However, in accord with several models, it operates mainly in the intermediate term, pending the consolidation of the relevant information in those neocortical-BG networks.

Key words Conditional motor learning · Frontal cortex · Premotor cortex · Basal ganglia · Hippocampus

E.A. Murray (✉) · T.J. Bussey
Laboratory of Neuropsychology,
National Institute of Mental Health,
Building 49, Room 1B80, 49 Convent Drive, Bethesda,
MD 20892, USA
e-mail: eam@ln.nimh.nih.gov
Tel.: +1-301-4965625, Fax: +1-301-4020046

S.P. Wise
Laboratory of Systems Neuroscience,
National Institute of Mental Health, Bethesda,
MD 20892, USA

Introduction

Imagine a door knob located just above waist level and slightly to your right. When you reach toward the door knob, you automatically transform the relevant visuospatial information into a motor program that directs the forelimb toward the target of reach, in this case the door knob. This action is based on what has been termed *standard* visuomotor mapping, through which the central nervous system transforms the targets of action into motor coordinates (Wise et al. 1996a, 1997). Often, this class of visuomotor guidance involves the movement of the hand to a visible target.

Contrasting forms of visuomotor guidance depend on *nonstandard* mapping (Wise et al. 1996a), which comes in at least two categories. In one, termed *transformational* mapping, an algorithm relates visuospatial information to the direction of movement. For example, one might be required to direct a movement at a 90° clockwise deviation from the visual stimulus. The transform is generally, but not necessarily, the same for all stimulus locations. In the other class of nonstandard visuomotor mapping, which is the topic of this paper, the relationship between the visual stimulus and the movement is arbitrary. The location of a visual stimulus does not indicate the direction of movement to be made, nor is there any algorithm that relates stimulus location to movement direction. Instead, the central nervous system maps the relevant visual information onto an action or set of actions. The system that performs this function appears to have highly general capabilities within its information-processing domain: any visual input that can be detected and discriminated from any other can apparently be mapped onto any movement within a learned motor repertoire.

In a typical *arbitrary* mapping task, nonspatial aspects of a visual stimulus, such as color, instruct a movement direction or target. Returning to our door-knob example, imagine now that you are in a strange building in which amber rooms require that the door knobs be twisted clockwise, but red rooms require a twist in the counter-clockwise direction. And to open a door, you only get one chance to choose which action to perform. You would reach toward the door knob using a standard mapping mechanism, but would have to compute an arbitrary visuomotor mapping to open the doors. Although our door-knob dilemma is contrived, arbitrary visuomotor mapping has *bona fide* applications in everyday life. Most signal-guided behavior, including almost all language-guided behavior, depends on arbitrary mapping abilities. This includes such behaviors as stopping at a red light or at the sound of the word "stop."

Much of the neural network that underlies arbitrary visuomotor mapping has been identified in macaque monkeys and rats. In this article, we review evidence implicating parts of the prefrontal cortex (PF), premotor cortex (PM), basal ganglia (BG), and hippocampal system (HS) in arbitrary visuomotor mapping. We will show, partly based on preliminary results from our own laboratories, that damage to any one of those four structures causes a deficit in some aspect of arbitrary visuomotor mapping. Thus, we will make reference to a distributed PF-PM-BG-HS network. In addition, we will review evidence that each of these structures contains neurons that systematically alter the pattern and level of their discharge modulations during the learning of such mappings. We will neglect the brain-imaging literature (see, for example, Passingham et al. 1998), which is discussed elsewhere in this volume (Passingham et al. 2000).

Our thesis does not imply that arbitrary visuomotor mapping encompasses the main function of the PF-PM-BG-HS network or that mapping visual inputs onto spatially directed motor outputs has any special prominence over other forms of associative learning. Visual-to-visual mappings, mappings involving other sensory modalities, and those involving reinforcement depend on many of the same structures. Nor does this network operate in a vacuum. The arbitrary visuomotor mapping functions of PF, PM, BG, and HS depend on interactions with the visual cortex and a motor-control network, at a minimum. Nevertheless, arbitrary visuomotor mapping tasks serve as a valuable laboratory tool, one that incorporates clearly observed responses with the rigorous sensory and motor control needed for behavioral neurophysiology. As such, it may serve as a paradigm for progress in understanding the general mechanisms underlying associative learning and memory. Finally, we note that in this article there is no attempt to distinguish between visuomotor and visuospatial mapping.

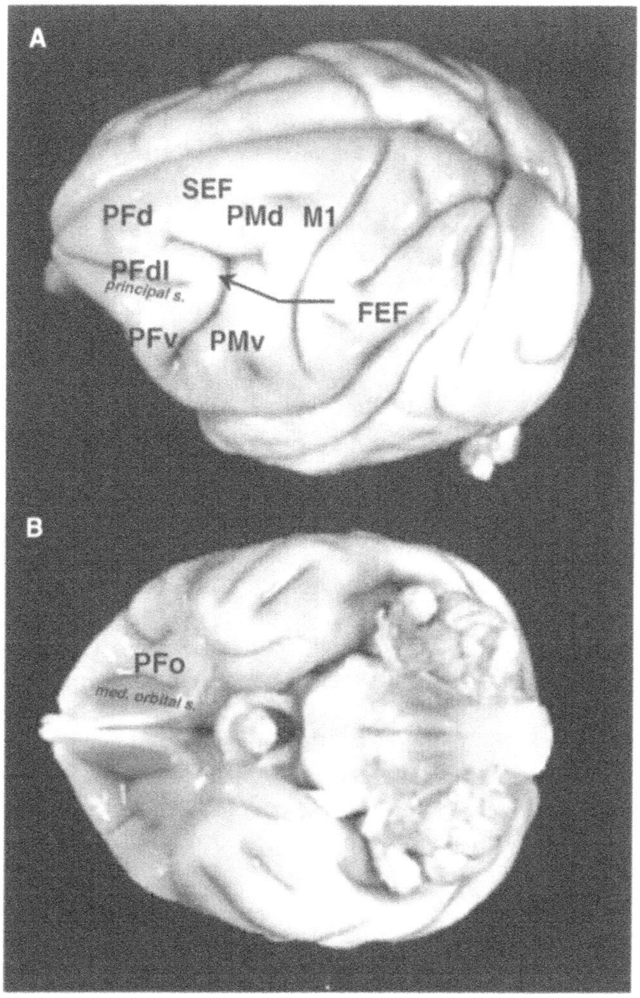

Fig. 1A, B Two surface views of the cerebral cortex of a macaque monkey. **A** Dorsolateral view of the left hemisphere. Rostral is to the left, dorsal is up. **B** Ventral view, rostral is to the left. Photographs from Noe et al. (1999). *PF* Prefrontal cortex, *PM* premotor cortex, *SEF* supplementary eye field, *FEF* frontal eye field, *M1* primary motor cortex, *d* dorsal, *dl* dorsolateral, *v* ventral, *o* orbital, *s* sulcus, *med* medial

Terminology

Figure 1 shows the nomenclature we will use in referring to the various parts of the frontal cortex and the approximate locations of those regions. For example, the general region on the lateral convexity of the hemisphere ventral to the principal sulcus will simply be termed PFv, for ventral prefrontal cortex. Similarly, the orbital prefrontal cortex will be designated PFo. When we want to refer to more than one region, we will use a notation such as PFv+o, which is meant to include both the orbital and ventral prefrontal cortex.

Neuropsychology

Interruption of the basal ganglia outputs at the level of the thalamus (Canavan et al. 1989) and damage to the hippocampal system (Rupniak and Gaffan 1987; Murray and Wise 1996) cause profound impairments in arbitrary visuomotor mapping in monkeys. Canavan et al. (1989) found that monkeys with radiofrequency lesions centered in the ventral anterior nucleus of the thalamus could not retrieve or relearn preoperatively learned (i.e., familiar) visuomotor mappings. Because the monkeys could not relearn the familiar mappings postoperatively, it seems relatively unlikely that they could master novel ones, although that proposition remains to be tested experimentally. Hippocampal-system lesions that include the hippocampal formation as well as the underlying parahippocampal cortex, or in some experiments consist of fornix transection, have little effect on preoperatively learned visuomotor mappings, but severely disrupt the ability to acquire novel mappings. Frontal cortex lesions have effects on both previously learned and postoperatively acquired mappings (Murray and Wise 1997; Petrides 1997).

The hippocampal data have been reviewed recently (Wise and Murray 1999), and there is little to add to what is stated above for BG, at least for primates. Accordingly, we will focus the present discussion on the effects of frontal cortex damage in primates. We will then review some of the relevant literature derived from studies of rats.

Clinical studies

In clinical studies, patients with large excisions of either left or right prefrontal cortex, often including portions of PM, were found to be significantly impaired in learning a visuomotor mapping task in which different colored lights instructed different hand postures (Petrides 1985). More recently, Vriezen and Moscovitch (1990) suggested that this impairment was due to deficits in the application of strategies, which would presumably be taxed by the noncorrection trial-and-error training method that was used, as opposed to deficits in visuomotor mapping *per se*. To address this possibility, Petrides (1997) trained subjects with similar excisions on the same task, but unlike the original study, he first showed the subjects the correct stimulus-response pairings. During learning, he offered subjects immediate correction after errors. As in the earlier study, the patients with excisions of the left or right frontal lobe were impaired in learning the arbitrary visuomotor mapping task. These findings support the view that the impairment reflects a failure to compute the mapping between stimulus and action. As is often the case in clinical studies, it is not possible to state with confidence whether the lesions involved PF, PM, or some combination.

Premotor cortex in primates

In monkeys, Petrides and, separately, Passingham and his colleagues have examined the effects of frontal cortex ablations on the acquisition and retention of arbitrary visuomotor problems, respectively. Petrides (1982) found that monkeys with ablations including the dorsal aspect of PM were severely impaired relative to control monkeys in learning to emit different responses in the presence of two different visual cues. In his experiment, the monkeys were required to grasp a rod in the presence of object A and to touch a button in the presence of object B. Normal monkeys learned this problem in about 300 trials. The operated monkeys were unable to learn this task within the training limit of roughly 1000 trials, although the same monkeys could learn a visual discrimination problem at a normal rate. The latter observation rules out the possibility that the impairment was due to visual deficits *per se*. Halsband and Passingham (1982) found that monkeys with bilateral removals of PM, but not those with ablations of the frontal eye field, were severely deficient in the retention and relearning of a preoperatively learned visuomotor mapping problem. By contrast, the monkeys with PM lesions were able to learn new movements and to learn color discriminations as rapidly as control subjects. Taken together, these findings strongly suggest that the deficit after PM lesions was specific to mapping visual cues onto an appropriate action.

Prefrontal cortex in primates

Gaffan and Harrison (1989) showed that ablations of the dorsolateral prefrontal cortex (PFdl in Fig. 1) caused mild impairments in learning novel visuomotor mappings. Other studies have found either a mild deficit (Petrides 1982) or no deficit (Petrides 1987) on visuomotor conditional tasks after lesions that included some of PFdl. There is also evidence that interactions of inferior temporal cortex (IT) with PF are important for arbitrary visuomotor mapping, which would be expected on anatomical grounds. The two general regions of temporal cortex that are most important in processing visual information about objects – area TE on the middle temporal gyrus and the perirhinal cortex on the inferior temporal gyrus (Meunier et al. 1993; Buckley et al. 1997; Buckley and Gaffan 1997, 1998a, 1998b; Murray and Bussey 1999) – both project to frontal cortex with axons that terminate in PFv+o (Pandya and Kuypers 1969; Webster et al. 1994; Carmichael and Price 1996). Gaffan and Harrison (1988) made lesions of IT and PF in different hemispheres, combined with transection of the corpus callosum. They found that disconnecting IT from PF in this way caused a deficit in the acquisition of arbitrary visuomotor mappings. Interruption of the uncinate fascicle, the fiber bundle which connects much of IT with PF, also caused a mild deficit on this task (Eacott and Gaffan 1992).

Given the foregoing data, we found it surprising that there was no direct evidence in primates showing that bilateral ablations of ventral or orbital portions of prefrontal cortex caused deficits on arbitrary visuomotor mappings. To test the prediction that such effects should be observed, we used the same experimental design as in an earlier study that examined the role of the amygdala and hippocampus in arbitrary mapping (Murray and Wise 1996). The results of this experiment have been reported only in abstract form (Murray and Wise 1997). In brief, rhesus monkeys were seated in a primate chair in front of a video monitor and were required to move a joystick in a specific direction, according to an arbitrary visual instruction stimulus (IS) that appeared on the monitor screen. The joystick was constrained to move in only three directions in the horizontal plane. The monkeys were required to learn several new problems within their daily sessions and were always required to learn three arbitrary visuomotor mappings concurrently (e.g., if stimulus A, move the joystick to the left; if stimulus B, to the right; if stimulus C, pull the joystick). A correct response led to delivery of juice or applesauce reward and termination of the trial. An incorrect response led only to a blank intertrial interval followed by up to two additional presentations of the trial for correction. Just as for the original trial, a correct response on a correction trial led to delivery of reinforcement and termination of the trial. Each monkey was given 50 trials (not counting the correction trials) to learn a set of three arbitrary visuomotor mappings, after which it was presented with a new set of problems, and so on, until the monkey had completed eight such sets (for a total of 24 mapping problems) per day. After a long training period, we found that only one of the first two monkeys studied (Murray and Wise 1997) was able to solve the visuomotor mapping problems rapidly (Fig. 2, preoperative data), and we will therefore present data for that subject only. We are currently studying additional monkeys, but the results from that one subject were sufficiently striking to warrant mention here.

With the exception of the first trial, all learning trials could be divided into two main types: trials on which the IS was the same as that on the previous trials, termed *repeat trials*, and trials on which the IS differed from that on the previous trial, termed *change trials*. From our initial study (Murray and Wise 1996), we knew that monkeys used at least two strategies in performing this task. On repeat trials, they exhibited a high level of performance even before much learning had occurred, indicating that they were simply remembering the stimulus and response from the previous trial and emitting the correct response again. Because the monkeys almost always got

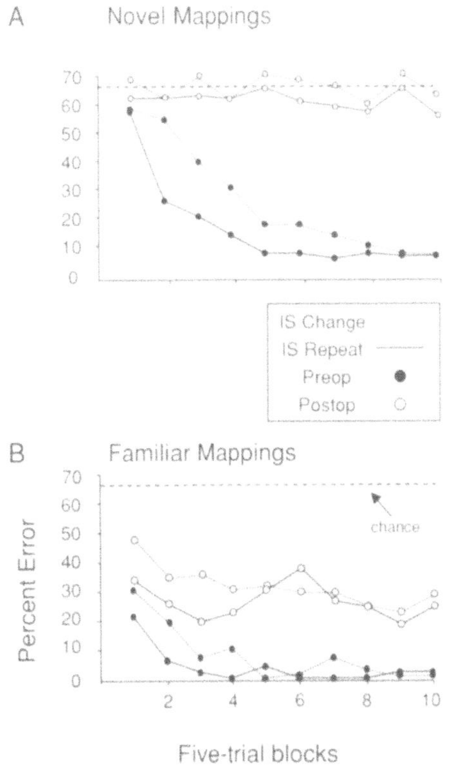

Fig. 2 Effect of bilateral prefrontal (PFv+o) ablation on learning novel mappings (**A**) and retrieval of familiar mappings (**B**). Data from one monkey. Each curve shows the average learning rate for the monkey, pre- (*Preop*) and post-operatively (*Postop*), for repeat and change trials. Data are means for performance over 5 days of testing for novel mappings, 3 days for familiar mappings. *IS Change* Those trials in which the instruction stimulus changed from the previous trial, *IS Repeat* those trials in which the instruction stimulus was the same as in the previous trial

a trial correct, either on the original presentation or on one of the two correction presentations, and because roughly one-third of the trials were repeat trials, use of this *Repeat-Stay* strategy proved beneficial to the monkey's overall performance. In addition, on change trials, it turned out that monkeys avoided the previously emitted response in favor of one of the two remaining possibilities. Application of this *Change-Shift* strategy effectively reduced the three-choice problem to a two-choice problem. On change trials, then, initial performance was roughly 50% in experienced monkeys. Together, we refer to these two aspects of the monkey's performance as the Repeat-Stay/Change-Shift strategy (Wise and Murray 1999). We note that this strategy is related to, but different from, a Win-Stay/Lose-Shift strategy. According to the Win-Stay/Lose-Shift strategy, a new response is selected only after an error, i.e., after failure to obtain reward on the previous trial. By contrast, in the Change-Shift strategy, the change in response is driven not by a failure to obtain reward but, rather, by the knowledge that a different stimulus requires a different response.

After the monkey had learned the task, PFv was ablated from just below the principal sulcus (see Fig. 1A) ventrally to the junction with orbital prefrontal cortex,

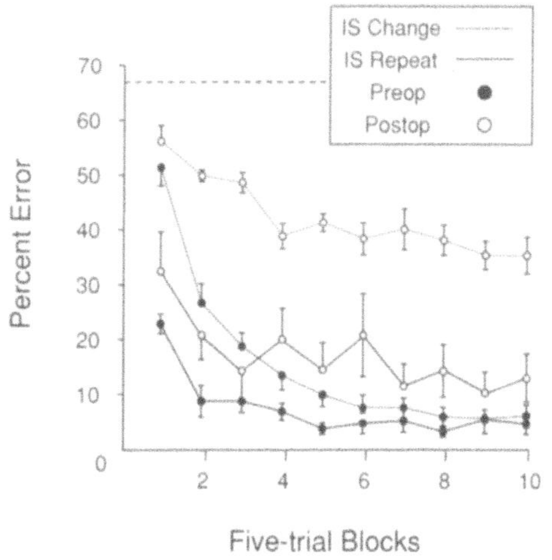

Fig. 3 Effect of bilateral removal of hippocampal formation plus underlying parahippocampal cortex (n=4) on learning novel mappings. The task was the same as that used for the monkey with a bilateral prefrontal (PFv+o) lesion, illustrated in Fig. 2. Curves show means (±SEM; abbreviations as in Fig. 2). Data from Murray and Wise (1996)

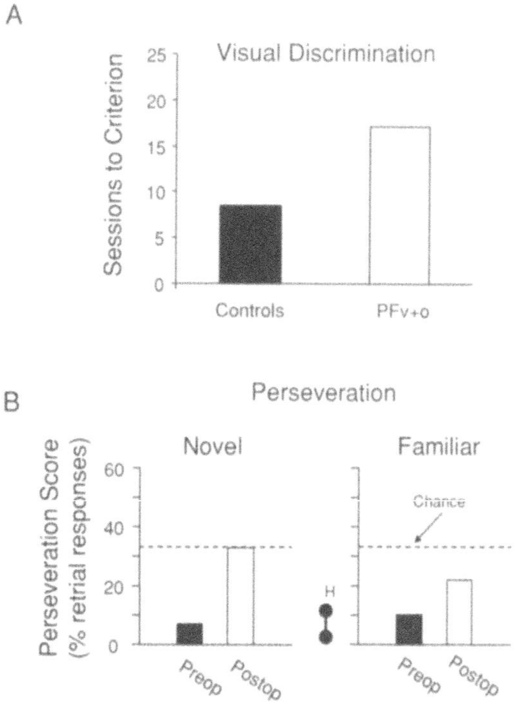

Fig. 4 A Visual discrimination learning. The number of sessions to criterion (90% correct) on a set of two-choice visual-discrimination problems. Monkeys were trained on 20 problems concurrently at the rate of 20 trials (one per problem) per daily session. Control monkeys (n=13) versus one with bilateral prefrontal (*PFv+o*) removal (the same monkey on which Fig. 2 is based). **B** Perseveration scores for the same monkey. The *left panel* shows perseveration, defined as the immediate repetition of a previously unreinforced response, during novel mapping problems. The *right panel* shows comparable data for familiar mapping problems. Between the two panels, for comparison, are perseveration scores from the four monkeys with "hippocampal" (*H*) ablations (see Fig. 3). *Preop* Pre-operatively, *Postop* post-operatively

and PFo was removed from its lateral junction with PFv to the medial orbital sulcus (see Fig. 1B). After this single-stage, bilateral removal of PFv+o, the monkey was no longer capable of learning new mappings within sessions or of applying the Repeat-Stay/Change-Shift strategy (Fig. 2A). The monkey showed no place (or response) preference, i.e., it distributed its correct and incorrect responses roughly equally among the three response choices. For comparison, Fig. 3 shows previously published data for monkeys with removals of the HS. These animals were severely impaired in learning new mappings, but exhibited slow postoperative learning within the 50-trial training blocks on change trials and were virtually normal in their ability to perform the same task according to familiar (i.e., preoperatively learned) mappings (Wise and Murray 1999). By contrast, the monkey with a bilateral PFv+o lesion showed no evidence of learning within the 50-trial blocks (Fig. 2A) and was substantially impaired in performance for familiar mappings (Fig. 2B). However, performance of arbitrary visuomotor mappings for familiar stimuli was clearly above chance levels, so the prior experience or, alternatively, the accumulated experience across sessions, did benefit performance. We focus the remainder of this section on the dramatic deficit in learning novel, arbitrary visuomotor mappings that follows the bilateral PFv+o lesion.

Several accounts of the deficit appear plausible. First, the mapping deficit could have been due to an inability to discriminate the stimuli from each other. Such a deficit in what is often termed perceptual learning could be due to the postulated role of PFv in top-down attention and a loss of the mechanism for biasing specific feature or object representations in IT. To test that possibility, the monkey with a PFv+o lesion was trained postoperatively on a visual discrimination task. Figure 4A shows that, in accord with previous results after PF lesions (Passingham 1972; Gaffan et al. 1993), the monkey had a mild deficit, but was clearly able to reach criterion performance (>90% correct). Because the monkey required approximately twice the number of sessions to learn as did the unoperated control monkeys, we cannot rule out the possibility that a deficit in learning to discriminate visual stimuli contributed to the deficit in visuomotor mapping. However, the fact that the monkey seemed virtually unable to learn the visuomotor mappings suggests that sensory deficits alone do not explain the impairment. Clearly, a more detailed examination of this question is indicated, and we can reject the "sensory" interpretation of the deficit only provisionally.

The deficit could conceivably have resulted from response perseveration, which has been reported to follow PF lesions. Figure 4B shows the results from one analysis of perseveration: the repetition of a previously unreinforced response on correction presentations. Data from the HS-lesion group are also shown in Fig. 4B, between the two graphs. Preoperatively and after HS ablations, there was minimal perseveration. Instead, the monkey showed a Lose-Shift strategy, in which the repetition of an unreinforced response was relatively unlikely (see also Chen and Wise 1996). After PFv+o lesions, relative to before surgery, the monkey was more likely to repeat a previously emitted incorrect response (unfilled bars in Fig. 4B), but appeared to be no more likely to do so than to emit any alternative response. We also searched for, and failed to find, any tendency to repeat incorrectly a previously rewarded response on change trials. Thus, these types of perseveration cannot account for the profound deficits in learning the arbitrary mappings.

Another possible cause of the deficits involves a failure of working memory. A detailed discussion of this issue is beyond the scope of the present paper and was not the focus of the experiment described here. Taking only the present results into account, we cannot rule out an interpretation in terms of working memory. However, the recent results of Rushworth et al. (1997a) show that the PFv, at least, is not necessary for the short-term storage of nonspatial visual information. In their study, monkeys with removals of PFv were able to store visual stimuli for up to 8 s, as measured in a delayed matching-to-sample task using familiar stimuli. We also note that not all the deficits that followed a PFv lesion in their monkeys could be accounted for in terms of working-memory dysfunction. The findings of Rushworth et al. thus falsify the widely promoted hypothesis that the sole specialized function of PF, as a whole, is the mediation of working memory. Furthermore, in the present experiment, demands for storage or manipulation of stimulus information were minimal. The instruction stimulus was present on the video screen throughout the time that the choice of response was made and the response was executed. Accordingly, we are inclined to dismiss the possibility that arbitrary mapping deficits after PFv+o lesions reflect problems with working memory.

We are thus left with two interpretations of the deficit, which are not mutually exclusive. First, PFv+o may compute and store the arbitrary mappings, as well as the strategies and rules that facilitate the network's acquisition of those mappings. Second, the deficit may be due to the disruption of routes by which information is transferred from IT to PM. These interpretations will be discussed in more detail in the section entitled Conclusions and interpretations, below.

A comparable network in rats

The rat frontal cortex consists of several distinct regions, and it appears that at least some play a role in arbitrary visuomotor mapping. As in monkeys, BG and HS appear to do so as well.

Passingham et al. (1988) trained rats preoperatively to pull open a black door, and to push open a white door, in order to gain food reward. In a second experiment, rats were trained either to lift up or to push down a lever, depending on the ambient lighting conditions. Lesions of the medial agranular cortex, termed AGm by some researchers (Donoghue and Wise 1982) or Fr2 by others (Zilles 1985), disrupted the postoperative performance of both of these arbitrary visuomotor tasks. Lesions of approximately the same area caused disruption in the acquisition of a similar visuomotor mapping task (Winocur and Eskes 1998). In that task, the rat faced two levers and instruction lights were placed both to the left and right of center in an operant chamber. When the lights to the left of center were illuminated, they served as an instruction that depressing the left lever was appropriate on that trial and vice versa. However, because the location of a correct response was related to the location of the instruction stimulus, the mapping was not arbitrary in the sense used here. If taken as an example of visuomotor mapping more generally, these data would extend those of Passingham et al., which suggested a role for AGm in the retrieval and retention of familiar (i.e., preoperatively learned) mappings, to indicate a role in acquisition of novel mappings as well. More recently, Quirk et al. (1999) found that AGm lesions slowed the acquisition of a different arbitrary visuomotor mapping task, one in which the frequency at which a light flashes maps onto the direction of response. Rats learned a rule of the type "if lights flash slowly, then go left; if lights flash rapidly, then go right." For convenience, we term this a frequency-motor mapping task. Lesions of the agranular insular cortex (AGi) also impaired acquisition of this task and did so without causing deficits on a visual discrimination problem or on familiar (i.e., preoperatively trained) frequency-motor mappings. Thus, parts of what is often termed prefrontal cortex in rats, AGi and AGm, appear to be important for the acquisition of arbitrary visuomotor mappings.

Other experiments have examined the involvement of rat frontal and cingulate cortex in learning novel visuomotor mappings. Medial frontal cortex lesions, including the prelimbic cortex and the anterior cingulate cortex rostral to the genu of the corpus callosum, had no effect on acquisition of frequency-motor mapping (Bussey 1996) or on acquisition of another arbitrary visuomotor mapping task. In the latter, a nose-poke to targets on the left or right of a computer screen was instructed by a shape presented in the center (Bussey et al. 1997). Surprisingly, excitotoxic lesions of the anterior cingulate cortex caudal to the genu actually facilitated this type of learning, at least in the early stages of learning (Bussey et al. 1996), as did cholinergic denervation of cingulate cortex via lesion of the vertical limb of the diagonal band of Broca (Muir et al. 1996). By contrast, posterior cingulate cortex lesions led to impairments in acquisition, but only in the latest stages of learning, on both of the arbitrary mapping tasks described above (Bussey et al. 1996, 1997). A similar result, for frequency-motor mapping, has been reported to follow lesions of the infralimbic cortex (Quirk et al. 1999).

Taken together, the available data suggest an involvement of parts of the rat frontal cortex in arbitrary visuomotor mapping, with differential involvement of various frontal regions in acquisition and retention/retrieval. However, a general statement about these areas is under-

Table 1 Summary of results from ablation studies (in monkeys) that examined the neural basis of arbitrary visuomotor mapping. *BG output* Basal ganglia output to cortex through thalamus, *HS* hippocampal system, *PFv+o* ventral and orbital prefrontal cortex, *PFdl* dorsolateral prefrontal cortex, *PM* premotor cortex

Site of lesion	Higher-order rules and strategies	Lower-order rules, specific mappings, and exemplars	
		Familiar mappings (retention, relearning)	Fast novel mappings (learning)
PFv+o	lost	partially preserved or relearned across sessions	lost
PFdl	?	preserved	partially disrupted
PM	?	lost	lost
BG output	?	lost	?, presumably lost
HS	preserved	preserved	severely disrupted

mined by the difficulty in identifying homologous frontal areas in rats and monkeys (Preuss 1995).

Lesions in the BG can also affect visuomotor mapping in rats. Dorsal striatal lesions yield deficits on the visuomotor mapping task used by Winocur and Eskes (1998), which, as pointed out above, does not necessarily involve an arbitrary mapping. However, dopamine depletions in a similar region did have disruptive effects on a genuinely arbitrary visuomotor mapping task (Robbins et al. 1990). Reading et al. (1991), using selective excitotoxic lesions, found that damage to the lateral, but not the medial striatum impaired performance on the frequency-motor mapping task. Lesions of the nucleus accumbens also impaired acquisition of this task, but Reading et al. attributed that effect to an attentional deficit. More recently, Quirk et al. (1999) have reinvestigated the involvement of the BG in arbitrary visuomotor mapping. Using the frequency-motor mapping task, they found that lesions of neither the dorsolateral nor ventrolateral striatum caused a deficit. However, lesions of the core (but not the shell) of the nucleus accumbens did lead to impairment (Quirk et al. 1999).

As for the HS, both Winocur (1997) and Sziklas et al. (1998) have reported data from hippocampectomized rats that are consistent with a role in visuomotor mapping. Other studies of rats with hippocampal (Marston et al. 1993) or fornix lesions (Bussey et al., 2000), however, have failed to find an effect on acquisition of visuomotor mapping. We cannot resolve this discrepancy at the present time. However, as emphasized above, in two-choice mapping tasks, animals can perform exceptionally well by employing strategies such as the Repeat-Stay/Change-Shift strategy. Only when the task requires three or more responses can acquisition of the stimulus-response mapping be dissociated from the use of such a strategy. It is therefore conceivable that, in some of the above studies, negative results were obtained because the rats adopted such a strategy. Indeed, this possibility applies to all of the studies carried out so far in rats, which invariably used two stimuli mapped onto two responses. Reconciliation of the foregoing discrepancies may thus require further investigation, including the use of three-choice arbitrary mapping tasks (Wise and Murray 1999) and an explicit evaluation of learning strategy (Parker and Gaffan 1997; Collins et al. 1998; Wise and Murray 1999).

Summary of the neuropsychological data

The data reviewed thus far indicate that a distributed network including PF, PM, BG, and HS underlies arbitrary visuomotor mapping in primates. A summary of the cited results is provided in Table 1. A similar network appears to underlie arbitrary visuomotor mapping in rats, with the qualification that the identification of PF and PM remains uncertain in rodents.

Other brain structures in monkeys appear to contribute little, if anything, to the computations underlying arbitrary visuomotor mapping. For example, lesions of the medial premotor cortex in monkeys, including supplementary motor and anterior cingulate areas, have little or no effect on the retention and retrieval of arbitrary visuomotor mappings (Chen et al. 1995; Thaler et al. 1995). There is a report that lesions to the dorsal prefrontal cortex (PFd in Fig. 1) result in similarly negative results (Passingham 1987). Parts of the posterior parietal cortex also appear to contribute little to the retention of familiar mappings (Rushworth et al. 1997b). As for subcortical structures, notwithstanding some clinical evidence suggesting involvement of cerebellum in arbitrary mappings of various kinds in humans (Bracke-Tolkmitt et al. 1989; Canavan et al. 1994; Tucker et al. 1996; Drepper et al. 1999), lesions of the deep cerebellar nuclei in monkeys do not appear to cause deficits in learning visuomotor mappings (Nixon and Passingham 1999). Complete bilateral ablation of the amygdala likewise has no effect on the rapid acquisition of arbitrary mappings (Murray and Wise 1996).

In rats, damage to brain regions outside the PF-PM-BG-HS network also yield few, if any, deficits in arbitrary visuomotor mapping. Burns et al. (1999), for example, report no effect on visuomotor mapping of excitotoxic lesions of the amygdala. Y. Chudasama, T. Bussey, and J. Muir (unpublished results) found no effect on visuomotor mapping of excitotoxic lesions of the mediodorsal nucleus of the thalamus, the anterior group of thalamic nuclei, or the prelimbic cortex. As noted above, Bussey et al. (1997) reported similar sparing after excitotoxic lesions of medial frontal or anterior cingulate cortex. In addition, Bussey et al. (2000) found no effect on visuomotor mapping of combined excitotoxic lesions of the perirhinal and postrhinal cortex. This sparing may be due to the stimuli being discriminable on the basis of simple features such as luminance, thus failing to require access to the complex visual representations in perirhinal cortex (Murray and Bussey 1999).

In summary, we conclude that parts of PF, PM, BG, and HS underlie both the acquisition and retention of arbitrary visuomotor mappings and probably form the bulk of the network that subserves these mappings. As we will discuss in the next section, each of the four brain regions implicated by the ablation studies contains neurons that show dramatic and systematic changes in activity as monkeys learn visuomotor mappings.

Neurophysiology

Premotor areas

The first systematic study of the neural correlates of learning arbitrary mappings was that of Mitz et al. (1991) in PM. The experimental design was much like that described above for the ablation study involving PFv+o, with the exception that an *instructed delay period* of one to several seconds was inserted between the stimulus presentation and the choice of response. As in the lesion study, the monkey selected one of three possible joystick movements based on nonspatial information in a visual instruction stimulus. A fourth possible response was to refrain from moving the joystick (no go). Mitz et al. found that more than half of the sample of neurons in PM showed a systematic change in activity as the monkeys learned novel, arbitrary mappings. In that early study, most changes consisted of increases in discharge rate as the monkeys learned. Averaged over the entire population of PM neurons, the time-course of activity increases corresponded very closely with the animals' improvement in performance. Changes during learning were later confirmed with a very different experimental design (Germain and Lamarre 1993), in a study that emphasized the relative lack of such learning-dependent changes in the primary motor cortex (M1 in Fig. 1).

However, the complexity of limb movement in the study by Mitz et al. (1991) led to potential problems in interpreting the results. For example, it was conceivable that the monkey performed the joystick movement differently once the mapping had been learned. Perhaps such a change in the movement could account for the evolution of PM activity during learning. In addition, the monkeys' eye positions were not controlled, which led to possible interpretations of the data in terms of either the retinocentric or craniocentric location of the visual stimuli. This variable could also change systematically as the monkeys mastered the arbitrary mappings. For example, early in the process of learning, the monkeys may have scrutinized the stimulus carefully with foveal vision and done so for a protracted period of time. Later, when the mapping had been mastered, a brief glance could have been sufficient, given that the instruction could be rapidly recognized and "prospectively coded" into action (Gaffan 1977).

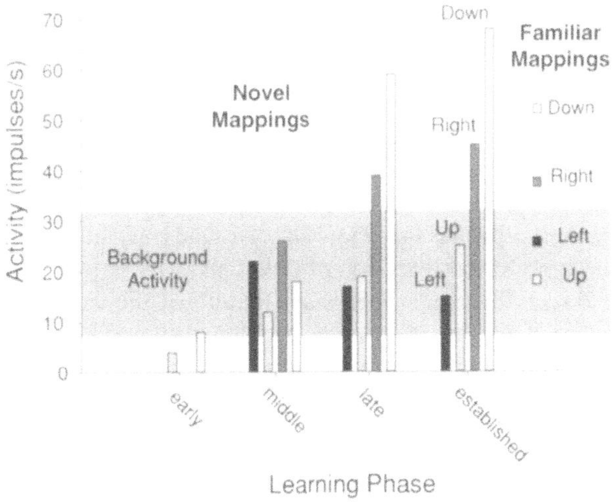

Fig. 5 Development of directional selectivity during learning, from one neuron in the supplementary eye field (SEF). Learning is divided into four phases (*early, middle, late, established*). The cell's activity (measured in the period in which the instruction stimulus was presented) is plotted separately for stimuli (trials) instructing each of the four possible response directions (*up, down, left, right*). All data are from correctly executed trials. The *rightmost column* shows the activity of the same cell during performance of arbitrary visuomotor mappings according to four familiar instruction stimuli. The *shaded area* shows the background activity level ±SD for the familiar-mapping trials. Adapted from Chen and Wise (1996)

Accordingly, Chen and Wise (1995) redesigned the experiment to address those problems. Instead of moving a joystick, the monkeys responded to the visual stimulus by shifting gaze to one of four potential eye-movement targets. This change in task design helped rule out the possibility that any changes in neural activity during learning were related to variations in the way the movement was being performed, because the responses were highly stereotyped saccades. To avoid the problems resulting from the stimulus tracking across or lying on different parts of the retina, the monkeys were required to maintain central fixation before, during, and after the presentation of the visual instruction stimulus. Because eye movements were studied, the recordings were made in the supplementary eye field (SEF in Fig. 1), which is treated here as an oculomotor part of PM.

Each trial unfolded as follows: after a brief presentation of the instruction stimulus, the fixation point remained on the screen and four potential targets appeared in the cardinal directions from screen center. When the fixation point disappeared a few seconds later, the monkey was required to make a saccadic eye movement to one (and only one) of the four targets within about half a second and to maintain fixation of that target for about the same amount of time. We intermixed familiar and novel instruction stimuli in the same stimulus set.

Figure 5 shows the evolution of activity in one SEF neuron as the monkey learned four novel visuomotor mappings, one each for upward, leftward, rightward, and downward saccade targets. The activity was measured in the period that the instruction stimulus was presented. The cell showed its greatest discharge rate for visuomotor mappings to the downward target. Significant activity, compared with that in a reference period, was also seen for mappings to the rightward target. No significant neuronal activity was observed for mappings to the leftward or upward targets. Thus, we can say that the cell had a preferred direction of down and to the right, mainly down. The most important feature of the data shown in Fig. 5 is that, for novel problems, the cell's activity evolved during learning, only becoming significantly different from background levels of activity during the later stages of learning.

It is important to emphasize that the data shown in Fig. 5 were taken exclusively from trials on which the monkey executed the correct response. Incorrect responses have been eliminated. The reason for the selection of "correct" trials is that, for any given direction of saccade, the monkey made the same response to the identical stimulus. This makes the physiological data much easier to interpret, since it rules out variation in motor or sensory factors as the cause of change in activity modulation. Because the stimulus changed on every trial, and remained present for only 0.5 s, we can be confident that the monkey not only attended to the stimulus in a general sense, but also attended to some of its nonspatial information at that time. Presumably, the monkey attended to some subset of features that distinguished the stimuli from each other, although in these complex, multi-dimensional stimuli we do not know which of the many stimulus features the monkey used. Nevertheless, we can be confident that, for each saccade direction, the stimulus was the same in all spatial coordinate frames and that it was attended on every correctly executed trial.

But there are other variables that could confound interpretation of the neurophysiological result. As the monkey learned, a variety of general factors changed in correlation with learning. For example, as the monkey mastered a novel visuomotor mapping, the reward frequency (rewards per minute) increased. It is reasonable to infer, and impossible to exclude, the possibility that reward expectation paralleled that increase. Furthermore, the monkeys may have changed their general level of motivation or arousal as they became more familiar with the initially novel mapping. However, none of these general factors can account for the evolution of activity illustrated in Fig. 5. The same changes in reward frequency, motivation, and arousal occurred for the visuomotor mappings to the upward and leftward targets as for the downward and rightward targets, but the neuronal activity did not increase significantly for the former. About half of the cells have sufficient directional selectivity to rule out general factors common to all mapping directions. Thus, the systematic change in discharge rate shown in Fig. 5 can be attributed to learning the arbitrary visuomotor mapping.

Figure 6 shows learning-related activity changes for a population of SEF cells. The panels on the left are aligned to the onset of the visual stimulus. Those on the right are aligned to the time that the monkey's saccade brought gaze into a window around the target. In each row, activity during a "background" reference period was subtracted from that in each of several successive time bins, averaged over the entire population for each of three phases of within-session learning. The row labeled "familiar" came from intermixed trials in which the monkey performed the task according to the familiar mappings. Early in learning (top row), there was little increase in activity over background levels for most of the trial. Note, however, that there was a significant burst of activity as the time of reinforcement approached, after target acquisition. Later in learning (second and third rows), the cells' activity increased throughout the trial to include significant stimulus-period, delay-period, presaccadic, and postsaccadic activity. By the end of the learning blocks (third row), activity levels typically exceeded that for the familiar stimuli, a phenomenon also seen for the single cell illustrated in Fig. 5.

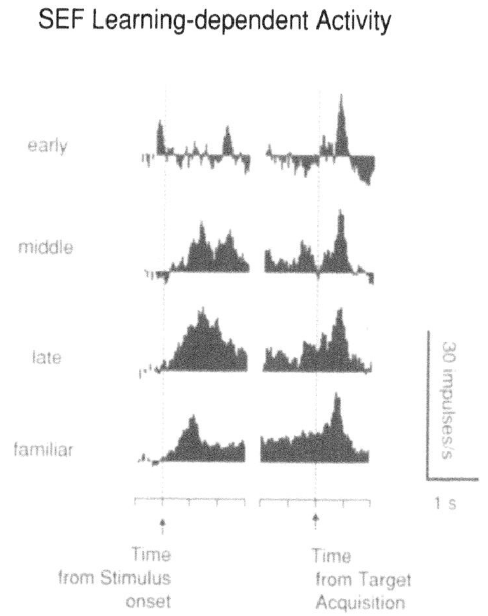

Fig. 6 Population histograms for a subpopulation of neurons in the supplementary eye field (*SEF*). The *left column* shows the neuronal-activity data aligned on the onset of the visual instruction stimuli. The *right column* shows data from the same neurons aligned on the acquisition of the eye-movement target. The *top three rows* show average activity for three phases of learning. The *bottom row* shows the average activity for performance according to familiar mappings. Note the development of activity during learning. Adapted from Chen and Wise (1995)

As illustrated in Fig. 7, three main types of learning-related activity were observed. The SEF population featured in Fig. 6 was termed learning-dependent activity (increasing), because the cells' modulation increased as the monkeys learned the arbitrary mapping (Fig. 7A). These cells had activity at the end of the learning block that was generally similar to that observed when familiar stimuli instructed the same action. Another kind of activity was only observed during the learning of novel map-

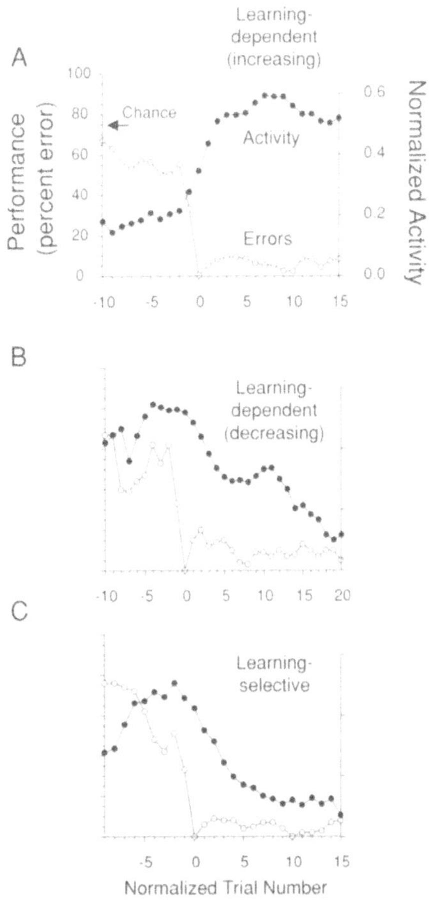

Fig. 7A–C Three subpopulations of supplementary eye field (SEF) cells, showing their evolution of activity during learning in relation to the rate of learning. **A** Learning-dependent activity, with increasing discharge rates (see also Fig. 6). *Unfilled circles* show mean error rate (moving average of three trials), as the monkey learns new mappings, aligned on the first occurrence of three consecutive correct responses. *Filled circles* show the three-point moving average of the subpopulation's activity, aligned on the same trial as the corresponding behavioral data point. **B** Learning-dependent activity, with net decreasing discharge rates. **C** Learning-selective activity. Adapted from Chen and Wise (1995)

pings and not for performance according to the familiar mappings. Accordingly, we termed this pattern of activity "learning-selective" (Fig. 7C). The third pattern of activity (Fig. 7B) was classed as learning-dependent (decreasing) by Chen and Wise (1995) because the cells showed a significant task relationship for the familiar mapping problems, which was the basis for their definition of learning dependency. In general, however, this pattern appeared more similar to learning-selective activity (Fig. 7C). These three patterns appeared to be completely intermixed within the SEF. The majority (55%) of SEF neurons showed either learning-dependent or learning-selective activity. From a population of 101 SEF neurons, 37% were classed as learning dependent (like those in Fig. 7A and B) and 18% as learning selective (like those in Fig. 7C).

Prefrontal cortex

Watanabe (1990) reported changes in the activity of PFdl neurons during an arbitrary stimulus-stimulus mapping task, but reported on the activity of only three cells during learning. No systematic work had been done on learning-related neurons until very recently. For PFv and PFdl (see Fig. 1), Asaad et al. (1998) studied the changes in the directional selectivity of PF neurons as monkeys learned arbitrary mappings in an oculomotor paradigm similar to that described above for the SEF study. They found a systematic shift in the development of directional selectivity as the monkeys mastered the arbitrary mappings. Changes in activity during learning have also been reported by Tremblay and Schultz (1996) in PFo and by Li et al. (1997) in PFv. Asaad et al. (1998) confirmed a finding for PF that was originally made for SEF: activity for novel mappings, once learned, exceeded that for familiar ones (see Figs. 5 and 6). In their analysis, Asaad et al. were able to estimate the relative sensitivity of PF neurons to three different factors: the instruction stimulus, the direction of a saccade, and the mapping. First, they taught the monkey two mappings, e.g., stimulus A instructed a saccade to the left (A-left) and stimulus B instructed a saccade to the right (B-right). Then they reversed the mappings (to A-right and B-left). For many PF neurons, Asaad et al. recorded activity as the monkey performed the task according to both the original and the reversed mappings. They found that some PF neurons were selective for the stimulus, especially relatively early in a trial. An example would be a cell with activity that was greater for A-left and A-right than for B. That percentage decreased from 45% in the stimulus period, to 32% in the delay periods, to 21% in the presaccadic period. A smaller percentage of PF neurons was selective for saccade direction. An example would be a cell with greater activity for A-left and B-left than for right. That percentage increased from 14% during the stimulus period, to 21% and 34% in the delay and presaccadic periods, respectively. However, a large population of PF neurons reflected the specific mapping. In a typical example, a PF neuron had activity for one combination of stimulus and response, e.g., B-left, that was greater than for any other combination. The percentage of cells showing this property ranged from 41% to 47% in the various periods of the trial.

Hippocampus

Cahusac et al. (1993) reported changes in activity levels during the learning of arbitrary visuomotor mappings. They found neurons that corresponded to both the learning-selective and learning-dependent activity changes reported for SEF. Learning-selective activity appeared to be more prominent than learning-dependent activity, 45% to 22%, and most of the latter took the form of increasing activity during learning. The changes in activity observed in hippocampus were relatively weak. This observation may reflect differences in the experimental design, of course. However, it is tempting to interpret the small hippocampal activity changes as a characteristic of a sparsely coded network like the hippocampus. Because the hippocampus represents so many different kinds of information, any given type is likely to be distributed over several neurons, which comprise only a relatively small percentage of the overall hippocampal network. By contrast, premotor areas like SEF represent only a limited kind of information, much of it having to do with eye movements and the sensory signals that guide such movements. The robust activity changes seen in SEF during learning may be representative of a densely coded network. This view corresponds with a role for the hippocampus in many information-processing domains, compared with a role for each individual neocortical area in relatively few domains.

Basal ganglia

Tremblay et al. (1998) studied neuronal activity in the striatum that was associated with arbitrary visuomotor learning. They compared activity for novel mappings with activity in the same neurons during familiar mappings. About one-third of the striatal neurons they studied had firing rates that differed between the novel and familiar mappings, despite the similarity of the response and stimulus material. In addition, they noted a much higher incidence of learning-related changes immediately after the instruction stimulus relative to that observed after other task events (such as the movement). Tremblay et al. also concluded that, compared with PM, SEF, and PFo (Tremblay and Schultz 1996), the striatum had fewer neurons that showed learning-related activity evolution.

Conclusions and interpretations

It seems unlikely that all parts of the PF-PM-BG-HS network make the same contribution to arbitrary visuomotor mapping. In discussing potential specializations within the network, we will make use of the concept of distributed information-processing architectures spanning several neural structures, especially as applied to the frontal cortex and basal ganglia (Houk and Wise 1995). In this view, recurrent neural networks include the neocortex, basal ganglia, and thalamus, and each cortical area participates in a large number of such cortical-BG modules, operating largely in parallel.

We propose that several interacting capabilities, supported by cortical-BG modules, contribute to arbitrary visuomotor learning. The central ability, of course, consists of acquiring the specific mappings. However, underlying and speeding that process is the ability to learn higher-order rules (defined below), to learn and apply strategies for problem solving and to transfer processed information from cortical-BG modules in one area to those in another. We further propose, in accord with several other models, that HS stores mappings, rules, and strategies over the intermediate term pending their consolidation into frontal cortical-BG modules. Our conclusions and interpretations are summarized in Table 2.

Higher-order rules

In the section entitled Prefrontal cortex in primates, we suggested two interpretations of the deficit in arbitrary visuomotor mapping that followed bilateral ablation of PFv+o. The first involved disruption of rules and strategies; the second invoked the concept of a disconnection. The latter interpretation is taken up below in the section titled Disconnection. We distinguish between higher-order rules and lower-order rules (Wise et al. 1996b). Lower-order rules are equivalent to exemplars and specific mappings, for example, when a red square maps onto a leftward joystick movement. A higher-order rule deals with the same kinds of information as a lower-order rule, but at a more abstract level. For arbitrary visuomotor mappings, one important higher-order rule is that colors and shapes instruct a particular action or target of action. The disruption of higher-order rules, which we suppose to be encoded in PF cortical-BG modules, could have contributed to the deficit observed after PFv+o lesions. Of course, a role for PF in learning higher-order rules does not preclude a role in learning lower-order rules (i.e., exemplars) as well. However, once PFv+o is removed, its contribution to both would be eliminated.

Failure to learn or apply the higher-order rule that nonspatial visual information guides action could have devastating effects on arbitrary visuomotor learning, but only on the assumption that higher-order rules are necessary for learning lower-order ones. That assumption is doubtful, however. Each exemplar could be learned, one by one, without ever encoding the general rule that nonspatial visual information always provided the critical signal. Accordingly, this factor alone does not explain the severe deficit that follows PFv+o lesions (Fig. 2A). Nevertheless, the ability to learn and apply higher-order rules may increase the speed and efficiency of learning.

Strategy

A strategy can be considered to be a plan or method for solving a problem, and evidence obtained in monkeys implicates PF in the learning and implementation of strategies (Parker and Gaffan 1997; Collins et al. 1998). The Repeat-Stay/Change-Shift strategy is particularly effective in a three-choice visuomotor mapping task because, as noted above, it reduces a three-choice problem to a two-choice problem for change trials and solves the problem completely for repeat trials. Despite their marked deficit in new learning, monkeys with HS lesions continued to apply the Repeat-Stay/Change-Shift

Table 2 Summary of conclusions and interpretations (*italic text*) regarding the effects of brain damage on arbitrary mapping abilities in monkeys. *BG* Basal ganglia, *M1/BG* cortical-BG modules of the primary motor cortex, *PM/BG* premotor cortex cortical-BG modules, *PF/BG* prefrontal cortex cortical-BG modules, *HS* hippocampal system, *PFv+o* ventral and orbital prefrontal cortex, *PFdl* dorsolateral prefrontal cortex, *BG output* basal ganglia output through thalamus

Ability after lesion	Higher-order rules and strategies	Lower-order rules, specific mappings, and exemplars	
		Familiar mappings (retention, relearning)	Fast novel mappings (learning)
Relatively spared	**After HS lesion** *due to preserved PF/BG*	**After HS, PFv+o, or PFdl lesion**[a] *due to preserved PM/BG and PF/BG*[b]	
Lost or almost lost	**After PFv+o lesion** *due to lost PF/BG*	**After PM lesion** *due to: i) lost PM/BG, ii) disconnection of PF from motor output*[c] **After BG-output lesion** *due to lost PM/BG and/or PF/BG*	**After PFv+o lesion** *due to: i) lost PF/BG for strategy and/or rules*[d], *ii) disconnection of PM/BG from visual input*[e] **After PM lesion** *due to lost PM/BG and/or lost motor input to PF*[f] **After HS lesion** *due to lost intermediate-term, fast-mapping network*[g]

[a] Partial retention or relearning across sessions after PFv+o ablations (see Fig. 2B)
[b] For PFv+o and PFdl lesions, those PF cortical-BG modules not removed by the ablation
[c] PF/BG→PM/BG→M1/BG
[d] Lower-order rules as well as higher-order rules
[e] IT→PF/BG→PM/BG
[f] PM/BG→PF/BG
[g] Slow encoding into long-term mapping network preserved (Fig. 3), but HS needs PF/BG and/or PM/BG to effectuate learned actions, hence the deficits after PM or PFv+o lesions

strategy (Fig. 3). However, a different result followed PFv+o removals. That lesion eliminated the strategy as well as learning (Fig. 2A), at least within the 50-trial blocks we examined. This finding indicates that PFv+o is necessary for implementation of the Repeat-Stay/Change-Shift strategy, and we attribute the loss of this ability to the elimination of cortical-BG modules that include neurons in this region.

Although PFv+o lesions abolished the Repeat-Stay/Change-Shift strategy, it seems unlikely that this factor alone accounts for the dramatic deficit observed in Fig. 2A. In a three-choice task, perfect application of the Repeat-Stay/Change-Shift strategy decreases the initial error rate, when faced with a set of novel mapping problems, from 67% to 33% (0% on the repeat trials and 50% on the change trials, which occur twice as often). After the PFv+o removals, the percentage of errors on initial choices was, therefore, increased to ~ 67%. Still, that does not explain why the visuomotor mappings that were reinforced were not learned at all over the 50-trial block. As with higher-order rules, the ability to learn and to apply problem-solving strategies may contribute to the speed and efficiency with which arbitrary visuomotor mappings can be learned.

Disconnection

PFv+o may support arbitrary visuomotor mapping through either or both of two mechanisms. One mechanism could involve computing and storing the mappings within its cortical-BG modules. However, this mechanism cannot account for all the evidence, because PF is insufficient to support learning in the absence of PMd. This finding points to a possible second mechanism, namely, that fast, novel visuomotor mappings may depend on PFv+o providing a route by which visual information reaches PMd. More specifically, it seems likely that the PFv+o lesion interrupted the flow of information from nonspatial visual areas (particularly IT, including perirhinal cortex) to PM cortical-BG modules. PFv+o receives most of the frontal lobe's input from IT, which does not project directly to PM (Pandya and Kuypers 1969; Webster et al. 1994; Carmichael and Price 1996). Thus, a lesion of PFv+o could effectively disrupt the transmission of information between IT and PM. This disconnection could involve corticocortical pathways, projections through the basal ganglia, or both. By cutting off the route of nonspatial visual information to PM and the parts of the basal ganglia interconnected with PM, the ability of PM cortical-BG modules either to acquire or execute mappings would be undermined. Taken together, the direct effects of PFv+o lesions (including the loss of rules and strategies) and the disconnection could account for the devastating deficit in fast, new learning that we observed after PFv+o removal.

Similarly, the ability of PF cortical-BG networks to encode specific mappings and to produce motor outputs could have been compromised by lesions of PM. Such lesions could deprive PF networks of information about the movements that are being prepared and executed on each trial. The lack of such information, especially at the time of the occurrence or absence of reward, could prevent the encoding of exemplars into PF cortical-BG modules as well as the extraction of higher-order rules based on those exemplars. In addition, PM lesions could disrupt the flow of information from PF cortical-BG modules to the motor output structures of the caudal frontal lobe.

Long- versus intermediate-term memory

It appears that HS supports specific mappings or exemplars in the intermediate term, pending consolidation of that information into a long-term memory store involving both PM and PF *cortical-BG* modules. We suggest that HS also supports, in parallel, higher-order rules and strategies in the intermediate term pending their consolidation into PF *cortical-BG* modules.

Lesions of HS (Rupniak and Gaffan 1987; Gaffan and Harrison 1989; Murray and Wise 1996), PFdl (Gaffan and Harrison 1989) and PFv+o (described above) cause a deficit in learning novel mappings, but have much less dramatic effects on familiar (i.e., preoperatively learned) mappings. The relative sparing of preoperatively learned mappings could arise in either of two ways. First, preserved performance might be due to repeated presentation of the same stimulus-response mappings over several days. [For the data presented here (Fig. 2A), novel stimuli were presented on one day only, but familiar stimuli reappeared across days.] Preliminary data suggest that this interpretation may apply to the effects of PFv+o lesions (T. Bussey, S.P. Wise and E.A. Murray, unpublished observations). However, there is a second possibility, one that would lead to an even more dramatic preservation of familiar mappings. If the networks storing exemplars in the long term were preserved, then excellent performance on familiar-mapping problems should emerge quickly after surgery, without requiring days of repeated experience with specific mappings. The HS-lesion data support this interpretation (E.A. Murray and S.P. Wise, unpublished observations). In accord with several models of hippocampal function, we suppose that HS functions as the intermediate-term storage network, whereas frontal cortical-BG modules store the same information in the long term.

Generality and advantages of arbitrary mapping

How general is the capability of this distributed neural network, and is it specific to mapping visual inputs onto action? There is reason to believe that at least part of the network is involved in mapping functions of a more general nature. An interaction of IT with PF supports other types of mapping, for example, when a visual stimulus maps onto another visual stimulus (also known as visual paired-associate learning or arbitrary visuovisual mapping). Transection of the uncinate fascicle causes a dramatic impairment in that task (Eacott and Gaffan 1992; Gutnikov et al. 1997). Using a crossed-lesion disconnection approach, Parker and Gaffan (1998) have also pointed to IT/PF interactions as important in arbitrary mapping. In their study, food rewards mapped onto visual stimuli. Specifically, the arrival or nonarrival of a food-pellet reward served as an instruction cue, signaling which one of two visual stimuli was correct on that trial. These data thus support a more general role for these parts of the network in arbitrary mappings involving visual information, one not restricted to arbitrary visuomotor mapping.

In contrast to its role in arbitrary mapping, IT/PF interaction does not appear to be necessary for other tasks involving visual information, such as visual discrimination and configural learning (Eacott and Gaffan 1992; Gutnikov et al. 1997; Parker and Gaffan 1998). These problems could be solved by an arbitrary mapping mechanism, but they are probably not. We think that discrimination learning is more akin to standard mapping than to arbitrary mapping. Solving the discrimination problem only requires "approach" to a visible target of relatively high affective valence. Some configural learning tasks could have a similar solution. For example, a typical configural discrimination problem might involve AB+ or CD+ versus BC– or AD–, where + indicates a rewarded configural stimulus and – an unrewarded one. This problem could be solved by approaching AB and CD, but avoiding BC and AD. When sample and choice stimuli occur at different times or are in different spatial locations, animals could be biased toward solving the problems through arbitrary mapping (Holland 1991). However, if the features are always temporally and spatially contiguous, as they were in the monkey experiments (e.g., Gutnikov et al. 1997), animals may be biased toward learning these by approaching configurations with high affective valence. Thus, the lack of deficits observed after PF/IT disconnections in either discrimination or configural learning tasks does not rule out the possibility that these structures underlie arbitrary mapping of visual information in some general sense.

Could an arbitrary mapping ability, assuming it is highly general and arbitrary, have some bearing on the search for precursors to human language? Both Lieberman (1991) and Bickerton (1992) have emphasized that, in an attempt to understand the evolution of language, some attention should be paid to capabilities that could be "co-opted" by the language system once it evolved. This view should not be construed as antithetical to current conceptualizations of a language module specific to humans; it holds only that the nervous system would not dispense with an information-processing capacity that could be marshaled in the service of language, merely because it evolved before language. In visuomotor mapping, the relationship between visual stimuli and the actions that they map upon is arbitrary, and so is the relationship of words to the information they represent.

A characteristic of "arbitrariness" in vocal communication is shared by human language and nonhuman primate vocalization (Hockett 1960). Furthermore, "fast mapping" is a key concept in the psycholinguistics of word learning and the learning of other information as well (Markson and Bloom 1997). Of course, both arbitrary-mapping ability and vocalizations in monkeys lack many of the other essential features of language, to say nothing of syntax. Nevertheless, it is of some interest that the regions involved in subserving arbitrary mapping in monkeys (PM/PF anterior to orofacial M1 cortex, BG and HS) are all thought to have an important role in language (Heit et al. 1988; Pickett et al. 1998). The neocortical components of this network are closer, in anatomical terms, to human language areas (e.g., Broca's area) than to the medial motor and auditory areas usually put forward as precursors to human language areas (Sutton and Jürgens 1988). Like human language areas, they are situated on the lateral convexity of the frontal lobe, generally rostral to the orofacial and forelimb representations of the primary motor cortex.

Even if the ability to acquire arbitrary mappings was a precursor to one aspect of language, it would do macaque monkeys no good. The ability of monkeys to acquire arbitrary visuomotor mappings is, in itself, an adaptive advantage. Arbitrary visuomotor mapping allows the ability to select any action within an already learned behavioral repertoire in response to any environmental context that can be detected and discriminated from any other. This rapid, arbitrary mapping provides nothing less that the ability to learn, in the short term, the behavioral significance of stimuli, places, and events, enabling monkeys to respond flexibly to challenging and changeable circumstances.

Acknowledgment The authors thank Dr. David Gaffan for his comments on an earlier version of this paper.

References

Asaad WF, Rainer G, Miller EK (1998) Neural activity in the primate prefrontal cortex during associative learning. Neuron 21:1399–1407

Bickerton D (1992) Language and species. University Chicago Press, Chicago

Bracke-Tolkmitt R, Linden A, Canavan AGM, Rockstroh B, Scholz E, Wessel K, Diener H-C (1989) The cerebellum contributes to mental skills. Behav Neurosci 103:442–446

Buckley MJ, Gaffan D (1997) Impairment of visual object-discrimination learning after perirhinal cortex ablation. Behav Neurosci 111:467–475

Buckley MJ, Gaffan D (1998a) Perirhinal cortex ablation impairs configural learning and paired-associate learning equally. Neuropsychologia 36:535–546

Buckley MJ, Gaffan D (1998b) Perirhinal cortex ablation impairs visual object identification. J Neurosci 18:2268–2275

Buckley MJ, Gaffan D, Murray EA (1997) Functional double dissociation between two inferior temporal cortical areas: perirhinal cortex versus middle temporal gyrus. J Neurophysiol 77:587–598

Burns LH, Everitt BJ, Robbins TW (1999) Effects of excitotoxic lesions of the basolateral amygdala on conditional discrimination learning with primary and conditioned reinforcement. Behav Brain Res 100:123–133

Bussey TJ (1996) Functions of the cingulate cortex in learning and memory in the rat. Doctoral dissertation, University of Cambridge, Cambridge, U.K.

Bussey TJ, Duck J, Muir JL, Aggleton JP (2000) Distinct patterns of behavioral impairments resulting from fornix transection or neurotoxic lesions of the perirhinal and postrhinal cortices in the rat. Behav Brain Res (in press)

Bussey TJ, Muir JL, Everitt BJ, Robbins TW (1996) Dissociable effects of anterior and posterior cingulate cortex lesions on the acquisition of a conditional visual discrimination: facilitation of early learning vs. impairment of late learning. Behav Brain Res 82:45–56

Bussey TJ, Muir JL, Everitt BJ, Robbins TW (1997) Triple dissociation of anterior cingulate, posterior cingulate, and medial frontal cortices on visual discrimination tasks using a touchscreen testing procedure for the rat. Behav Neurosci 111:920–936

Cahusac PMB, Rolls ET, Miyashita Y, Niki H (1993) Modification of the responses of hippocampal neurons in the monkey during the learning of a conditional spatial response task. Hippocampus 3:29–42

Canavan AGM, Nixon PD, Passingham RE (1989) Motor learning in monkeys (*Macaca fascicularis*) with lesions in motor thalamus. Exp Brain Res 77:113–126

Canavan AGM, Sprengelmeyer R, Diener HC, Homberg V (1994) Conditional associative learning is impaired in cerebellar disease in humans. Behav Neurosci 108:475–485

Carmichael ST, Price JL (1996) Connectional networks within the orbital and medial prefrontal cortex of macaque monkeys. J Comp Neurol 371:179–207

Chen LL, Wise SP (1995) Neuronal activity in the supplementary eye field during acquisition of conditional oculomotor associations. J Neurophysiol 73:1101–1121

Chen LL, Wise SP (1996) Evolution of directional preferences in the supplementary eye field during acquisition of conditional oculomotor associations. J Neurosci 16:3067–3081

Chen Y-C, Thaler D, Nixon PD, Stern C, Passingham RE (1995) The functions of the medial premotor cortex (SMA). II. The timing and selection of learned movements. Exp Brain Res 102:461–473

Collins P, Roberts AC, Dias R, Everitt BJ, Robbins TW (1998) Perseveration and strategy in a novel spatial self-ordered sequencing task for nonhuman primates: effects of excitotoxic lesions and dopamine depletions of the prefrontal cortex. J Cogn Neurosci 10:332–354

Donoghue JP, Wise SP (1982) The motor cortex of the rat: cytoarchitecture and microstimulation mapping. J Comp Neurol 212:76–88

Drepper J, Timmann D, Kolb FP, Diener HC (1999) Non-motor associative learning in patients with isolated degenerative cerebellar disease. Brain 122:87–97

Eacott MJ, Gaffan D (1992) Inferotemporal-frontal disconnection: the uncinate fascicle and visual associative learning in monkeys. Eur J Neurosci 4:1320–1332

Gaffan D (1977) Response coding in recall of colours by monkeys. Q J Exp Psychol 29:597–605

Gaffan D, Harrison S (1988) Inferotemporal-frontal disconnection and fornix transection in visuomotor conditional learning by monkeys. Behav Brain Res 31:149–163

Gaffan D, Harrison S (1989) A comparison of the effects of fornix transection and sulcus principalis ablation upon spatial learning by monkeys. Behav Brain Res 31:207–220

Gaffan D, Murray EA, Fabre-Thorpe M (1993) Interaction of the amygdala with the frontal lobe in reward memory. Eur J Neurosci 5:968–975

Germain L, Lamarre Y (1993) Neuronal activity in the motor and premotor cortices before and after learning the associations between auditory stimuli and motor responses. Brain Res 611:175–179

Gutnikov SA, Ma YY, Gaffan D (1997) Temporo-frontal disconnection impairs visual-visual paired association learning but

not configural learning in macaque monkeys. Eur J Neurosci 9:1524–1529
Halsband U, Passingham RE (1982) The role of premotor and parietal cortex in the direction of action. Brain Res 240: 368–372
Heit G, Smith ME, Halgren E (1988) Neural encoding of individual words and faces by the human hippocampus and amygdala. Nature 333:773–776
Hockett CF (1960) Principles of animal communications. In: Lanyon WF, Tavolga WN (eds) Animal sounds and communication. Am Inst Biological Sci Washington, DC, pp 392–430
Holland PC (1991) Transfer of control in ambiguous discriminations. J Exp Psychol: Anim Behav Processes 17:231–248
Houk JC, Wise SP (1995) Distributed modular architectures linking basal ganglia, cerebellum, and cerebral cortex: their role in planning and controlling action. Cereb Cortex 5:95–110
Li BM, Inase M, Takashima T, Iijima T (1997) Potentiation of neuronal responses to well-learned cues in the inferior prefrontal cortex during conditional visuomotor learning. Soc Neurosci Abstr 23:1615
Lieberman P (1991) Uniquely human: the evolution of speech, thought, and selfless behavior. Harvard University Press, Cambridge
Markson L, Bloom P (1997) Evidence against a dedicated system for word learning in children. Nature 385:813–815
Marston HM, Everitt BJ, Robbins TW (1993) Comparative effects of excitotoxic lesions of the hippocampus and septum/diagonal band on conditional visual discrimination and spatial learning. Neuropsychologia 31:1099–1118
Meunier M, Bachevalier J, Mishkin M, Murray EA (1993) Effects on visual recognition of combined and separate ablations of the entorhinal and perirhinal cortex in rhesus monkeys. J Neurosci 13:5418–5432
Mitz AR, Godschalk M, Wise SP (1991) Learning-dependent neuronal activity in the premotor cortex of rhesus monkeys. J Neurosci 11:1855–1872
Muir JL, Bussey TJ, Everitt BJ, Robbins TW (1996) Dissociable effects of AMPA-induced lesion of the vertical limb diagonal band of Broca on performance of the 5-choice serial reaction time task and on acquisition of a conditional visual discrimination. Behav Brain Res 82:31–44
Murray EA, Bussey TJ (1999) Perceptual-mnemonic functions of the perirhinal cortex. Trends Cogn Sci 3:142–151
Murray EA, Wise SP (1996) Role of the hippocampus plus subjacent cortex but not amygdala in visuomotor conditional learning in rhesus monkeys. Behav Neurosci 110:1261–1270
Murray EA, Wise SP (1997) Role of orbitoventral prefrontal cortex in conditional motor learning. Soc Neurosci Abstr 23:11
Nixon PD, Passingham RE (1999) The cerebellum and cognition: cerebellar lesions impair sequence learning but not conditional motor learning in monkeys. Neuropsychologia 11: 4070–4080
Noe A, Welker W, Johnson JI (1999) Comparative mammalian brain collection. http://www.neurophys.wisc.edu/brain/
Pandya DN, Kuypers HGJM (1969) Cortico-cortical connections in the rhesus monkey. Brain Res 13:13–36
Parker A, Gaffan D (1997) Frontal/temporal disconnection in monkeys: memory for strategies and memory for visual objects. Soc Neurosci Abstr 23:11
Parker A, Gaffan D (1998) Memory after frontal/temporal disconnection in monkeys: conditional and non-conditional tasks, unilateral and bilateral frontal lesions. Neuropsychologia 36: 259–271
Passingham RE (1972) Non-reversal shifts after selective prefrontal ablations in monkeys (*Macaca mulatta*). Neuropsychologia 10:41–46
Passingham RE (1987) From where does the motor cortex get its instruction? In: Wise SP (ed) Higher brain functions. Wiley, New York, pp 67–97
Passingham RE, Toni I, Rushworth MFS (2000) Specialisation within the prefrontal cortex: the ventral prefrontal cortex and associative learning. Exp Brain Res DOI 10.1007/s002210000405
Passingham RE, Myers C, Rawlins N, Lightfoot V, Fearn S (1988) Premotor cortex in the rat. Behav Neurosci 102:101–109
Passingham RE, Toni I, Schluter N, Rushworth MF (1998) How do visual instructions influence the motor system? Novartis Symposium. In: Goode J (ed) Sensory guidance of movement. Wiley, Chichester, pp 129–141
Petrides M (1982) Motor conditional associative-learning after selective prefrontal lesions in the monkey. Behav Brain Res 5: 407–413
Petrides M (1985) Deficits on conditional associative-learning tasks after frontal- and temporal-lobe lesions in man. Neuropsychologia 23:601–614
Petrides M (1987) Conditional learning and the primate frontal cortex. In: Perecman E (ed) The frontal lobes revisited. IRBN Press, New York, pp 91–108
Petrides M (1997) Visuo-motor conditional associative learning after frontal and temporal lesions in the human brain. Neuropsychologia 35:989–997
Pickett ER, Kuniholm E, Protopapas A, Friedman J, Lieberman P (1998) Selective speech motor, syntax and cognitive deficits associated with bilateral damage to the putamen and the head of the caudate nucleus: a case study. Neuropsychologia 36: 173–188
Preuss TM (1995) Do rats have prefrontal cortex? The Rose-Woolsey-Akert program reconsidered. J Cogn Neurosci 7: 1–24
Quirk RH, Parkinson JA, Everitt BJ, Robbins TW (1999) Prefrontal and ventral striatal lesions produce dissociable deficits on a conditional learning task in the rat. Soc Neurosci Abstr 25:890
Reading PJ, Dunnett SB, Robbins TW (1991) Dissociable roles of the ventral, medial and lateral striatum on the acquisition and performance of a complex stimulus-response habit. Behav Brain Res 45:147–161
Robbins TW, Giardini V, Jones GH, Reading P, Sahakian BJ (1990) Effects of dopamine depletion from the caudate-putamen and nucleus accumbens septi on the acquisition and performance of a conditional discrimination task. Behav Brain Res 38:243–261
Rupniak NMJ, Gaffan D (1987) Monkey hippocampus and learning about spatially directed movements. J Neurosci 7:2331–2337
Rushworth MFS, Nixon PD, Eacott MJ, Passingham RE (1997a) Ventral prefrontal cortex is not essential for working memory. J Neurosci 17:4829–4838
Rushworth MFS, Nixon PD, Passingham RE (1997b) Parietal cortex and movement. I. Movement selection and reaching. Exp Brain Res 117:292–310
Sutton D, Jürgens U (1988) Neural control of vocalization. Comp Primate Biol 4:625–647
Sziklas V, Lebel S, Petrides M (1998) Conditional associative learning and the hippocampal system. Hippocampus 8:131–137
Thaler D, Chen Y-C, Nixon PD, Stern C, Passingham RE (1995) The functions of the medial premotor cortex (SMA). I. Simple learned movements. Exp Brain Res 102:445–460
Tremblay L, Schultz W (1996) Neuronal activity in primate orbitofrontal cortex during learning. Soc Neurosci Abstr 22: 1388
Tremblay L, Hollerman JR, Schultz W (1998) Modifications of reward expectation-related neuronal activity during learning in primate striatum. J Neurophysiol 80:964–977
Tucker J, Harding AE, Jahanshahi M, Nixon PD, Rushworth M, Quinn NP, Thompson PD, Passingham RE (1996) Associative learning in patients with cerebellar ataxia. Behav Neurosci 110:1229–1234
Vriezen ER, Moscovitch M (1990) Memory for temporal order and conditional associative-learning in patients with Parkinson's disease. Neuropsychologia 28:1283–1293
Watanabe M (1990) Prefrontal unit activity during associative learning in the monkey. Exp Brain Res 80:296–309

Webster MJ, Bachevalier J, Ungerleider LG (1994) Connections of inferior temporal areas TEO and TE with parietal and frontal cortex in macaque monkeys. Cereb Cortex 5:470–483

Winocur G (1997) Hippocampal lesions alter conditioning to conditional and contextual stimuli. Behav Brain Res 88:219–229

Winocur G, Eskes G (1998) Prefrontal cortex and caudate nucleus in conditional associative learning: dissociated effects of selective brain lesions in rats. Behav Neurosci 112:89–101

Wise SP, Murray EA (1999) Role of the hippocampal system in conditional motor learning: mapping antecedents to action. Hippocampus 9:101–117

Wise SP, di Pellegrino G, Boussaoud D (1996a) The premotor cortex and nonstandard sensorimotor mapping. Can J Physiol Pharmacol 74:469–482

Wise SP, Murray EA, Gerfen CR (1996b) The frontal cortex – basal ganglia system in primates. Crit Rev Neurobiol 10:317–356

Wise SP, Boussaoud D, Johnson PB, Caminiti R (1997) The premotor and parietal cortex: corticocortical connectivity and combinatorial computations. Annu Rev Neurosci 20:25–42

Zilles K (1985) The cortex of the rat: a stereotaxic atlas. Springer, Berlin Heidelberg New York

T.W. Robbins

Chemical neuromodulation of frontal-executive functions in humans and other animals

Published online: 16 May 2000

Abstract Neuromodulation of frontal-executive function is reviewed in the context of experiments on rats, monkeys and human subjects. The different functions of the chemically identified systems of the reticular core are analysed from the perspective of their possible different interactions with the prefrontal cortex. The role of dopamine in spatial working memory is reviewed, taking account of its deleterious as well as facilitatory effects. Baseline-dependent effects of dopaminergic manipulation are described in rats on an attentional task, including evidence of enhanced function following infusions of D1 receptor agonists into the prefrontal cortex. The precise nature of the cognitive task under study is shown to be a powerful determinant of the effects of mesofrontal dopamine depletion in monkeys. Parallels are identified in human subjects receiving drugs such as the indirect catecholamine agonists L-dopa, methylphenidate and the dopamine D2 receptor blocker sulpiride. The effects of these drugs on different types of cognitive function sensitive to frontal lobe dysfunction are contrasted with those of a manipulation of 5-HT function, dietary tryptophan depletion. Hypotheses are advanced that accord the ascending systems a greater deal of specificity in modulating prefrontal cortical function than has hitherto been entertained, and clinical and theoretical implications of this hypothesis are discussed.

Key words Prefrontal cortex · Orbitofrontal cortex · Dorsolateral prefrontal cortex · Dopamine · Serotonin · Noradrenaline · Acetylcholine · Methylphenidate · Executive function · Working memory · Planning · Set shifting

T.W. Robbins (✉)
Department of Experimental Psychology,
Downing St., Cambridge CB2 3EB, UK
e-mail: twr2@cus.cam.ac.uk
Tel.: +44 1223 333558, Fax: +44 1223 314547

Introduction

Mapping the functions of the prefrontal cortex (PFC) onto the richness and heterogeneity of its constituent anatomical regions poses a major conceptual problem. The prefrontal cortex is often said to have 'executive functions', which can be defined as that set of cognitive control processes that serve to optimize performance in complex tasks engaging the dedicated processing modules (for example, within the posterior cerebral cortex). The anatomical relationships of the prefrontal cortex are characterized by its contribution of inputs to several levels of the neuraxis, which presumably enable this region to participate in many aspects of control. These prefrontal outputs include backprojections to the posterior cortex and projections to the striatal feedback loop circuitry, the hypothalamus and the brain stem (Goldman-Rakic 1987; Pandya and Yeterian 1995). However, of especial relevance to the present chapter, the prefrontal cortex also targets the main sources of the forebrain monoaminergic and cholinergic neurotransmitter systems – including dopamine-containing cells of the ventral tegmental area, noradrenergic neurons of the locus coeruleus, serotoninergic neurons of the raphé nuclei, and the cholinergic basal forebrain (Goldman-Rakic 1987). Presumably, therefore, through their diffuse ascending inputs, these projections enable the prefrontal cortex to exert profound control over global influences such as arousal, stress, reinforcing feedback and mood, on processing within all of the main telencephalic structures, including the limbic system, thalamus and striatum, as well as the cortical mantle itself. Specific functions such as error signals in reinforcement learning (Schultz et al. 1997), and selective attention and vigilance (Aston-Jones et al. 1991), have also been proposed. The theoretical challenge therefore is to understand the nature of these global and specific influences and their functional significance.

Dissociable effects of manipulations of the chemically defined systems of the reticular core and their possible relationship to frontal cortex function in the rat

Clues about the functions of the monoaminergic and cholinergic pathways have accrued from a number of studies using electrophysiological and neurochemical as well as pharmacological and behavioural methodologies (see Robbins and Everitt 1995). Our own approach has been to compare the effects of relatively specific neurotoxins to effect changes in each of these systems on performance in common behavioural paradigms. One example is our version of the five-choice reaction time task used to assess attentional performance in rats. We have manipulated different parameters of this task in order to define distinct profiles of deficit following neurochemical lesions. Thus, for example, 6-hydroxydopamine (6-OHDA) lesions of the dorsal noradrenergic pathway, emanating from the locus coeruleus, produce impairments in the accuracy of stimulus detection, but only under certain conditions, in which the stimuli are presented unpredictably in time, or bursts of loud white noise are interpolated to disrupt performance (Carli et al. 1983). Excitotoxic (Muir et al. 1994) or immunotoxic (McGaughy et al. 1999) lesions of the cholinergic nucleus basalis produce deficits in the accuracy of stimulus detection even under baseline conditions (see Everitt and Robbins 1997). By contrast, profound depletion of mesolimbic dopamine (Cole and Robbins 1989) and forebrain serotonin (Harrison et al. 1997) mainly serve to affect the general vigour (speed and probability) of responding without affecting accuracy, and mesostriatal dopamine loss again only leads to significant deficits in accuracy under certain conditions (Baunez and Robbins 1999). Whilst it requires evidence from other, independent procedures to begin to make firm conclusions about the psychological nature of these deficits, the fact that they are distinct is consistent with the notions that these neurochemical systems are all implicated in the efficient performance of this task, and that they modulate performance in different ways. The functions of the chemical ascending systems are often referred to as *neuromodulatory*: the term 'neuromodulation' here is taken to mean the enhancement, reduction, prolongation or curtailment of information processing by activity within these systems, often with only their minor participation in the computations of the neural networks they innervate. The ascending systems appear to effect different forms of neuromodulation, which interact in complex ways. This is consistent with previous theorizing that unitary theories of arousal have become outmoded (e.g. Robbins 1984), and must be replaced by more detailed specifications of the roles of these systems.

To what extent the effects of the rather gross manipulations of subcortical neurotransmitter function actually depend on the altered neuromodulation of processes occurring in the prefrontal cortex remains unclear. It is, however, the case that the effects of the basal forebrain cholinergic lesions do somewhat resemble those following excitotoxic lesions of the prefrontal cortex, and also that the effects of forebrain 5-HT depletion to increase premature or 'impulsive' responding are matched by similar excitotoxic lesions of the anterior cingulate cortex (Muir et al. 1996). Finally, the effects of catecholamine depletion in the prefrontal cortex on the five-choice task are largely manifest as impaired accuracy under conditions of temporal unpredictability – resembling therefore the effects of depletion of catecholamines from the cerebral cortex (Robbins et al. 1998a). Thus, some of the effects of neurochemical lesions of the ascending monoaminergic and cholinergic systems might serve to alter the neuromodulation of functions of the prefrontal cortex. What is less clear is how prefrontal cortical manipulations regulate these systems, although there is evidence for example that they influence each of the ascending dopamine (Roberts et al. 1994; Wilkinson et al. 1997; Dalley et al. 1999: see Moore et al. 1999 for a review), noradrenaline (Arnsten and Goldman-Rakic 1984; Jodo et al. 1998) and serotonin (Hajos et al. 1998) systems.

The role of prefrontal dopamine in working memory and other cognitive functions in rats and monkeys

There is also considerable evidence that manipulations of prefrontal dopamine systems have seemingly specific effects on working memory processes. This evidence begins with the work of Brozoski et al. (1979), who showed convincingly that 6-OHDA lesions of the prefrontal cortex of macaques impaired their accuracy of performance on a delayed response type test. These deficits could be remediated by dopaminergic agents, indicating that they were mediated largely by dopamine. The evidence was extended and refined further by later demonstrations that iontophoretic applications of dopamine (DA) D1 receptor antagonists to the principal sulcus of the PFC produced similarly specific impairments in performance in delayed saccade tasks. However, since these seminal observations, further behavioural and electrophysiological evidence has shown that the relationship between working memory function and dopaminergic mechanisms of the PFC is far from simple. Thus, for example, Williams and Goldman-Rakic (1995) have shown that low doses of DA receptor antagonists sharpen the firing patterns of prefrontal cortical 'memory' cells, predicting that this might lead to behavioural improvements rather than deficits. A number of studies in the rat have suggested that high levels of prefrontal cortical DA activity are associated with poorer delayed alternation performance in the rat (Sahakian et al. 1985; Murphy et al. 1996; Zahrt et al. 1997). These results suggest that the relationship between mesofrontal DA function and efficiency of working memory might be characterized by an inverted U-shaped function, with extreme low and high levels of DA activity being associated with impaired performance (Robbins 1985; Arnsten 1998; Zahrt et al. 1997). This relationship begs the question of what the

Table 1 Summary of effects of mesofrontal dopamine depletion on functions sensitive to frontal lobe lesions in monkeys

Function	Effect	References
Spatial working memory (delayed response)	Impaired	Brozoski et al. 1979; Roberts et al. 1994; Collins et al. 1998
Extra-dimensional set-shifting	Enhanced	Roberts et al. 1994
Spatial sequencing	No effect	Collins et al. 1998
Reversal learning	No effect	Roberts et al. 1994

fluctuations in frontal dopamine activity might reflect in terms of normal physiological processes, a clear possibility being the relationship of mesofrontal DA function to increasing levels of 'stress'.

In recent work (Granon et al. 2000), we have been able to show that intra-PFC infusions of the partial D1 receptor agonist SKF-38393 can improve the accuracy of performance of rats in the five-choice task. However, these effects depended on the baseline levels of performance. In those rats performing at a lower level of performance (around 70% correct), there was an improvement in accuracy, whereas in rats performing at a superior level (80%), though still well below the maximum, the drug had no effect. The DA D1 receptor antagonist SCH-233890 had opposite effects, impairing performance at the elevated, but not the lower, level of performance. Such effects were not observed with the DA D2 receptor antagonist sulpiride. Several conclusions can be reached. The mesofrontal DA system is clearly implicated in those processes by which performance reaches a high level of accuracy, with the D1 receptor agonist apparently providing the necessary DA receptor activity for reaching the elevated baseline, and the DA receptor antagonist presumably damping such activity in the high performing rats to reduce performance to the lower level. This appears to reflect a clear modulation of attentional performance by dopaminergic activity. However, such modulation may well depend on the nature of the task under study, presumably reflecting its component processes. The clear possibility exists that DA receptor stimulation sufficient to improve performance on the attentional task may actually be detrimental to performance on other tasks, if for example they require different degrees of dopamine activity for optimal performance. There may thus be costs as well as benefits to cognitive performance following treatment with dopaminergic agents. This notion is consistent with the classic Yerkes-Dodson principle suggesting that undemanding, 'easy' tasks are performed optimally at higher levels of 'arousal' than more 'difficult' ones. This hypothesis remains to be tested directly in the present case, although it might predict that the presumably more effortful task of holding a stimulus 'online' once it has been attended to might well be impaired, consistent with the data reviewed above. On the other hand, it is the more difficult attentional task which seems to respond better to effects of agonists or to resist DA receptor blockade, and so the dimension of task difficulty per se may not be the relevant one. Rather, as suggested by Granon et al. (2000), the relevant factor may be one of individual differences in rats in their capacity to perform accurately on the five-choice task.

A series of studies that have employed 6-OHDA-induced lesions of the mesolimbic DA system in marmosets also support the notion that different effects may be obtained following such depletion depending on the nature of the task (Table 1). In this case, performance in the spatial delayed response task was compared in two separate experiments with (1) an extra-dimensional shift learning task, modelled after the Wisconsin Card Sort Test used clinically for humans (Roberts et al. 1994), and (2) a spatial sequencing task in which marmosets had to monitor their generation of a spatial sequence of responses performed on a computerized touch-sensitive screen (Collins et al. 1998). Each of these tasks is seriously impaired by lesions of the prefrontal cortex itself (Dias et al. 1996a, 1996b; Collins et al. 1998); however, the effect of mesocortical DA depletion varied as a function of the task. In both cases, acquisition of the spatial delayed response task was seriously impaired, consistent with the evidence of Brozoski et al. (1979) mentioned above. However, the performance of the spatial sequencing task was unaffected by the mesofrontal DA depletion (Collins et al. 1998), and performance of the extra-dimensional shift task was actually apparently facilitated (Roberts et al. 1994). A parsimonious conclusion is that the frontal DA deletion had the effect of placing the animal into a state that is detrimental to spatial delayed response performance but at the same time beneficial to the demands of making an extra-dimensional shift (in which the animal has to cease responding to one perceptual dimension that characterizes a complex object and to respond instead to another one that has previously been irrelevant). It is possible that a change in attentional lability, or distractibility, might explain the pattern of results. The effects of enhanced dopamine activity in the prefrontal cortex may make the animal focus more effectively on the stimuli currently controlling performance. This would also help to explain the beneficial effects of D1 agonists in the divided attentional task in rats (Granon et al. 2000).

Cross-species behavioural homology: comparisons with human studies

There is also evidence for a role for dopamine in human working memory functions; although progress has been beneficial, effects have been shown under certain circumstances of low doses of the DA D2 receptor agonist bromocriptine (Luciana et al. 1992, 1998). Follow-up studies have proven rather contradictory in nature, although they all serve to show that DA agonists can have beneficial effects on cognitive performance in certain circumstances. For example, Muller et al. (1998) have demonstrated performance-enhancing effects of the mixed D1–D2 agonist pergolide on spatial working memory performance, but no effect of bromocriptine. This result may thus possibly indicate a role for D1 rather than D2 receptors. Kimberg et al. (1997) were successful in showing some beneficial effects of bromocriptine on several aspects of executive performance, but only in subjects with low levels of working memory performance, the results being thus reminiscent of those described above for rats in response to DA D1 receptor agonist treatment.

In fact, we have observed that bromocriptine can enhance short term spatial memory performance in humans (Mehta et al., unpublished results), and we have also studied in depth the effects of the DA D2 receptor antagonist sulpiride (Mehta et al. 1999), as outlined below. However, in general we have sought indirect means of assessing the possible role of dopamine in cognitive function, for example by focusing especially on tasks that are known to be sensitive to frontal lobe dysfunction, and also on patient groups with profound dopaminergic dysfunction, as occurs for example in Parkinson's disease. Finally, we have also examined the effects of the stimulant drug methylphenidate (Ritalin), an agent which potentiates catecholaminergic neurotransmission, and which has been used in the treatment of attention deficit and hyperactivity disorder (ADHD).

For cognitive tests we have used those tests from the CANTAB battery that seem especially sensitive to frontal lobe dysfunction, including a test of self-ordered spatial working memory, a test of spatial planning, using a computerized form of the Tower of London task, and the CANTAB 'ID/ED' attentional set-shifting paradigm described above (see Robbins et al. 1998b). At least two of these tasks (spatial working memory and ID/ED) have clear analogues in the animal literature (see Robbins 1998). In fact the ID/ED task employs exactly similar stimulus dimensions and exemplars as for the marmoset version (Roberts et al. 1994). Whether these tasks, despite their obvious superficial similarity across the human and animal versions, do engage similar cognitive processes across species is a debatable point. One way of testing for 'behavioural homology' is to demonstrate that the paradigms show similar qualitative effects when factors of importance to psychological theory are manipulated in parallel across species (e.g. the advantage for IDS performance over EDS performance that has been shown for monkeys as well as humans: Downes et al. 1989; Robbins 1998; Weed et al. 1999). A converging test for behavioural homology is to identify which neural systems are recruited by the tasks in both humans and monkeys. If they too are similar, it would seem reasonable to infer that similar functions are being studied (see Robbins 1998).

Each of the three tasks has been employed in functional neuroimaging studies in normal volunteers using positron emission tomography (PET) to index changes in regional cerebral blood flow (Baker et al. 1996; Owen et al. 1996a, 1996b). The self-ordered spatial working memory task produces activations in both the ventrolateral and dorsolateral prefrontal cortex (Owen et al. 1996a). This pattern may be consistent with Petrides' (1996) two-stage model which proposes that the function of holding memories 'online' depends on the ventrolateral prefrontal cortex, whereas the task of monitoring choices (for example, the strategy by which they are sequenced and their association with reinforcement) may recruit additional dorsolateral prefrontal activation. The pattern of activation is quite similar for the Tower of London test of planning, which also, however, exhibited considerable parieto-occipital activation. However, this similarity is consistent with evidence of psychometric associations between the two tasks (Robbins 1996). The Tower of London task was also shown to activate the caudate nucleus upon a later analysis (Elliott et al. 1997b). Finally, the attentional set-shifting task, in a modified form in which three (rather than the usual two) perceptual dimensions were employed, produced significant changes in regional cerebral blood flow in the right dorsolateral prefrontal cortex and the left frontal pole for the extra-dimensional shift compared with the intra-dimensional shift control condition (Rogers et al. 2000).

Effects of dopaminergic agents on tests sensitive to frontal lobe dysfunction in humans

In the absence of very specific DA receptor agonists for use in human subjects, it has proven necessary, but productive, to investigate the dopaminergic modulation of cognitive function by relatively indirect means, including patient groups such as Parkinson's disease, as well as examining effects of less specific agents in healthy volunteers. Comparison of patients with Parkinson's disease at various stages of the disease, including the early-in-the-course, never previously medicated condition, provides some clues. For example, the extra-dimensional set-shifting deficit seen early in the disease in unmedicated patients seems less severe later in the course when patients have been stabilized on medication (Downes et al. 1989). A similar picture is evident for the one-touch Tower of London task (Owen et al. 1995a). On the other hand, severely affected patients, later in the course of the disease, seem to lose the beneficial effects of medication (Owen et al. 1992, 1995a).

The critical study is to withdraw L-dopa in a controlled, but double-blind manner. This has been done by Lange et al. (1992), but only for relatively severely affected Parkinson's disease patients. The results were quite clear cut in showing selective deficits in the tests sensitive to frontal lobe dysfunction, but no effect on visual recognition memory or visuospatial paired associate learning tasks. Unfortunately, the effects for the extra-dimensional set shifting task were ambiguous, as the deficit under placebo was so profound for the earlier discriminations in the series that it precluded a meaningful analysis of the effects of L-dopa withdrawal on extra-dimensional shifting itself. The results are consistent with other clinical studies of the effects of L-dopa medication. For example, Growdon et al. (1998), in a longitudinal clinical study of a large number of patients, concluded that medication had no major effect on cognitive function, but that it improved performance on certain tests of executive function that would be sensitive to frontal lobe dysfunction. What is not yet apparent is at which neural locus dopaminergic agents might exert their effects on cognition, as it is difficult, on present evidence, to distinguish between possible targets in the striatum or the prefrontal cortex.

Some converging evidence has come from a recent study of the effects of the dopamine D2 receptor antagonist sulpiride in normal healthy volunteers, which showed that the drug generally simulated the pattern of cognitive deficits seen in Parkinson's disease, including impairments in certain forms of spatial working memory, attentional set-shifting and planning, though not visual recognition memory (Mehta et al. 1999). As dopamine D2 receptors greatly predominate in the striatum as compared with the prefrontal cortex, it can be assumed that the effects probably reflect an action within the former structure, rather than a modulation of prefrontal cortex. The possibility of effects via D1 receptors in Parkinson's disease, possibly at the level of the prefrontal cortex, can, however, not be excluded.

In order to test the possibility of improvements in aspects of cognitive function sensitive to frontal lobe lesions, following treatment with compounds that might modulate function in the prefrontal cortex via catecholamine receptors, we have resorted to testing the effects of the psychomotor stimulant drug methylphenidate, which is much used in the treatment of ADHD, but potentiates noradrenergic as well as dopaminergic transmission. An acute dose of methylphenidate (40 mg p.o.) produced significant improvements in the self-ordered spatial working memory task as well as in spatial span, and in two forms of the Tower of London planning task, when compared with placebo in a double-blind crossover design (Elliott et al. 1997b). The performance-enhancing effects were generally seen on the first session, but the significance of this selectivity is not yet totally clear. It might, for example, simply reflect a less sensitive baseline on session 2 for exhibiting drug-induced improvement because of practice effects carrying over from session one. On the other hand, some aspects of performance appeared to worsen after methylphenidate on session 2. This was mainly evident for the easier form of the Tower of London planning task, where subjects produce the actual move sequences. Performance was faster in terms of more rapid initiation times, but less accurate after methylphenidate. These results were interpreted in terms of a model which suggests that performance on this task might reflect a balance between cortical and striatal function, with methylphenidate affecting the neuromodulation (by dopamine and noradrenaline) of the cortical monitoring of performance accuracy and also, via effects on striatal dopamine, the speed and vigour of performance. This pattern of results emphasizes the costs, as well as the benefits, inherent in the effects of catecholaminergic agents.

Methylphenidate also has striking, mixed effects on performance of a difficult version of the ID/ED attentional set-shift task, with three perceptual dimensions. Rogers et al. (1999a) have shown that methylphenidate, while tending to impair performance at the intradimensional shift (IDS) stage, actually reduces errors made at the extra-dimensional shift (EDS) stage – and generally lengthens response latencies. The most obvious interpretation of this pattern of results, which generally mirrors the effects of the D2 receptor antagonist sulpiride, described above, is that Ritalin increases distractibility, possibly both at the level of attending to the perceptual dimensions in the compound stimuli – and also to extra-task stimuli, thus accounting for the lengthier latencies. The results are of considerable interest for the studies reviewed above in non-human primates in the context of the improvements in performance produced by Ritalin on tests such as the self-ordered spatial working memory task. In those studies (Roberts et al. 1994), impaired spatial delayed response was accompanied by enhanced extra-dimensional shift learning. Presumably, it can be concluded that methylphenidate is not simply mimicking the effects of the altered cortical/striatal balance in dopaminergic activity that accompanies mesofrontal dopamine loss (cf. Roberts et al. 1994).

Another example of mixed effects of dopaminergic drugs on cognitive function comes from certain effects of dopamine agonist therapy in Parkinson's disease (L-dopa, bromocriptine and pergolide) (Swainson et al. 2000). These authors reported results that could be construed as showing a deficit in the learning of a difficult, probabilistic reversal task, following dopaminergic therapy in patients with Parkinson's disease whose spatial working memory function, according to certain measures, was enhanced under drug treatment. The deficits in reversal learning were significantly correlated with the dose of the mixed D1/D2 agonist pergolide for these patients. The results are reminiscent of an earlier study of L-dopa withdrawal, in which Gotham et al. (1988) found that certain tests sensitive to frontal lobe dysfunction were improved following L-dopa, whereas others were impaired. Those authors speculated that the dopaminergic therapy repleted certain corticostriatal circuits (notably the putamen) but effectively 'overdosed' others (e.g. the caudate nucleus) that had been less affected by the disease. Swainson et al. (2000) make a parallel suggestion that the ventral striatum might be more selectively implicated in reversal learning (for which there is some evidence in humans (Rogers et al. 2000), and so this circuitry, which is also relatively spared in the early stages of Parkinson's disease, would be relatively more susceptible to possible 'overdosing' effects of medication. Regardless of the actual neural mechanisms involved, these data do again demonstrate the varied effect of dopaminergic medication on cognitive function, while also showing how a Yerkes-Dodson-like function might reflect the engagement of circuitries with variably impaired neuromodulation, rather than simple effects on tasks with absolute and variable levels of difficulty. Task difficulty for patients will vary according to which systems are likely to be intact, rather than as a function of intrinsic 'task-difficulty'.

Effects of manipulation of brain serotonin (5-HT) on tests sensitive to frontal lobe dysfunction in humans

Investigation of the role of central serotonin receptors in cognition in humans is also handicapped by a lack of suitably selective agents. Grasby et al. (1992) have shown that buspirone, a rather non-specific 5-HT_{1A} agonist, impairs verbal learning in a functional neuroimaging context, the deficit correlating with changes in regional cerebral blood flow in the posterior neocortex. Another popular method has been the tryptophan depletion technique. By giving food-deprived humans or rats a diet deficient in the amino acid tryptophan, it is possible to produce a transient depletion of the indoleamine 5-HT, and presumably deficient serotoninergic activity, because tryptophan is a necessary precursor of 5-HT synthesized in the brain (Young et al. 1985).

An early study of the effects of tryptophan depletion on cognitive function in humans found that there was rather little effect on many tests sensitive to frontal lobe dysfunction. For example, performance on the Tower of London test of planning and self-ordered spatial working memory were both unaffected (Park et al. 1994), in marked contrast to the effects of the catecholaminergic agents sulpiride, methylphenidate and also the noradrenergic agents clonidine and idazoxan (Middleton et al. 1999). Learning of the paired associates task was retarded, an interesting parallel to the effects seen on verbal learning by Grasby et al. (1992). The paired associates learning deficit may have been due to actions of 5-HT in posterior cortical memory circuits, for example in the parietal or temporal lobe, although the task is also sensitive to frontal cortical damage (Owen et al. 1995b).

The low tryptophan treatment did impair performance on the CANTAB attentional set-shifting paradigm, although the effects were more evident at the extra-dimensional reversal stage than the extra-dimensional shift condition, which immediately precedes it. Reversal learning is another example of shift learning in which the discriminative stimuli remain the same, but identity of the reinforced stimulus (or 'object') is switched. Thus the subject has to desist responding to the previously reinforced stimulus and begin responding to the previously non-reinforced stimulus in order to gain reward. The capacity to show reversal can be partialled into two main components: the ability to inhibit responding to the previously reinforced stimulus; and the ability to learn which stimulus is now rewarded. Marmosets with lesions of the lateral and orbitofrontal cortex exhibit differential impairments on reversal learning as compared with extra-dimensional shift learning. Animals with lateral lesions are impaired in the extra-dimensional shift learning task, whereas those with the orbitofrontal lesions are impaired specifically at extra-dimensional reversal learning (Dias et al. 1996a). This result can be characterized as a double dissociation of effects of prefrontal lesions on two forms of shift learning – shift learning at the level of single stimuli or objects, and learning at the more abstract level of entire stimulus dimensions. Given the strong anatomical connections of the orbitofrontal cortex with limbic structures such as the anterior cingulate and the amygdala, it is perhaps not surprising that the orbitofrontal lesion should impair the specific stimulus-reward learning required in reversal. Further evidence for a specific role of the orbitofrontal cortex in reversal learning comes from human studies. Rolls et al. (1994) have found that patients with closed head injuries producing brain damage that includes the orbitofrontal cortex are impaired in forms of reversal learning. Rahman et al. (1999) have recently shown using the CANTAB suite of visual discriminations that includes reversal learning, as well as extra-dimensional set shifting, that patients with dementia of the frontotemporal type (where the initial neurodegeneration affects the orbitofrontal cortex) have greater problems with the reversal, rather than the non-reversal, stages of the task. Consequently, it appears that there may be functional commonalities between the effects of orbitofrontal lesions and procedures affecting 5-HT function in humans.

In order to test further the hypothesis that reductions in central 5-HT may selectively impair reversal learning, Rogers et al. (1999a) used the same, three-dimensional discrimination learning and shifting paradigm as was employed to test the effects of methylphenidate. It was anticipated that this more difficult form of the two-dimensional version of the task might lead to more clear-cut findings than were apparent in the Park et al. study, where effects appeared to be limited largely to the first session in a crossover design. Significantly, the results of Park et al. (1994) were extended and confirmed, reversal learning being much more impaired than non-reversal learning at several of the stages of the task – contrasting also with the effects of both methylphenidate (described above) and clonidine (Rogers et al. 1999a).

In order further to test the hypothesis that the serotoninergic manipulation might be affecting functions controlled by the orbitofrontal cortex to a greater extent than those of the dorsolateral prefrontal cortex, we have also compared the effects of the catecholaminergic agent methylphenidate with those of tryptophan depletion on performance in another paradigm that we have showed to be sensitive to orbitofrontal dysfunction. This task is modelled after the 'gambling task' sensitive to orbitofrontal damage in humans reported by Bechara et al. (1998) and is described in greater detail in a recent paper (Rogers et al. 1999b). Briefly, subjects are required to make probabilistic decisions and then assign proportions of their previously earned reward to those decisions. This decision-making task is also sensitive to damage of the orbitofrontal cortex, whether produced by lesions (Rogers et al. 1999b) or by neurodegeneration (Rahman et al. 1999). Importantly, in the present context, tryptophan depletion produced effects on performance which mimicked some of those produced by orbitofrontal lesions (Rogers et al. 1999b). On the other hand, the same dose (40 mg p.o.) of methylphenidate previously shown to affect many of the other tasks described above that depended on dorsolateral prefrontal cortical functioning had no effects on the decision-making task. Given the relative lack of effect of tryptophan depletion on performance on the spatial working memory task and the Tower of London planning task, in relation to its significant effects on reversal learning and the decision-making task – and the opposite effects on these of the indirectly acting catecholaminergic agonist methylphenidate, we appear to have provided evidence, summarized in Table 2, for a double dissociation of effects on tasks controlled by different sectors of the prefrontal cortex.

Synthesis and implications

We have reviewed the effects of manipulations of the main monoaminergic systems in the context of frontal lobe functions in rats, monkeys and humans. The main points to have emerged are as follows:

1. Drugs or manipulations affecting the central catecholamine (noradrenergic and dopaminergic) systems specifically affect certain tasks sensitive to frontostriatal dysfunction.
2. Performance on such tasks can be improved or impaired in experimental animals, healthy human volunteers, or patients, for example with Parkinson's disease, depending on such factors as the dose of drug, level of baseline performance, and individual differences.
3. An especially important factor is probably the nature of the task under study. This may in turn depend on the neural circuitry that underlies different tasks: those exhibiting improvement following catecholamine agonists appear to be more dependent for example on the dorsolateral rather than the orbitofrontal cortex.
4. Manipulations of other neurotransmitter systems, for example, serotonin (and also acetylcholine; see Roberts et al. 1992) appear to affect tasks mediated by rather different frontal circuitry that includes the orbitofrontal rather than the dorsolateral prefrontal cortex.
5. The implication is that the different chemically defined systems of the reticular core do have different functions. This conclusion is apparent from the effects of gross manipulations to the different systems in a common task requiring attentional processing, as in the case of the studies of the five-choice task in the rat, but also when more local manipulations are made into these systems projecting into a common terminal field, in this case the prefrontal cortex.

From the perspective purely of neurochemical anatomy, these conclusions may perhaps be surprising, as there is very little evidence of major differences in the pattern of innervation of different regions within the prefrontal cortex for any of the four main systems considered. Further research is required to explain this apparent mismatch between function and anatomy: there is apparently much more specificity than at first would have appeared likely from the details of the neurobiological organization of the monoamine systems.

The results have many theoretical and clinical implications. In the latter case, we can begin to make predictions about which types of function are likely to respond to pharmaceutical treatment in different disorders. We can also make more precise conclusions about the types of function that are vulnerable to malfunction in particular neurotransmitter systems, for example, serotoninergic abnormalities in depression. Finally, we can speculate about the adaptive significance of the types of functional relationships we have seen between neurotransmitter function and behaviour, in terms of the natural influences that affect the functioning of these chemically identified systems. Most of them have been implicated in such general functions as stress and arousal, although little is known about the precise pattern or sequence of changes of state in these systems. However, it is evident that a single inverted U-shaped Yerkes-Dodson-like function is

Table 2 Summary of effects of catecholamine (dopamine, noradrenaline) versus indoleamine (serotonin) manipulations on cognitive functions sensitive to frontal lobe dysfunction

Function and putative PFC domain	Catecholamine (DA and NA)	Indoleamine (5-HT)
Tasks implicating dorsolateral or rostrolateral PFC		
Spatial working memory	Improved[a,b] or impaired[c]	No effect[d]
Tower of London planning	Improved[a,b] or impaired[a,c]	No effect[d]
Extra-dimensional shift	Improved[e] or impaired[c]	No effect[e]
Tasks implicating orbitofrontal PFC		
Reversal shifts	No effect[e] or impaired[f]	Impaired[e]
Decision-making	No effect[g]	Impaired[h]

[a] Elliott et al. 1997b, [b] Lange et al. 1992, [c] Mehta et al. 1999, [d] Park et al. 1994, [e] Rogers et al. 1999a, [f] Swainson et al. 2000
[g] Rogers et al., unpublished, [h] Rogers et al. 1999b

inadequate to account for all of these effects. The different states in which the fluctuating levels of neurotransmitter activity place the prefrontal neuronal circuitry would seem to allow a much greater flexibility in facilitating those sets of 'cognitive control processes' most adaptive to the situation at hand, for example, working memory, response inhibition, response sequencing, and 'somatic marking'. The current working hypothesis is therefore:

That chemically selective neuromodulation of executive functioning can serve to optimize performance of certain types of task or operations, but not others, related to the adaptive imperative to engage processing that is appropriate to both the current environmental setting (including the presence of stressors) and the internal state (e.g. fluctuations in mood and arousal).

What now has to be determined, however, is a greater understanding of what constitutes these optimal allocations of resources and how they are facilitated by the neuromodulatory systems we have investigated.

Acknowledgements This work was supported by a Programme grant from the Wellcome Trust to T.W. Robbins, B.J. Everitt, A.C. Roberts and B.J. Sahakian. I thank my collaborators for their contributions to the studies reviewed.

References

Arnsten AFT (1998) Catecholamine modulation of prefrontal cortical cognitive function. Trends Cog Sci 2:436–447

Arnsten AFT, Goldman-Rakic PS (1984) Selective prefrontal cortical projection to the region of the locus coeruleus and raphe nuclei in the rhesus monkey. Brain Res 306:9–18

Aston-Jones G, Chiang C, Alexinsky T (1991) Discharge of noradrenergic locus coeruleus neurons in behaving rats and monkeys suggests a role in vigilance. Prog Brain Res 88:521–532

Baker SC, Rogers RD, Owen AM, Frith CD, Dolan RJ, Frackowiak RSJ, Robbins TW (1996) Neural systems engaged by planning: a PET study of the Tower of London task. Neuropsychologia 34:515–526

Baunez C, Robbins TW (1999) Effects of dopamine depletion of the dorsal striatum and further interaction with subthalamic nucleus lesions in an attentional task in the rat. Neuroscience 92:1343–1356

Bechara A, Damasio H, Tranel D, Anderson SW (1998) Dissociation of working memory from decision making within the human prefrontal cortex. J Neurosci 18:428–437

Brozoski T, Brown RM, Rosvold HE, Goldman PS (1979) Cognitive deficit caused by regional depletion of dopamine in prefrontal cortex of rhesus monkey. Science 205:929–931

Carli M, Robbins TW, Evenden JL, Everitt BJ (1983) Effects of lesions to ascending noradrenergic neurones on performance of a 5-choice serial reaction task in rats; implications for theories of dorsal noradrenergic bundle function based on selective attention and arousal. Behav Brain Res 9:361–380

Cole BJ, Robbins TW (1989) Effects of 6-hydroxydopamine lesions of the nucleus accumbens septi on performance of a 5-choice serial reaction time task in rats: implications for theories of selective attention and arousal. Behav Brain Res 33:165–179

Collins P, Roberts AC, Dias R, Everitt BJ, Robbins TW (1998) Perseveration and strategy in a novel spatial self-ordered sequencing task for non-human primates: effects of excitotoxic lesions and dopamine depletions of the prefrontal cortex. J Cog Neurosci 10:332–354

Dalley JW, Thomas K, Howes SR, Tsai TH, Aparicio-Legarza MI, Reynolds GP, Everitt BJ, Robbins TW (1999) Effects of excitotoxic lesions of the rat prefrontal cortex on CREB activation and presynaptic markers of dopamine and amino-acid function in the nucleus accumbens. Eur J Neurosci 11:1265–1274

Dias R, Roberts A, Robbins TW (1996a) Dissociation in prefrontal cortex of affective and attentional shifts. Nature 380:69–72

Dias R, Robbins TW, Roberts AC (1996b) Primate analogue of the Wisconsin Card Sort Test: effects of excitotoxic lesions of the prefrontal cortex in the marmoset. Behav Neurosci 110:870–884

Downes JJ, Roberts AC, Sahakian BJ, Evenden JL, Robbins TW (1989) Impaired extra-dimensional shift performance in medicated and unmedicated Parkinson's disease: evidence for a specific attentional dysfunction. Neuropsychologia 27:1329–1344

Elliott R, Sahakian BJ, Matthews K, Bannerjea A, Rimmer J, Robbins TW (1997a) Effects of methylphenidate on spatial working memory and planning in healthy young adults. Psychopharmacology 131:196–206

Elliott R, Baker SC, Rogers RD, O'Leary DA, Paykel ES, Frith CD, Dolan R, Sahakian BJ (1997b) Prefrontal dysfunction in depressed patients performing a planning task: a study using positron emission tomography. Psychol Med 27:931–942

Everitt BJ, Robbins TW (1997) Central cholinergic systems and cognition. Ann Rev Psychol 48:649–684

Goldman-Rakic PS (1987) Circuitry of primate prefrontal cortex and the regulation of behaviour by representational memory. In: Plum F, Mountcastle V (eds) Handbook of physiology, vol 5. American Physiological Society, Bethesda, MD, pp 373–417

Gotham AM, Brown RG, Marsden CD (1988) 'Frontal' cognitive function in patients with Parkinson's disease 'on' and 'off' levodopa. Brain 111:299–321

Granon S, Passetti F, Thomas KL, Dalley JW, Everitt BJ, Robbins TW (2000) Enhanced and impaired attentional performance following infusion of D1 dopaminergic receptor agents into rat prefrontal cortex. J Neurosci 20:1208–1215

Grasby PM, Friston KJ, Bench CJ, Frith CD, Paulesu E, Cowen PJ, Liddle PF, Frackowiak RSJ, Dolan R (1992) The effect of apomorphine and buspirone on regional cerebral blood flow during the performance of a cognitive task – measuring neuromodulatory effects of psychotropic drugs in man. Eur J Neurosci 4:1203–1212

Growdon JH, Kieburtz K, McDermott MP, Panisset M, Friedman JH, Shoulson I, et al. (1998) Levodopa improves motor function without impairing cognition in mild nondemented Parkinson's disease patients. Neurology 50:1327–1331

Hajos M, Richards CD, Szekely AD, Sharp T (1998) An electrophysiological and neuroanatomical study of the medial prefrontal cortical projection to the midbrain raphe nuclei in the rat. Neuroscience 87:95–108

Harrison AA, Everitt BJ, Robbins TW (1997) Central 5-HT depletion enhances impulsive responding without affecting the accuracy of attentional performance: interactions with dopaminergic mechanisms. Psychopharmacology 133:329–342

Jodo E, Chiang C, Asron-Jones G (1998) Potent excitatory influence of prefrontal cortex on noradrenergic locus coeruleus. Neuroscience 83:63–79

Kimberg DY, D'Esposito M, Farah MJ (1997) Effects of bromocriptine on human subjects depends on working memory capacity. Neuroreport 8:3581–3585

Lange K, Robbins TW, Marsden CD, James M, Owen A, Paul GM (1992) L-Dopa withdrawal selectively impairs performance in tests of frontal lobe function in Parkinson's disease. Psychopharmacology 107:394–404

Luciana M, Depue RA, Arbisi P, Leon A (1992) Facilitation of working memory in humans by a D2 dopamine receptor agonist. J Cog Neurosci 4:58–68

Luciana M, Collins PF, Depue RA (1998) Opposing roles for dopamine and serotonin in the modulation of human spatial working memory functions. Cereb Cortex 8:218–226

McGaughy J, Dalley JW, Everitt BJ, Robbins TW (1999) Behavioural and neurochemical effects of cholinergic de-afferentation on visual attention in a 5-choice serial reaction time task. Soc Neurosci Abstr 25:1376, Abstr 554.1

Mehta MA, Sahakian BJ, McKenna PJ, Robbins TW (1999) Systemic sulpiride in young adult volunteers simulates the profile of cognitive deficits in Parkinson's disease. Psychopharmacology 146:162–174

Middleton HC, Sharma A, Agouzoui D, Sahakian BJ, Robbins TW (1999) Idazoxan potentiates rather than antagonizes some of the cognitive effects of clonidine. Psychopharmacology 145:401–411

Moore H, West AR, Grace AA (1999) The regulation of forebrain dopamine transmission: relevance to the pathophysiology and psychopathology of schizophrenia. Biol Psychiatry 46:40–55

Muir JL, Robbins TW, Everitt BJ (1994) AMPA-induced lesions of the basal forebrain: a significant role for the cortical cholinergic system in attentional function. J Neurosci 14:2313–2326

Muir JL, Everitt BJ, Robbins TW (1996) The cerebral cortex of the rat and visual attentional function: dissociable effects of mediofrontal, cingulate, anterior dorsolateral and parietal cortex lesions on a five choice serial reaction time task in rats. Cereb Cortex 6:470–481

Muller U, von Cramon DY, Pollmann S (1998) D1 – versus D2 – receptor modulation of visuospatial working memory in humans. J Neurosci 18:2720–2728

Murphy BL, Arnsten AFT, Goldman-Rakic PS, Roth RH (1996) Increased dopamine turnover in the prefrontal cortex impairs spatial working memory performance in rats and monkeys. Proc Natl Acad Sci U S A 93:1325–1329

Owen AM, James M, Leigh PH, Summers BA, Marsden CD, Quinn NP, Lange KW, Robbins TW (1992) Fronto-striatal cognitive deficits at different stages of Parkinson's disease. Brain 115:1727–1751

Owen AM, Sahakian BJ, Hodges JR, Summers BA, Polkey CE, Robbins TW (1995a) Dopamine-dependent fronto-striatal planning deficits in early Parkinson's disease. Neuropsychology 9:126–140

Owen AM, Sahakian BJ, Semple J, Polkey CE, Robbins TW (1995b) Visuospatial short term recognition memory and learning after temporal lobe excisions, frontal lobe excisions or amygdala-hippocampectomy in man. Neuropsychologia 33:1–24

Owen AM, Evans AC, Petrides M (1996a) Evidence for a two stage model of spatial working memory processing within the lateral frontal cortex: a positron emission tomography study. Cereb Cortex 6:31–38

Owen AM, Doyon J, Petrides M, Evans AC (1996b) Planning and spatial working memory: a positron emission tomography study in humans. Eur J Neurosci 8:353–364

Pandya DP, Yeterian EH (1995) Morphological correlations of human and monkey frontal lobe. In: Damasio AE, Damasio H, Christen Y (eds) Neurobiology of human decision making. Springer, Berlin Heidelberg New York, pp 13–46

Park SB, Coull JT, McShane RH, Young AH, Sahakian BJ, Robbins TW, Cowen PJ (1994) Tryptophan depletion in normal volunteers produces selective impairments in learning and memory. Neuropharmacology 33:575–588

Petrides M (1996) Specialized systems for the processing of mnemonic information within the primate frontal cortex. Philos Tran R Soc Lond B Biol Sci 351:1455–1461

Rahman S, Sahakian BJ, Hodges JR, Rogers RD, Robbins TW (1999) Specific cognitive deficits in mild frontal variant frontotemporal dementia. Brain 122:1469–1493

Robbins TW (1984) Cortical noradrenaline, attention and arousal. Psychol Med 14:13–21

Robbins TW (1985) Neuropsychological evaluation of higher cognitive function in animals and man: can psychopharmacology contribute to neuropsychology? In: Iversen SD (ed) Psychopharmacology: recent advances and future prospects. Oxford University Press, Oxford, pp 155–169

Robbins TW (1996) Dissociating executive functions of the prefrontal cortex. Philos Trans R Soc Lond Biol 351:1463–1471

Robbins TW (1998) Homology in behavioural pharmacology: an approach to animal models of human cognition. Behav Pharmacol 9:509–520

Robbins TW, Everitt BJ (1995) Arousal systems and attention. In: Gazzaniga M, et al. (eds) The cognitive neurosciences. MIT Press, Cambridge, MA, pp 703–720

Robbins TW, Granon S, Muir JL, Durantou F, Harrison A, Everitt BJ (1998a) Neural systems underlying arousal and attention. In: Harvey JA, Kosofsky BE (eds) Cocaine: effects on the developing brain. Ann N Y Acad Sci 846:222–237

Robbins TW, James M, Owen AM, Sahakian BJ, Lawrence AD, McInnes L, Rabbitt PMA (1998b) A study of performance on tests from the CANTAB battery sensitive to frontal lobe dysfunction in a large sample of normal volunteers: implications for theories of executive functioning and cognitive aging. J Int Neuropsychol Soc 4:474–490

Roberts AC, Robbins TW, Everitt BJ, Muir JL (1992) A specific form of cognitive rigidity following excitotoxic lesions of the basal forebrain in monkeys. Neuroscience 47:251–264

Roberts AC, De Salvia MA, Wilkinson LS, Collins P, Muir JL, Everitt BJ, Robbins TW (1994) 6-Hydroxydopamine lesions of the prefrontal cortex in monkeys enhance performance on an analogue of the Wisconsin Card Sorting test: possible interactions with subcortical dopamine. J Neurosci 14:2531–2544

Rogers RD, Blackshaw AJ, Middleton HC, Matthews K, Deakin JFW, Sahakian BJ, Robbins TW (1999a) Tryptophan depletion impairs stimulus-reward learning while methylphenidate disrupts attentional control in healthy young adults: implications for the monoaminergic basis of impulsive behaviour. Psychopharmacology 146:482–491

Rogers RD, Everitt BJ, Baldacchino A, Blackshaw AJ, Swainson R, Wynne K, Baker NB, Hunter J, Carthy T, Booker E, London M, Deakin JFW, Sahakian BJ, Robbins TW (1999b) Dissociable deficits in the decision-making cognition of chronic amphetamine abusers, opiate abusers, patients with focal damage to prefrontal cortex, and tryptophan depleted normal volunteers: evidence for monoaminergic mechanisms. Neuropsychopharmacology 20:322–339

Rogers RD, Andrews TC, Grasby PM, Brooks D, Robbins TW (2000) Contrasting cortical and sub-cortical PET activations produced by reversal learning and attentional-set shifting in humans. J Cog Neurosci 12:142–162

Rolls ET, Hornak J, Wade D, McGrath J (1994) Emotion-related learning in patients with social and emotional changes associated with frontal lobe damage. J Neurol Neurosurg Psychiatry 57:1518–1524

Sahakian BJ, Sarna GS, Kantamaneni BD, Jackson A, Hutson PH, Curzon G (1985) Association between learning and cortical catecholamines in non-drug-treated rats. Psychopharmacology 86:339–343

Sara SJ, Herve-Minivielle A (1995) Inhibitory influence of frontal cortex on locus coeruleus. Proc Natl Acad Sci U S A 92:6032–6036

Schultz W, Dayan P, Montague PR (1997) A neural substrate of prediction and reward. Science 275:1593–1598

Swainson R, Rogers RD, Sahakian BJ, Summers BA, Polkey CE, Robbins TW (2000) Probabilistic learning and reversal deficits in patients with Parkinson's disease or frontal or temporal lobe lesions: possible adverse effects of dopaminergic medication. Neuropsychologia 38:596–612

Weed MR, Taffe MA, Polis L, Roberts AC, Robbins TW, Koob GF, Bloom FE, Gold LH (1999) Performance norms for a rhesus monkey neuropsychological testing battery: acquisition and long term performance. Cogn Brain Res 8:185–201

Wilkinson LS, Dias R, Thomas KL, Augood J, Everitt BJ, Robbins TW, Roberts AC (1997) Contrasting effects of excitotoxic lesions of the prefrontal cortex on the behavioural response to *d*-amphetamine and presynaptic and postsynaptic measures of striatal dopamine function in monkeys. Neuroscience 80:717–730

Williams GV, Goldman-Rakic (1995) Modulation of memory fields by dopamine D1 receptors in prefrontal cortex. Nature 376:572–575

Young SN, Smith SE, Phil PO, Ervin FR (1985) Tryptophan depletion causes a rapid lowering of mood in normal males. Psychopharmacology 87:173–177

Zahrt J, Taylor JR, Mathew RG, Arnsten AFT (1997) Supranormal stimulation of D1 dopamine receptors in the rodent prefrontal cortex impairs working memory performance. J Neurosci 17:8528–8535

GPSR Compliance

The European Union's (EU) General Product Safety Regulation (GPSR) is a set of rules that requires consumer products to be safe and our obligations to ensure this.

If you have any concerns about our products, you can contact us on ProductSafety@springernature.com

In case Publisher is established outside the EU, the EU authorized representative is:

Springer Nature Customer Service Center GmbH
Europaplatz 3
69115 Heidelberg, Germany

Batch number: 10755910

Printed by Printforce, the Netherlands